PATIENT Heal Thyself

**A Remarkable Health Program Combining
Ancient Wisdom with Groundbreaking Clinical Research**

by Jordan Rubin, N.M.D., Ph.D.

Disclaimer: This information is presented by an independent medical expert whose sources of information
include studies from the world's medical and scientific literature, patient records, and other clinical and anecdotal
reports. The material in this book is for informational
purposes only and is not intended for the diagnosis or
treatment of disease. Please visit a medical health professional for specific diagnosis of any ailments mentioned or
discussed in this material.

Cover design by Phil Glenn
Book design by Bonnie Lambert

ISBN 1-893910-24-5
Eighth printing
Printed in the United States
Published by Freedom Press
1801 Chart Trail
Topanga, CA 90290
Bulk Orders Available: (800) 959-9797
E-mail: info@freedompressonline.com

"Straight is the gate and
narrow is the path that leads to life
and there are few who find it"
Matthew 7:14

Dedication

To all people afflicted with illnesses that leave them fearful and hopeless and who suffer needlessly and don't experience the abundant life we were all meant to enjoy. This book and my prayers go out to each and every one of you.

Acknowledgements

I guess one never realizes how lucky he is to have so many wonderful people in his life until he is asked to thank those who have helped him become who he is today.

I would first like to thank the Lord my God for turning my mourning into gladness and giving me more than I could ever ask for or imagine. You are my Rock and my Salvation.

To my wife of three years Nicki. Every time I look into your eyes, I realize the man I was created to be. Your help and support means more to me than you can ever imagine. And baby, the best is yet to come!

To my mother, who always made me believe that I could accomplish anything I set my mind to. In a dictionary defining the words "a mother's love" there displays your picture.

To my father, who laid for me a foundation in natural health that would one day become my life's work. You always knew there was an answer for me. Dad, we found it!

To my grandmother Rose, you are my great champion. Thank you for always being there for me and also for being a model patient.

To all of my close friends, if a man ever wonders what kind of person he is, he needs to look no further than the men of valor that surround him. Thank you for sticking with me through thick and thin, and agreeing to help me to "never grow old."

To my great team at Garden of Life, your support makes this all worthwhile.

I would like to thank my editor and publisher David Steinman and the great people at Freedom Press. Thank you for believing in me and my message and giving me the opportunity to write my first book.

Lastly, I would like to thank William "Bud" Keith, who once told a sick, emaciated young man that "the answer to all of your health problems is found in the Bible." Bud, wherever you are, I hope you receive extra jewels on your crown in heaven.

Contents

Foreword by Garry Gordon, M.D., M.D.(H.), D.O. 9
Introduction 11

Part I—PATIENT Heal Thyself!
1. The Journey 15
2. I've Got A Gut Feeling 31

Part II—Enter the Garden of Life
3. Beyond Probiotics 38
4. Mankind's Most Powerful Immune Enhancer 66
5. Attacking the Seven Causes of Inflammation 84
6. You're Not What You Eat, But What You Digest 89
7. Capture the Power of the Sun 95
8. The Healing Power of Green Foods 101

Part III—The Garden of Life Healing Program
9. Return to the Maker's Diet 112
10. The Maker's Diet in Your Daily Life 148
11. The Maker's Diet Recipes 164

Part IV—Health & Healing
12. Healing Protocols 170

Part V—Resources
Appendix A: Recommended Food Sources 274
Appendix B: Recommended Supplements 277
Appendix C: Lifestyle Recommendations 280
Appendix D: Educational Materials 281

References 283
Index 286

Foreword

The Jordan Rubin story ranks as one of the most dramatic natural healing stories ever told. Although Jordan came from a family that stressed a healthy diet (his father is a naturopath and chiropractor), his own deteriorating dietary habits while an athletic scholarship student at Florida State University, coupled with stress and receiving the measles, mumps and rubella (MMR) vaccine at age 15, may have all contributed to the onset of his nearly terminal case of Crohn's disease. Once the diagnosis had been made, initial medical treatments, which consisted of massive doses of intravenous and oral antibiotics and anti-inflammatory drugs, only exacerbated his condition.

Crohn's disease nearly cost Jordan his life. Only natural healing could save him. Faced with his own near death battle, Jordan was forced to search the world for answers. He learned the amazing dietary secrets employed by our ancestors that allowed them to live long disease-free lives. Most of all, he returned to health, thanks to his use of ancient soil organisms (his now world famous homeostatic soil organisms), beneficial microbes found in pristine soils that are as necessary to health as any known vitamin or mineral.

But even greater than his own healing journey are the secrets of health and longevity that Jordan has gathered together for the benefit of all humanity. Through this book, Jordan is bringing to us the secrets of ancient healing that have been lost through time and modernity, but that are absolutely essential to our becoming, and staying, well.

There's so much more I want to tell you about this amazing person. Let me say this: Jordan is one of the most brilliant new voices in the fields of medicine and nutrition, and I don't say this lightly. The experts tell us "there is nothing new under the sun," but Jordan's discovery of the ancient healing secrets contained in this important book is, indeed, revolutionary—at least to modern men and women. Not only are they new to modernity, but they are also essential to good health.

In Jordan's prescription for health, you will find nutritional treasures far more powerful than simply your run-of-the-mill vitamins and minerals. Primitive dietary essentials such as health-giving phytochemicals found in herbs and whole foods, the ever important essential fats (including some that you probably thought were forbidden if you've been listening to our so-called modern dietary experts), and of course, homeostatic soil organisms—these are all part of the healthy diet enjoyed by our ancestors. Jordan calls his eating program The Maker's Diet, which will be explained in detail in this profound work.

Though his secrets are culled from ancient wisdom, it is, ironically, science at the cutting edge that tells us Jordan's message is solid. Preliminary findings from recently concluded clinical trials published in the peer-reviewed medical journal *Progress in Nutrition* demonstrate when patients, with a wide-range of modern illnesses, follow Jordan's healing guidelines they truly get better, and they stay better—even when their doctor's medications and procedures have failed to yield health.

I truly believe the information in this book will form the foundation program for your journey to super health or recovery from disease. Based on work with my own patient load, I personally can attest to the solid results health-conscious consumers can expect. As an example, we all know that intestinal illnesses, chronic fatigue syndrome, and rheumatoid arthritis are complex, debilitating, expensive diseases to treat. With Jordan's healing secrets, we have not found a panacea but are so close to it that I feel compelled to make this exciting information known to you now. No one needs to suffer from these or any other seemingly incurable conditions anymore—if they merely follow the simple principles and guidelines detailed in this book.

I will also tell you this—anyone who takes to heart what Jordan tells us can expect to improve virtually any health problem. I truly believe through work with my own patients, who have implemented Jordan's healing program, that this book will bring all of us into a nutritionally and spiritually rich land of health—a true garden of life.

I encourage you to enjoy this book and to pay close attention. Your health and the health of your loved ones may depend on it.

—*Garry Gordon, M.D., D.O., M.D.(H.),*
Board of Medical Examiners for Alternative and
Homeopathic Medicine in the State of Arizona,
Director of Peer Review for Chelation Therapy for the State of Arizona.
Payson, Arizona, November 1, 2002

Introduction

Everyone flocks to see today's heroes play music to thousands of adoring fans, or dunk a basketball with thunderous power, or glide their way to Olympic gold in the downhill skiing finals. We see these modern day heroes, musicians, athletes, and actors at their best, at their shining moments, standing on the crest of the mountain looking down at the rest of us. But think for a moment. These heroes each put in thousands of hours of sweat, toil and failures with no screaming fans to encourage them. They made sacrifices far beyond what any of us have made. They swam hundreds of laps in cold pools in the wee hours of the morning while we were still asleep. They played music in dingy clubs to a handful of people who weren't even paying attention to them. They practiced day in and day out, even when their friends were out having fun. The common denominator in the lives of these superstars was an insatiable drive and determination to succeed. The truth is that the chance of any one of us becoming a rock star, or an all-star basketball player or an Olympic gold medalist is smaller than winning the lottery.

I believe that the process of overcoming an incurable illness is much the same as training for and winning the Olympics. The individuals who have the courage to take charge of their own health, have the unending determination and make the near impossible sacrifices it takes to be one of the select few who beat illness and choose life are today's true heroes.

My own healing journey from death's door to a return to super health was not an easy one. I made a lot of mistakes along the way. But I know in the end that my journey produced lasting changes in my life, and I hope that by sharing what I have learned with you, you can take charge of your own health and realize your body's phenomenal potential.

In the midst of life's trials and tribulations, we often ask why God would allow us to go through such ordeals. But I now know more than ever, God would never allow anyone to suffer like I did without a divine plan.

The fact is, I went through a real life "hell" and nearly died. And I truly believe that this was part of God's plan so that I might become your teacher and show you, as well as others, how to regain your birthright of great health.

In the pages that follow, you will learn the health secrets that allowed our ancestors to live long, disease-free lives. You will learn how to regain your health if you've lost it or how to maintain the excellent health that you currently enjoy and even slow premature aging.

But let me warn you. Some of the recommendations in this book may surprise you. In fact, many of my instructions fly in the face of what "they" are telling you. The "they" I'm referring to are the American Medical Association, American Heart Association, American Cancer Society, American Dietetic Association, and many governmental agencies. If a politically correct approach to health and nutrition is what you're looking for, you've come to the wrong place. If you're looking for an optimal health plan for you and your family that is validated by history, science and our Creator, then buckle up; you're in for a wild ride!

If I had to boil my message down to one sentence, it would be this: *No matter what health challenges plague you today, there is hope for an answer.* It's time to get armed with powerful truths from our Creator. It's time to provide your body with the nutritional tools it needs to regenerate from head to toe. The time is now. *Patient, heal thyself!*

—*Jordan Rubin, N.M.D., Ph.D.*
Jupiter, Florida, October 1, 2002

Part I–
Enter the
Garden of Life

The Journey

There I was, standing on the field at Doak Campell Stadium at Florida State University doing the tomahawk chop with my fellow cheerleaders and 80,000 screaming fans as our Seminoles marched their way to their first ever National Championship. Life couldn't have been better. I was an 18-year-old freshman on an academic and athletic scholarship, with more friends than I could spend time with and a member of a great fraternity. In my spare time, I was a soloist in a traveling singing group and a quarterback for my intramural football team. I lived with seven of my friends in a house just outside of campus. Life was great.

Then, it happened.

It was 1994, the summer after my freshman year, and I was working as a counselor at a day camp to earn extra money. I remember the afternoon I first started getting sick. I was riding on a bus with the kids at camp. I was feeling sleepy which was very unusual for me. I usually had an energy level that rivaled the Energizer Bunny. I just kept going, and going and going. At one point, while riding on the bus, I actually fell asleep. "Jordan, Jordan! Wake up!" One of the kids was shaking me to wake me up, which was embarrassing. Unfortunately, falling asleep at inopportune times such as this became a regular occurrence for me. I also became frequently tired during the day and lacked energy.

Shortly after my noticeable loss of energy, I remember getting terrible stomach cramps that had me running to the bathroom several times a day with diarrhea. Before long, frequent trips to the toilet were routine for me. But even though I was feeling lousy, I didn't want to admit it to myself. Getting sick didn't really fit into my schedule, if you know what I mean. In fact, I even decided to attend a week-long overnight camp, in spite of my need to be close to a toilet. What was I thinking! Camping out in the summer heat of Florida is tough enough on a healthy person. My nausea was making me feel even worse, and the usual camp "chow" wasn't helping. I found myself gulping iced tea and beating a well-worn path to the outdoor bathrooms.

The next fact I want to tell you is quite startling. In seven days, I lost twenty pounds. That's *twenty* pounds in *seven* days. For some people, losing twenty pounds in a week could be a dream come true. But for me, it was a nightmare. I remember trying to tackle a friend of mine during a camp football game, and getting trampled. I realized how much weaker I had become. At this point, I had to face reality to a certain extent. Something was really wrong with me.

Like a seasick passenger on a long bumpy boat ride, my upset stomach was now constant. I became completely dehydrated; my mouth felt like I had a large ball of cotton stuffed in it, and my gums were riddled with canker sores and ulcers.

I had become so sick and fatigued that I couldn't even make it through one week of overnight camp. I had to have someone drive me four hours home to Palm Beach Gardens. When I got there, I was in denial. I hugged my mom and dad and did a darn good job of hiding my illness from my parents (which was sort of dumb since my father is a doctor). Actually, I *had* to hide my illness. If my parents had any idea how sick I really was, they would have made me go to the hospital. Or worse, they would not have let me go back to school, and the new semester started in only ten days. This was my sophomore year, and I wasn't about to start late. I was sure that if I could hang on until school started, everything would be fine. I just needed to get back into the swing of things.

Without telling my parents, I visited a family doctor in our community on my own. I detailed my symptoms—the nausea, constant diarrhea, weight loss, cotton-mouth, and fatigue. That was just the beginning of my list.

The doctor put me through a series of tests looking for viruses, including the AIDS virus; none were detected. He ordered a stool culture that came back negative and prescribed a course of antibiotics for me to take. Neither the doctor nor I ever asked why I had developed these severe digestive problems. Looking back, I sure wish I or someone else had. I mean, I don't want to sound like a bad sport or an ungrateful patient, but when something goes wrong, it is often a good idea to find out *why*. I guess doctors are so busy these days just trying to get through their patient loads that they frequently prescribe whatever is covered by insurance and will get rid of the symptoms. It's sort of like putting a lot of make-up over a facial blemish. It works (sort of).

In any event, I took the antibiotics with me on my return to school and started taking them. Unfortunately, my condition only worsened, and I began experiencing even more severe gastrointestinal problems.

I did everything I could to ignore what was happening to my body. I kept busy by trying to go to class, but I had to discontinue all of my extracurricular activities. I was forced to quit the cheerleading squad and the fraternity. I also had to quit studying to pass my American College of Sports Medicine exam in preparation for becoming a fitness professional.

I weighed about 145 pounds at that time, down from my normal 175 to 180 pounds. As the days went by, things only worsened. I was falling apart. I was running fevers of 104 degrees every night. I barely slept because I was getting up to run to the bathroom all night.

To make matters worse, my gastrointestinal problems had become systemic, affecting my joints. My hip constantly popped out of its socket whenever I did anything. I would suffer minor dislocations even getting in and out of cars. I remember the situation became so severe that my hip popped out once as

I was walking to class. I was forced to turn around and go back to my house. At that point, leaving school seemed inevitable.

I mentioned previously that my father is a doctor. He is a naturopath and chiropractor who was in the first class of students at the National College of Naturopathic Medicine in Portland, Oregon. In fact, I've been told that I was the first child in the United States in the modern era to be delivered at home by naturopathic students. As a naturopath, my father was taught to work with the whole person and to use safe and natural, nontoxic healing methods.

My father had given me a cache of dietary supplements to take with me back to college. Exploring this collection one afternoon, I found probiotics, digestive enzymes, and many other herbal and nutritional dietary products. I didn't know much about nutritional supplements. I did, however, believe that these products would help me get well. I guess I made myself believe that.

That began my "magical mystery tour" of alternative medicine. These first nutritional supplements I started using were only the beginning for me. I also tried different diets. After I discovered that the cotton feeling in my mouth was oral thrush, which was linked with candida infection, I tried several anti-candida diets. My father also put me on the Specific Carbohydrate Diet. It has been purported to have been used successfully by many people to treat Crohn's disease, ulcerative colitis, irritable bowel syndrome, celiac disease, cystic fibrosis, and chronic diarrhea.

The premise of the diet is that damage done to intestinal walls by bacterial/fungal overgrowth is part of a vicious cycle that wreaks havoc with the body's health and immunity. The diet attempts to eliminate the type of carbohydrates such as grains, sugar, dairy, corn and potatoes that tend to nourish these "bad" bacteria and fungal species. This diet often helps to lower their populations and restores the body's balance or inner ecology. I tried to stop eating sugar, molasses, sucrose, high fructose corn syrup, or any other processed sugars. I tried to avoid corn, wheat, barley, oats, rye, rice, and other grains. I tried to avoid starchy foods such as potatoes, yams, and parsnips. I was told to forget milk and certain cheeses. Pasta was also a food of my past. That was just the beginning of the dietary restrictions.

The Specific Carbohydrate Diet may have helped some. Trouble was, I didn't have the self-discipline necessary to stay on a diet as rigorous as the Specific Carbohydrate Diet. Well, let me amend that statement. I could stay on the diet for periods of time—until my roommate who worked at a sorority house brought home leftovers from the kitchen—then, all of the sudden, I was not on a diet anymore (though promising to get back on it as soon as I was through pigging out).

I was hungry all the time. I had a ravenous appetite, but I only wanted to eat foods that tasted good to me which, of course, happened to not be healthy. Yet, no matter how much I ate, I continued to lose weight.

When you are as sick as I was, toilet locations become an obsession. No matter where I went, I had to know where the bathrooms were. Even if I felt well enough to go out with friends, I wouldn't go unless I knew that a toilet would be nearby. Long car rides were definitely out. Things can get kind of crazy when your daily plans are dominated by the question, "Where's the bathroom?" This may sound funny to most people, but not to the millions of people who suffer as I did.

I finally broke down and called my parents and told them how sick I really was. They were very concerned and made plans for me to fly home the next day. I walked in the door with a temperature of 105 degrees.

My dad took one look at me, packed the bathtub with ice cubes and dunked me in ice-cold water. I remember freezing in the ice water and overhearing my father crying out to my mother, "My God, I don't want my son to die."

I was confused. I didn't know what was happening. All I could think about was that I didn't want to die. I wanted to return to school. I wanted my old life back.

The very next morning, my father and mother took me to the emergency room. It was the first time I had ever been in a hospital. Unfortunately, it wouldn't be my last. I was hoping it would be a quick visit. I'd get some "cure all" medication and be on my way back to school.

My "quick visit" lasted two weeks. During this period, I would lie in bed with an IV pole attached to each arm, delivering intravenous antibiotics and nutrients, and watch TV. I got even more depressed because this was the time of the Oklahoma City bombing.

The doctors prescribed antibiotics and antiparasitic drugs that had to be given intravenously for maximum effect. To add to this, my body was so overridden by infection that it had become terribly inflamed. To combat this, I was prescribed two heavy-duty, highly toxic steroid medications, hydrocortisone and prednisone. I was given every kind of test imaginable. I got more x-rays in those two weeks than most people get in a lifetime. Both my upper and lower gastrointestinal tracts were scanned—and believe me, these weren't the usual short bursts of radiation you get with dental x-rays. I felt like radiologists were conducting an in-depth tour of my gut.

I was told that I had Crohn's colitis. Crohn's disease is a condition primarily involving the small bowel and proximal colon that causes the intestinal wall to thicken and cause narrowing of the bowel channel, blocking the intestinal tract. The result is abnormal membrane function, including nutrient malabsorption. I had an even worse variation of the disease. The doctors noted I had marked duodenitis, an inflammation of the duodenum, which is at the beginning of the small intestine, coupled with widespread inflammation through my large and small intestine. Although less than one percent of Crohn's disease patients specifically experience duodenitis, it appeared that I was one of the chosen few with both duodenal and total colonic inflammation.

At this point, the doctor ordered total parenterel nutrition (TPN). This is where nutrients are delivered intravenously directly into the bloodstream. I was rampant with infection, inflammation, and pain.

Crohn's disease was a much worse diagnosis than I had imagined. I was not in a very good state of mind at this point—especially when the doctor told me the disease was incurable. Patients with Crohn's disease experience frequent and progressive symptoms of abdominal pain, diarrhea, and extreme weight loss as seen in other wasting conditions such as cancer and AIDS. Many patients experience premature death. How's that for making you feel hopeful about your diagnosis! One thing was for sure, I was going to have to take medication if I wanted to stay alive. Yet, the side effects of the medications that keep you alive can be almost as bad as the disease itself.

Bowel diseases are on the rise. According to some literature, 85 percent of Americans have had a digestive problem of some kind. Crohn's disease, these experts argue, may eventually surpass ulcers as the number one digestive problem in the United States. The number of Americans who suffer from Crohn's disease has never been satisfactorily recorded, but is somewhere between 400,000 and 1,000,000. Each year, at least 20,000 Americans are clinically diagnosed as having Crohn's disease. Meanwhile, a good 20 percent of Americans have been diagnosed with irritable bowel syndrome. And, of course, we all know that sales of heartburn medications are booming.

Although today I can speak with experience and knowledge about bowel disease, at the end of 1994, I was just a 19-year-old suffering from a chronic disease I was told would require a lifetime of medication and who was very confused about how my entire life got so turned upside down in a matter of months. I didn't know anyone with this "Crohn's" disease and didn't even know where to go for help. I was too embarrassed to even tell my friends what my symptoms were. When they asked what was going on, I just told them I was sick. I refused to go into detail.

I left the hospital and returned home still desperately hoping to improve enough to return to school in a few weeks. I thought that there must be some kind of magic bullet that would get me well. But this new existence via medications was not a good one. True, I was no longer being given intravenous drugs, but this was only because the doctor now had my prednisone and other medications administered orally. What a dangerous drug prednisone is. That first day on it, I was hallucinating. I began crying. I was emotionally wrought. I also was taking asacol (Mesalamine), an anti-inflammatory used to treat ulcerative colitis, and two more antimicrobials, metronidazole (Flagyl) and fluconazole (Diflucan), for what had become a chronic case of thrush. To ensure I improved, the doctors also put me on ciprofloxacin (Cipro), which we now know is also prescribed for anthrax. Because a side effect of prednisone is heartburn, I had to be put on ranitidine (Zantac).

The worst part of this ordeal was that I wasn't getting better. I was still using the toilet a dozen to thirty times a day. Most of my stools were now bloody.

The nighttime was worse. You don't know what sleep deprivation is until you experience chronic nocturnal diarrhea. The trips to the bathroom began at about five every evening and went on all night every 45 minutes to an hour. If I got more than an hour of sleep during the entire night, it was a miracle. The cramps were often so intense that I wanted to pull my hair out or bang my head against the wall. I existed in a state of fatigue and exhaustion.

Not surprisingly, I almost completely lacked iron. In fact, at one point, I went more than an entire year with an almost unheard of serum iron level of 0. My serum levels of the blood protein albumin were so low they indicated my body was suffering from a severe wasting disease (cachexia). This was quite serious on both accounts. Iron is an essential component of hemoglobin, the oxygen-carrying protein in the blood. Iron is normally obtained through food in our diet and by the recycling of iron from old red blood cells. Iron deficiency or anemia means the tissues are receiving inadequate oxygen. Part of the cause was malabsorption syndrome. It was also a symptom of the polypharmacy approach to my condition the doctors had prescribed.

As for my albumin levels, this test helped to determine that not enough protein was being absorbed by my body. Albumin is the protein of the highest concentration in plasma. Albumin transports many small molecules in the blood (for example, bilirubin, calcium, progesterone, and drugs). It is also of prime importance in maintaining the oncotic pressure of the blood (that is, keeping the fluid from leaking out into the tissues). Low albumin levels also often indicate malnutrition. I was definitely malnourished.

Before my illness, I had never been hospitalized. Remember, I was born at home. In fact, I had never even set foot in a hospital until I got sick at age 19.

On a side note, I was vaccinated for the first time at age fifteen. I had the measles, mumps and rubella (MMR) vaccine. This vaccine had gone from a dead cell to a live cell vaccine sometime around 1987. The live measles vaccine has been suggested by some scientists to be linked to Crohn's disease (as well as autism and pervasive developmental disorder). In fact, a study by Dr. Andrew Wakefield and colleagues from the Royal Free Hospital, published in the February 28, 1998 issue of *The Lancet*, suggests there may be a link between the vaccine and Crohn's disease, as well as other inflammatory bowel conditions—and that even autism is linked with MMR. Perhaps the MMR vaccine was a cause of my illness. I will never know for sure.

As I recall my eating habits in the two years prior to my illness, I can say that I consumed more dairy products than I had previously in my life, including commercial frozen yogurt. I also ate my fair share of sugar. Of course, this seemed totally logical to me, since I believed that fat, not sugar, was the dietary culprit responsible for all manner of illness. Later on, I'm going to explain why I believe both cow's milk and over-consumption of carbohydrates are major causes of disease, though I do believe the properly prepared dairy products and high-quality carbohydrates that are part of the Maker's Diet, as described in this book, are invaluable to our health.

But, for now, let me say that most people are not aware that cow's milk-based dairy products can be contaminated with the *Mycobacterium avium subspecies paratuberculosis* (MAP) microorganism. Scientific research has been conducted in the United States and Europe that demonstrates that *Mycobacterium avium subspecies paratuberculosis* causes a chronic and fatal intestinal disease in a wide range of animal species. *Mycobacterium avium subspecies paratuberculosis* has, on at least one occasion, been suspected of crossing the species barrier to cause disease in a human. In fact, we now know that MAP has been implicated in causing human Crohn's disease.

But while the MMR vaccine or the consumption of large amounts of dairy may have played a role in the onset of my condition, I truly believe one of the exacerbating influences on my condition was my high carbohydrate, low fat diet. The body's gastrointestinal tract or gut is a key to optimum health. If your gastrointestinal tract isn't at optimal health, your overall health is compromised. This is true for everyone.

And the key to gastrointestinal health is our balance of good to pathogenic or bad bacteria. Put simply, bad bacteria in the gut love the types of sugary, high-carbohydrate and refined foods in the modern diet.

I had started eating large amounts of these kinds of foods when I went away to college. It was the bad bacteria that got the head start in repopulating the barren property within my gut that was left after my friendly bacteria were decimated by the large doses of antibiotics I had taken.

The growth of yeast, fungi, parasites and disease-causing bacteria within my gut had seriously damaged my gut lining, promoted absorption of internally produced toxins, and impaired absorption of nutrients. With this bacterial imbalance (dysbiosis) also came the breakdown of my body's immune barrier. You might not know that the gastrointestinal tract is critical to the body's immune function; yet, the gut is where most of the body's antibody-producing cells reside. To put it bluntly, my dysbiosis led to a host of debilitating illnesses. During my illness I had all of the following conditions:

- Chronic candidiasis (4+) (the absolute worst rating given for candida from the Great Smokies, Metametrix and Doctor's Data diagnostic laboratories, which test for such conditions). I also had an elevated candida titer, which is a measurement of blood levels of the yeast.
- Infestation by *Entamoeba histolytica*, also known as amebic dysentery.
- Cryptosporidiosis, yet another cause of intestinal illness, caused by a protozoa infection in the gastrointestinal tract.
- Incipient diabetes with extremely poor circulation (my whole lower leg was purple).
- Jaundice, besides other liver and gallbladder problems.
- Insomnia. The most I ever slept continuously was an hour and fifteen minutes.
- Hair loss. I was nineteen. (Need I say more?)
- Endocarditis (heart infection).
- Eye inflammation.
- Prostate and bladder infections.
- Chronic electrolyte imbalance due to dehydration. Electrolytes are salts in the body that conduct electricity and maintain healthy heart and kidney function.
- Elevated C-reactive protein, indicative of chronic inflammation and bacterial infection, as well as increased susceptibility to heart attack and stroke risk.
- Anemia. Anemia results when too few red blood cells are present in the bloodstream and insufficient oxygen reaches muscle tissues and organs.
- Chronic fatigue. I had all the symptoms of this mysterious, debilitating ailment—unceasing fatigue, headaches, weakness, aching in my muscles and joints, and the inability to concentrate.
- Arthritis. Arthritis inflames the joints and causes stiffness and pain. The disease in my case was autoimmune in origin—resulting from the immune system mistakenly attacking itself. (Not surprisingly, it is thought that Crohn's disease might also be autoimmune in origin and, perhaps, my body had begun attacking itself in the joints.)
- Leukocytosis. This is caused by an abnormal increase in white blood cells. There are various types of white blood cells that normally appear in the blood. While each has a unique immune function, the take-home message here is that any inflammatory condition, such as Crohn's or rheumatoid arthritis

or an overall bodily state of infection or acute stress, will result in an increased production of white blood cells. This usually entails increased numbers of cells and an increase in the percentage of immature cells.

• Malabsorption syndrome. I could not assimilate the nutrients in the food I ate.

Because of my dad's naturopathy and chiropractic background, I had it in me to try natural methods that I hoped would turn on my body's healing response. So, not long after I was discharged from the hospital, my father and I made the decision to try to find natural pathways to do just that.

I tried everything. And I do mean *everything*. My getting well became an obsession for both my dad and me. Together we began a search around the world that took me to 70 health practitioners from seven different countries, including medical doctors, chiropractors, immunologists, acupuncturists, homeopaths, herbalists, nutritionists, and dieticians.

I mentioned my experience with the Specific Carbohydrate Diet. At this point I still believed that it could have helped me if I had stayed on it perfectly with no deviations. So I decided to try it one more time. I became a strict devotee and even consulted daily on the phone with Elaine Gottschall. She had worked with a physician, Elson Haas, to heal her own daughter of ulcerative colitis, a disease very similar to Crohn's disease. I stayed on the diet with fanatical adherence for three to six months, three different times. I was told it had helped a lot of people. But, unfortunately, it didn't work for me.

I must have tried every diet that has ever been written about. I consulted with some of the foremost practitioners and diet experts throughout the world. I visited Dr. Robert Atkins of the world famous Atkins Center in Manhattan and Atkins Diet. I met with California-based eicosanoid guru Barry Sears, Ph.D., author of *The Zone*. I contacted Jeffrey Bland, Ph.D., a highly regarded functional medicine expert and used his detoxification/elimination diet. No luck. Each of these health professionals was extremely knowledgeable and highly educated. They truly wanted to help. I knew they were sincere and that their diets had many solid underpinnings. But something was missing because none of them were able to help. I kept searching.

I estimate that over the course of about two years my father spent $150,000 on natural health treatments. I took dozens of probiotic formulas, as well as enzyme, fiber, anti-candida and antiparasitic formulas. At one point I was taking upwards of six bottles a day of extremely expensive probiotics; one of these products sold for two dollars a capsule and was delivered in a special oil matrix carrier. I remember using two bottles of powdered acidophilus a day, two bottles of bifidus, and two bottles of bulgaricus—mind you, every day. One product alone, the two-dollars-a-capsule oil matrix product, was at a dosage of thirty capsules a day. I wanted to get better. I wanted to end the pain. So I was willing to try anything and everything.

Someone told me my liver was the problem. I tried liver detoxification. I read about live cell therapy. I did cell therapy with injectable sheep cells taken from sheep embryos. The "health expert" who provided the products told me that in the United Kingdom he had cured some 250 Crohn's disease patients. The needles were huge. I read that cabbage juice was good for the gut and that it was rich in organic sulfur compounds, so I ingested large amounts of cabbage juice. I used more detoxification formulas. I did retention enemas and colonics and more liver detoxification, including several rounds on Dr. Bland's detoxification programs. I tried glandulars from every conceivable organ. I used injectable vitamins and minerals. For this regimen, I was instructed to inject myself *seven times a day*. I used a needle reserved for insulin injections. I had become so emaciated that when I injected myself in the shoulders and the sides of my hip, I could feel the needle hitting bone.

I used injectable thymus gland extract. I consumed wheat grass juice. I tried Chinese herbs, Peruvian herbs, Japanese kampo, olive leaf extract, and shark cartilage. I tried macrobiotics. I used nitrogenated soy. I visited alternative cancer clinics in Mexico and Germany. Often, I returned worse than when I began. Every doctor who treated me characterized my appearance as that of a "Nazi concentration camp survivor."

My search for an answer for my Crohn's disease sent me further and further from home. I traveled to clinics all over the world, oftentimes in a wheel chair. As I mentioned, I went to the offices of 70 health professionals from seven different countries—in Europe, South America, Mexico, and Canada. As my search grew more frantic and desperate, at times I was grasping for straws. I tried two or three treatments that no rational person would consider. I know what it's like to be desperate, willing to try anything. I tried almost 500 different "miracle" products. I was the victim—and I choose that word carefully—of many well-meaning network marketing distributors of health products who made outrageous and unfounded claims. So much of what passes for scientifically validated nutritional supplementation is shamelessly promoted through network marketing or multi-level marketing and truly has little, if any, scientific substance. The goal of too many of these companies is to brainwash their network into believing what they have will cure anything and everything—for a price. The companies fill their marketers' brains with outlandish claims from scientists for hire and know they can get away with it because they are usually operating well below the detection level of federal regulators. There's undoubtedly some good stuff out there. But there is also a lot of hype and flash that isn't worth your time or money and may actually be injurious to your health. I know from firsthand experience.

I did different IV treatments. I took something called adrenal cortical extract, or ACE, an extract of bovine adrenal gland that is thought to possess the powers of hydrocortisone and was once used extensively in medicine. Only belatedly did I learn many such batches were contaminated with *Mycobacterium abscessus*, a rapidly growing bacterium distantly related to the tuberculosis organism.

My dad, reading health magazines and calling colleagues, found all kinds of clinics and therapies for me to try. The number of machines that were hooked up to my body could fill a science fiction novel! I tried various forms of electro-dermal screening (EDS). Let me tell you about EDS. It is a form of computerized information gathering, based on physics. A blunt, noninvasive electric probe is placed at specific points on the patient's hands, face or feet, corresponding to acupuncture points at the beginning or end of the energy meridians. Minute electrical discharges from these points serve as information signals about the condition of the body's organs and systems. These signals are useful to the health practitioner in evaluating and developing a treatment plan. It is said that EDS can test for over 20,000 substances and find the underlying causes of illness and an appropriate treatment plan. Among these are: allergens, amino acids, botanicals, cosmetics, digestives, enzymes, essential oils, food additives, foods, geopathic stress, glandulars, hazardous wastes, heavy metals, herbicides, homeopathic remedies, household products, isotopes, miasmas (a vaporous exhalation formerly believed to cause disease), minerals, parasites, elements, pesticides, phenols, and pollutants, to name a few of the substances and causes of illness. Supposedly, according to one doctor who probed me with his EDS machine, my illness was due to electromagnetic fields in my house. I had to sleep in a steel cage that was put around my room. At night, I began to shut off the TV and clocks—all electrical devises. I don't need to tell you whether this worked. I think you know the answer.

This was all weird science, and it could only have come from the outer reaches of the alternative health field. Another so-called alternative health practitioner who treated me said I was sensitive to the movements of a certain satellite that orbited the Earth every ten years. He said I was one of the rare, unlucky people that the satellite influenced—and that I would have to wait a considerable period of time before the satellite left the Earth's orbit. Needless to say I was no longer a fan of the space program.

I tried applied kinesiology, a type of chiropractic where different tests for muscle strength and weakness are done on points of your body. I utilized acupuncture and homeopathy.

Taking various medications and supplements was my life. Unless I was visiting a doctor, which I did several times a week, I stayed home. I sat in my chair fantasizing by watching cooking shows. I felt a special bond with Chef Emeril.

I also read—just about every piece of literature and book about health that I could get my hands on. I read over 300 books on health and nutrition during my illness. I continuously puzzled over what products to use and which products could help me.

I didn't just read health books. I often went to the doctor who wrote the book and consulted in person with that doctor. If I couldn't get the top person, I wasn't interested. All the doctors and health practitioners I visited said they could cure me in a short period of time. They had never failed to cure their patients, they said. All of them made promises they couldn't keep. I'm not saying their claims were totally unfounded. I'm sure they believed in their work, but it turns out that very few of them have clinical validation to verify their claims. But my willingness to believe them and put all my faith in them demonstrates what people who are desperately ill go through.

Because I was so weak, traveling from clinic to clinic, especially by airplane, was an ordeal. I oftentimes got bladder as well as eye infections. At one point, as I sat in my seat waiting for an airplane to take off, I said to myself, "If this plane went down, it wouldn't be that bad." It was a sick thought, but it shows my mentality during the darkest days. I was not suicidal, but I just couldn't handle the pain anymore. I reasoned that, if I died, at least I could join my Creator.

I hit rock-bottom on a trip to Germany, where I went to take yet another herbal IV treatment. At that time, the U.S. Food and Drug Administration (FDA) did not permit this herb to be imported, so I had to go to Germany to take it. The timing for a trip to Germany couldn't have been worse. I was weaning myself from medications. I had gotten off prednisone, but I experienced a complete adrenal shock. I couldn't catch my breath. My mother accompanied me to the German clinic. All the way there, a 28-hour trip including planes and trains, one nightmare event after another occurred. I missed a train by a few minutes because my mom and I couldn't manage to drag our luggage through the station on time. Because we missed the train, we were stuck in the station for six hours. All the time I was running around looking for a bathroom.

The German doctor made an interesting diagnosis. He concluded that my problem rested with my immune system. Certain parts of my immune system were overactive and certain parts were underactive. My mom and dad still had to pay for my medical bills, so staying in Germany to care for me wasn't an option. My mother, a schoolteacher, had to return to work, and she left me in Germany.

I stayed in the clinic for six weeks. Not only did I get no results, the nurses were inattentive. After my six-hour IV treatment, no one would come to help me back to my room. Alone, sitting in an IV chair, shaking with cold chills, feeling like I was about to have a seizure, I waited for someone to help me. After about an hour of waiting with no help, I would then creep back to my room to sleep.

I certainly slept more while I was in Germany, because I was put on high doses of opium. In Germany, doctors prescribe tincture of opium to slow down peristalsis and keep patients from having to go to the bathroom so much. The doctor, like any good egotistical physician, decided that I wasn't getting well because I had mental problems.

I had reached rock-bottom. I was 19 years old. I had dropped out of college. I was far away from family and was without friends. My mother had left me in a German health clinic where nobody spoke English. My feeble attempts at German got me nowhere. I was imprisoned in my own body. I was miserable and constantly in pain. At the same time I was contemplating dark dreary thoughts, wondering if I would ever enjoy normalcy again, if ever I would simply wake up without pain, healthy like I once had been.

Finally, my parents and I decided it was time for me to come home. To catch my airplane, I had to leave at five a.m., but nobody in the clinic was awake that early. I was too frail and thin to carry my own luggage and I needed someone to help me but had no help. I couldn't find switches to turn on lights in the halls. I tripped down some stairs in the dark and finally managed to get my suitcases to the lobby. But when the taxicab showed up, I couldn't open the door. I was locked in. Finally I found a back entrance, managed to wheel my bags out, and tripped down another set of steps. I fell flat on my face.

Too weak to walk on my own, I had to be wheeled into the airport. At the ticket counter, they had to summon someone who spoke English, but he couldn't find any record of my ticket. I had no money. My credit card was declined. I was completely sick. I had a urinary tract infection in addition to my massive bowl problems. I was on opium. It appeared I wouldn't get home. I said a quick prayer: "Lord, I cannot do a single thing. Please help me get out of this situation. I feel completely hopeless." In a couple of minutes they told me that my ticket had been found. I got on the plane. I took a ten-hour flight to the United States, missed a connecting flight, and finally made it to Miami. Getting home had been a 30-hour ordeal.

I cannot describe how relieved I was to be home. I remember lying on the couch listening to "The Annette Funicello Story" on television. I had compresses over my eyes for double conjunctivitis. I had to run with my eyes closed to the bathroom either for a painful bowel movement or for burning urination. But in spite of my illness and pain, I was thrilled to be home again with my family—at least as thrilled as could be expected from someone who by now lacked hope of recovery from terminal illness.

Shortly after my return home from Germany, I was hospitalized a second time. I was now completely dehydrated and had a resting heart rate of between 160 to 180 beats per minute. I couldn't keep water down. My weight had dropped to 104 pounds, the lowest ever. The nurses tried to get IVs into me so I could be re-hydrated, but they couldn't get any blood return because my veins were so dry and tapped out. It took the nurses and doctors two and a half hours to get an IV into my body. The nurses started crying in the hallway. I heard one say, "That poor boy isn't going to make it through the night."

Feeling more hopeless than words can describe, I only knew to pray. I didn't blame God. Even while feeling grim and believing I was going to die, I always held a glimmer of hope that God would choose to cure me. If not, I was prepared to meet my Maker. I was disappointed that I had never fallen in love or married. But I had a great, great life. I trusted God's plan for my life, and put myself in the only capable hands I knew of—my heavenly Father's. I thanked my Creator for a wonderful life. I was grateful for every moment. That night, I lay in bed, alone in my room, prepared to die.

Then something happened. When I woke in the morning, my grandmother was there, her hand on my forehead. Soon, several nurses entered. They were elated when they were able to get a blood return and could hook me up to an IV. Overnight, I gained ten pounds of water weight. That's how dehydrated I was!

I felt a new resolve in my body. I wanted so badly to live. I felt a glimmer of sunshine entering my life, newfound hope, real hope. That is, until the doctors got hold of my body. Once again, I became a human drugstore. The doctors prescribed the same medications I had been given the first time I was hospitalized—the antibiotics, antifungals, antiparasitics and the steroids hydrocortisone and prednisone. When the time came to leave the hospital and they switched me once again from IV to oral medications, I had hallucinations. As baseball sage Yogi Berra likes to say: "It was déjà vu all over again."

Somehow I managed to break through the hallucinations to say something to my mom. I had an unusual demand. It completely startled her.

"I want you to take a picture of me."

She stammered and then refused. She couldn't fathom why anyone would want a picture to commemorate such a pathetic condition. But even with everything I had been through and all those doctors that failed to help me, I still had faith in my God's ability to deliver me from my despair.

I remember her asking, "Why in the world do you want me to take a picture of you?"

I answered with my best attempt at a smile, "Because no one will believe me when I get well. No one will believe that I was this sick. I'm getting out of bed and I need you to take my picture."

I nearly fell to the floor climbing out of bed. I needed help standing up and even then it was a struggle.

The picture you see on the cover of this book is the photograph my mother took. After a two week stint in the hospital, I had gained 10 pounds of water weight and weighed 114.

The skin on my body looked dead. People often compare my appearance in that photo to a concentration camp victim or prisoner of war. I had a beard because I was too weak to shave and couldn't afford to cut myself with my unsteady hand.

One doctor told me my only hope was to go to Cedars-Sinai in New York where surgeons would expertly remove all of my large and part of my small intestines. Alternatively, I could undergo another kind of surgery, experimental at the time, called a J-Pouch procedure. The surgery represented a way to try and preserve bowel function once I had my colon removed. Along with my family, I decided to go to Cedars-Sinai and get whatever surgery I needed. I read the doctors' transcripts of my medical records. My physician called my condition the worst case of Crohn's disease he had ever seen and doubted I would live to return home. It was crazy. The medications were only making me worse. At least their effects could probably be reversed, but surgery? That was permanent. Not only that, I have now learned that nearly 75 percent of people with Crohn's who have surgery must have a second surgery.

I had only a little bit of fight left, but enough to get myself into a wheelchair and out of the hospital. I left, scared, wounded, and not knowing what to do next.

So what else was new? It was early 1996. My father had just gotten through telling me he had spoken to an eccentric nutritionist on the phone. My father didn't want me to get my hopes up so he had investigated the man's program himself. The nutritionist told my father he believed I was ill because I was not eating the diet of my ancestors, based upon Biblical principles.

When my father told me about all of this, naturally, I was curious. Since I had opted not to have surgery and I was still alive, I decided to try this. It fit into my belief system.

In an effort to start all over, I took myself off all nutritional products and read the Bible to see what people ate thousands of years ago. I also learned that the longest living cultures in the world had one thing in common: they consumed living foods that abounded with beneficial microorganisms.

A few weeks later, I got on a plane, still bound to my wheelchair, and headed for southern California to live closer to the man who would teach me how to eat from the Bible. After integrating into that particular nutritionist's program some of my own findings about nutrition and health from the Bible I saw some improvement.

Most times promises are best kept, but, occasionally, times arise when a promise broken is best. It had been ten months since I had taken any supplements, and although my father had promised he wouldn't send me anything else to try, he decided to send me something anyway. It was a plastic bag containing black powder. I had already tried over thirty different probiotics. Now was I supposed to eat this stuff that looked like dirt?

"Forget it," I thought.

My dad called on the phone and urged me to give it a try.

"It may look like dirt, but it isn't," he said. "It contains healthy organisms from the soil."

An article that accompanied the package explained that these were the nutrients missing from today's pesticide-sterilized, barren soils—not only trace minerals but organisms (Homeostatic Soil Organisms™, or HSOs™, as I later named them).* These were living organisms that had been wiped out by the pesticide treatment of America's farm lands, pasteurization of foods, and modern man's disdain for all microorganisms—even those life-supportive bugs our bodies need for great health.

I decided to include these HSOs in my daily diet, which also included raw goat's milk in the form of fermented kefir, different organically grown free-range or grass-fed meats, natural sprouted or sourdough breads made from whole grains that were yeast-free, organic fruits and vegetables, raw sauerkraut, and carrot and other vegetable juices—all "live" foods with their beneficial enzymes and microorganisms intact.

Improvement didn't come immediately; I had somewhat of a Herxheimer reaction. Also referred to as "die-off," the Herxheimer reaction is an allergic response resulting from the death of large numbers of pathological organisms. Their cell-wall proteins become absorbed through the patient's chronically weakened mucous membranes which absorb toxic products from these dead organisms. The collective effects of organism die-off often temporarily worsen one's symptoms. Holistic physicians who practice environmental medicine believe this die-off reaction indicates that the patient is having an excellent backlash effect to good treatment. Since the time of Hippocrates it has been understood that symptoms of most diseases, other than degenerative disorders where irreversible organic damage has been sustained, represent the efforts of the body to eliminate toxins.[1] In 1848 Thomas Sydenham, the English Hippocrates, wrote, "[a] disease, however much its cause may be adverse to the human body, is nothing more than an effort of Nature who strains with might and main to restore the health of the patient by the elimination of the morbific matter."[2]

One month after adding the "black powder" to my diet, I noticed an elimination of "black, tar-like stuff." I also had newfound energy, and I went to the bathroom less frequently.

At this point, my father purchased a used motor home for me because he knew that staying close to the ocean and breathing the air would be good for me. In my motor home, I was something of a bum trying to find places to park at night—an unusual experience for an upper-middle-class kid like me. You may ask how on Earth I was able to drive a motor home in my condition. My answer is simply: Only the Lord knows. Different people stayed with me in the motor home to take care of me.

During my forty days and nights of parking my motor home close to the beach, I prayed, listened to music and planned everything around buying, preparing and eating my food. My weight went from 122 to 151 pounds. I gained 29 pounds in 40 days! The photograph of me on the beach that you see in this book

* Throughout the course of this book, I will refer to HSOs also as soil organisms.

was taken during this period. I was not completely well yet, but I had made miraculous strides toward full recovery. I continued to gain weight and strength, and by my twenty-first birthday, I weighed 170 pounds—practically my original weight before I got sick. I doubt if anyone in the world was happier than me.

The terrain of my body and my intestinal tract were being rebuilt, and it appeared that somehow the HSOs themselves were taking care of my underlying condition. After all, in three months, I had gained over 50 pounds.

The combination of the Biblical diet and the HSOs had restored my health. I still went through periods of detoxification every few months or so, but I continued to persevere. In December 1996, I came home to Florida. I was at my normal weight. I was ready to start my life again. I was finally healthy. Praise God!

I had done what hundreds of thousands of disease sufferers desperately want to do—I had recovered my health. My first idea was to go back to the many doctors who had treated me and tell them about the Biblical or Maker's Diet and the HSOs. I mailed my "before" and "after" pictures to the doctors I had consulted with. I thought everyone would be so eager to learn what had healed me. I thought the doctors would want to include the Maker's Diet and HSOs in their treatment programs. Some doctors were very excited. Elaine Gottschall, author of *Breaking the Vicious Cycle*, was very happy for me. The doctors all wanted to hear my story, but very few of them wanted to try the Maker's Diet and HSOs with their patients. I felt like I had something to help other sufferers of digestive disorders, especially other Crohn's disease sufferers. But no one wanted to hear about it.

Dr. Morton Walker, a medical journalist who had given me information for some of the clinics I visited, suggested that he write an article outlining my story for the *Townsend Letter for Doctors and Patients*, a prestigious health publication that focuses on alternative medicines and treatments. The article about my recovery generated over two thousand phone calls from doctors as well as individuals suffering from bowel disease.[3]

Literally overnight, I was forced to find a way to distribute the HSOs that had helped me get well. I started Garden of Life, a company that manufactures innovative products based on the dietary principles that helped me and are designed to help the body heal itself. In the ensuing years, I earned degrees in nutrition, sports medicine, and naturopathy.

My mission became helping people like myself who are ill to regain their health and helping people who are healthy flourish.

I believe I went through my ordeal for a reason. I consulted 70 doctors and took 500 health products for a reason. Because I have personally experienced and survived my walk through the valley of disease and death and because of my nutritional education, I can speak to you as an authority.

Today, I've been well for over seven years. I have been off medication for almost eight years. People say Crohn's disease is incurable, but from my experience, no disease is incurable. Some people may be too far gone and may not ever get completely well, but every single disease and every single state of health can be improved through whole-food nutrition and whole-food supplements that bring us back to a diet and a lifestyle that has been proven to work for thousands of years.

My goal after getting well was to create a vehicle whereby I could reach people who were suffering from digestive and immune system disorders. I began to design products based on the theory of anthropological nutrition or, simply, the nutrition of our history.

But now that I was better, I also wanted to know everything there is to know about *how* I got better. I wanted to design a program so that everyone who suffers from illness can take their health into their own hands.

Looking back on my illness, I think the one thing I and others missed most about my old self was laughter. I didn't laugh very much when I was ill. I'm usually a real clown, someone who likes good jokes and who enjoys telling them. I so much liked to make people laugh, and I like to laugh, too. But that part of my life had been sucked out of me by illness. I just wasn't myself. Now once again, I laugh. I tell jokes. I am an even better version of my old self. My bout with severe illness has made me stronger. Much like the story of Job in the Bible, the Lord had restored what was taken away and multiplied it more than I could have ever imagined.

CHAPTER TWO

I've Got A Gut Feeling

Why do we say when a performing artist, whose songs were so full of feeling, sang from his gut?

Why do performers get "butterflies in their stomach" before going on stage?

Why does indigestion produce nightmares?

Why are antidepressants now also being used for gastrointestinal ailments?

I like word games. I like definitions.

Here's one from *Merriam-Webster's Collegiate Dictionary*.

The etymology of the word *gut* leads us back to the Middle English word *guttas*, which then takes us to sometime before the twelfth century to the Old English word *gEotan*, meaning "to pour." Your gut, the dictionary says, is "the basic visceral or emotional part of a person," also "the alimentary canal or part of it (as the intestine or stomach)," or "the inner essential parts." As we go along, keep these definitions in mind.

It turns out that both our gut and our brain originate early in embryogenesis from a clump of tissue called the neural crest, which appears and divides during fetal development. While one section turns into the central nervous system, another piece migrates to become the enteric nervous system, and thus form both thinking machines. Only later are the two nervous systems connected via a cable called the vagus nerve, the longest of all the cranial nerves whose name is derived from Latin, meaning "wandering." In keeping with its etymological origins, the vagus nerve meanders from the brain stem through organs in the neck and thorax and finally ends up in the abdomen. There's the brain-gut connection.

So profoundly influential is the state of the gut upon people's health that I have coined the term—it's a tongue twister—gastro-neuro-immunology to try and capture the essence of the link between our two brains and even our immune function.

It is from the healthy gut that we enjoy neurological and psychological as well as immunological health. This is not to discount the highly important mass of gray between our ears—the human brain. This is simply to say that the body has two brains—the brain we all know of between our ears and the second brain, our gut.

GASTRO-NEURO-IMMUNOLOGY

No wonder why we talk so much about gut feelings.

Gut-wrenching feelings.

No wonder we tell people to trust their gut.

Are we living too much in our head? Should we think with our gut? Did you know that one half of all our nerve cells are located within the gut? Did you know that our capacity for feeling and emotional expression depends primarily on the gut and, to a lesser extent, the brain?

Did you know that your gastrointestinal health is a major key to your overall and total health?

Do you have a gut feeling where I'm headed with all of this?

Our journey has only begun.

We take our gastrointestinal tract or gut for granted. We really shouldn't. I was reading an article recently by Sandra Blakeslee, originally published in the January 23, 1996 issue of *The New York Times*. It tends to be widely circulated on the web and captured the link between our gut and brain perfectly:

Have you ever wondered why people get butterflies in the stomach before going on stage? Or why an impending job interview can cause an attack of intestinal cramps? And why do antidepressants targeted for the brain cause nausea or abdominal upset in millions of people who take such drugs? The reason for these common experiences is because each of us literally has two brains—the familiar one encased in our skulls and a lesser-known but vitally important one found in the human gut. Like Siamese twins, the two brains are interconnected; when one gets upset, the other does, too.

The gut's brain, known as the enteric nervous system (ENS), is located in sheaths of tissue lining the esophagus, stomach, small intestine and colon. (Enteric is derived from the *word* entera, simply meaning we also have a nervous system in our entera or intestinal tract.)

Considered a single entity, it is packed with neurons, neurotransmitters and proteins that zap messages between neurons, support cells like those found in the brain. It contains a complex circuitry that enables it to act independently, learn, remember and, as the saying goes, produce gut feelings, says the *Times* article.

In his book *The Second Brain* (HarperCollins 1998), Dr. Michael Gershon, a professor of anatomy and cell biology at Columbia-Presbyterian Medical Center in New York City, dubs the entire gastrointestinal system the body's second nervous system.

"The brain is not the only place in the body that's full of neurotransmitters," says Dr. Gershon. "A hundred million neurotransmitters line the length of the gut, approximately the same number that is found in the brain... The brain in the bowel has got to work right or no one will have the luxury to think at all."

The field of neurogastroenterology finds its start with the nineteenth century English investigators William M. Bayliss and Ernest H. Starling. Bayliss and Starling took anesthetized dogs and applied pressure to the intestinal lumen (i.e., the cavity of the tubular gastrointestinal organ). This pressure caused contraction and anal relaxation, followed by a propulsive wave. It is this propulsive wave or peristaltic reflex that scientists call the "law of the intestine." Peristalsis moves—rather, propels—food through the digestive tract. In experimental studies, even when all nerves connecting the bowel to the brain and spinal cord were severed, "the law of the intestine" prevailed and digestion continued. Thus, the scientists surmised the enteric nervous system to be independent from the central nervous system.

After the initial work of Bayliss and Starling and experiments some 18 years later conducted by German scientist Paul Trendelenburg, which confirmed their findings, science moved on. Researchers discovered other chemical neurotransmitters such as epinephrine and acetylcholine and lost interest in the law of the intestine. Exacerbating the situation, the publisher of Trendelenburg's results (reported in 1917) was John N. Langley who went on to author *The Autonomic Nervous System* in 1921. Langley was also editor and publisher of the *Journal of Physiology* and had over the years alienated many of his colleagues. Many of the theories that he popularized were ultimately trivialized in a case of wholesale scientific revenge. In a move involving an ultimate scientific insult, scientists at the Physiological Society, which took over the journal after Langley's death, reclassified the enteric nerves as simply part of the para-sympathetic nervous system.

It wasn't until the period between 1965 and 1967 that Dr. Gershon proposed, in a series of papers in *Science* and the *Journal of Physiology*, that there existed a third neurotransmitter, namely serotonin (5-hydroxytryptamine, 5-HT), that was both produced in and targeted to the ENS. Now we know this neurotransmitter is also found in the central nervous system. Details of how the enteric nervous system mirrors the central nervous system have been emerging in recent years. Nearly every substance that helps run and control the brain has turned up in the gut. In fact, many major neurotransmitters that until recently were usually associated with the brain, such as serotonin, dopamine, glutamate, norepinephrine and nitric oxide, we know now to be found in plentiful amounts in the gut. Some two dozen small brain proteins, called neuropeptides, are also found in relatively high amounts in the gut—as are major cells of the immune system. Enkephalins, one class of the body's natural opiates, are plentiful in the gut. And in a finding that confounds many researchers, the gut is a rich source of benzodiazepines—the family of psychoactive chemicals that includes such ever-popular drugs as Valium and Xanax, reports Blakeslee.

We all think that the brain in our skull is the "Big Cheese" or majordomo of the body, literally chief of the house. Trouble is, when you start counting nerve cells, as mentioned, we find some hundred million of them in the gut alone—about as many as in the spinal cord. Add in the esophagus, stomach and large intestine and suddenly we have more nerve cells in the gut than in the entire remainder of the peripheral nervous system.

Talk to people and most will tell you the brain determines whether you are happy or sad. But contrary to what most think, this may be all backward. Perhaps the gut is more responsible than we ever imagined for our mental well-being, how we *feel*.

No wonder Karl Lashley, generally considered the founder of neuropsychology, noted in 1951, "I am coming more and more to the conviction that the rudiments of every human behavioral mechanism will be found represented even in primitive activities of the nervous system."

As light is shed on the circuitry between the two brains, researchers are beginning to understand why people act and feel the way they do. The brain and gut are so much alike that during our sleeping hours both have natural 90-minute cycles. For the brain, this slow wave sleep is interrupted by periods of rapid eye movement sleep in which dreams occur. For the gut, the 90-minute cycles also involve slow waves of muscle contractions—but as with REM intervals—these are punctuated by short bursts of rapid muscle movement. Could it be that both brains influence each other? The answer is probably yes. REM sleep is a sleep phase characterized by arousal, altered activity of the autonomic nervous system and altered colon (large intestine) function.

We also know that patients with bowel problems tend to have abnormal REM sleep. Poor sleep has been reported by many, perhaps a majority of, patients with irritable bowel syndrome (IBS) and non-ulcerative dyspepsia—also known as "sour stomach"—who complain of awakening tired and unrefreshed in the morning. Even after patients awake from what they describe as a "sound sleep," they report a general feeling of tiredness and fatigue. Abnormal REM sleep is reduced by low-dose treatment with the antidepressant amitryptiline, which has also been shown to be effective in treating IBS and non-ulcerative dyspepsia. The sleep disturbance is likely to play an important role in the chronicity of symptoms by setting up a vicious cycle: pain, fatigue and emotional distress all alter the body's arousal systems during sleep. In turn, poor sleep quality increases sensitivity to bowel and somatic (skin and muscle) stimuli leading to more pain and distress. This finding supports traditional folk wisdom that indigestion produces nightmares. On a personal note, I believe that sleep is the single most important ingredient for digestive health. I believe that by getting enough sleep at the right time (sleep before midnight is much more valuable) you can do wonders for your digestion.

Many drugs designed to affect the brain also affect the gut. For example, the gut is loaded with the neurotransmitter serotonin. In fact, more serotonin is produced there than anywhere else in the body. Serotonin is linked with initiation of peristalsis.

About 25 percent of people taking fluoxetine (Prozac) and other types of similar-acting antidepressants experience gastrointestinal problems such as nausea, diarrhea and constipation. The problem with these drugs is that they prevent uptake of serotonin by cells that should be using it. While this enables the depressed person to have more serotonin in the brain, less is available for use by the cells of the gastrointestinal tract. "Serotonin is calming to the digestive tract, initiates peristaltic and secretory reflexes," notes nutritionist June Butlin, M.Sc., Ph.D. "Long-term use or the wrong dosage may cause fluctuations between nausea, vomiting, constipation and diarrhea, and can cause depression, anxiety, insomnia, and fluctuations in appetite."

In a study reported in *The New York Times* article, Dr. Gershon and his colleagues explain Prozac's side effects on the gut. They mounted a section of guinea pig colon on a stand and put a small pellet in the 'mouth' end. The isolated colon whips the pellet down to the 'anal' end of the column, just as it would inside an animal. When the researchers put a small amount of Prozac into the colon, the pellet "went into high gear," Dr. Gershon explained to the paper. "The drug doubled the speed at which the pellet passed through the colon, which would explain why some people get diarrhea," the paper says. "No wonder, in small doses, Prozac is used to treat chronic constipation.

"If a little is beneficial for constipation, a lot is not. When the Gershon team greatly increased the amount of Prozac in the guinea pig colon, the pellet stopped moving at all. Hence, a little cures constipation; a lot causes it. Prozac stimulates sensory nerves, thus can also cause nausea."

The gut has opiate receptors much like the brain. "Not surprisingly, drugs like morphine and heroin that are thought to act on the central nervous system also attach to the gut's opiate receptors, producing constipation," notes pain management specialist Michael Loes, M.D., M.D.(H.), author of *The Healing Response* (Freedom Press 2002) "Both brains," he says, "can be addicted to opiates."

Many Alzheimer's and Parkinson's disease patients are constipated. A sickness we think of as primarily affecting the brain or central nervous system also impacts the gut.

Our gut also helps us in some amazing ways. The gut also produces chemicals called benzodiazepines. These are the same chemicals found in antianxiety drugs like Valium, and these are the same chemicals that alleviate pain. Perhaps our gut is truly our body's anxiety and pain reliever. No wonder why when we're anxious we tend to overeat. Perhaps our body is trying to produce extra benzodiazepines.

While we are not sure whether the gut synthesizes benzodiazepine from chemicals in our foods, bacterial actions, or both, we know that in times of extreme pain, the gut goes into overdrive, delivering benzodiazepine to the brain. The result is to render the patient unconscious or at least reduce the pain, says Dr. Anthony Basile, a neurochemist in the Neuroscience Laboratory at the National Institutes of Health in Bethesda, Maryland.

Take care of your gut. It's taking care of you.

Dr. Gershon goes as far as to say that "the gut may be more intellectual than the heart and may have a greater capacity for feeling." He also believes that our society's many gastrointestinal problems originate from imbalances within the gut's brain.

"Throughout the world's healing and mystical traditions, the belly is seen as an important center of energy and consciousness," says Fernando Pagés Ruiz, a contributing editor to *Yoga Journal*. "You've probably noticed that many of India's great spiritual adepts sport prodigious bellies. These tremendous tummies are thought to be full of prana. Hence, Indian artists often depict their deities with a paunch.

"In China, the gentle art of tai chi emphasizes the lower abdomen as a reservoir for energy." In his online article, Pagés Ruiz quotes tai chi teacher Kenneth Cohen, author of *The Way of Qigong* (Ballantine Books, 1997) and says that, according to Cohen, "it's possible to strengthen the abdominals by learning how to compact qi (prana) into the belly." "From the Chinese viewpoint," he quotes Cohen, "the belly is considered the dan tian or 'field of the elixir,' where you plant the seeds of long life and wisdom."

Lastly, in Biblical times, the seat of emotion, which we call the heart, is actually referring to the bowels. That thought in itself conjures up an image of a young Romeo sending a love note to his girlfriend with the inscription, "Baby, you really move me."

The trouble with these modern times is that so many influences today are counterproductive to gastrointestinal health. I know: I was very likely one of the victims of one or more of these influences—including vaccinations; milk contaminated with *Mycobacterium avium subspecies paratuberculosis*; indiscriminate overuse of antibiotics; and poor diet—and that's just a few of our modern day enemies out to destroy our gastrointestinal health.

Many people are falling victim to these influences. As a result, they are experiencing health problems that could be overcome if they knew that they centered in their gut. No wonder so many of us have poor health. We've neglected the health of our gut for far too long.

Part II–
Enter the Garden
of Life

CHAPTER THREE

Beyond Probiotics

I mentioned that I started a nutrition company, Garden of Life. Many people far more expert in the business of natural health than I tell me Garden of Life is the fastest-growing nutrition company in the world today. If so, I believe that this is because everything we are doing now at Garden of Life is different than how it is being done currently and was done in the past in the field of nutritional supplements. That is because our theories of health are different than those of anyone else. For us, isolated vitamins and minerals are passé. We recognize their role in supplementing the diet, but they're so limited. Let me tell you, Nature has far more nutritional treasures than what have been isolated in the laboratory. The real goal ought to be to concentrate Nature's nutritional treasures as our Creator intended. (Besides, since almost everyone else is already manufacturing isolated, fractionated, and synthesized vitamin and mineral formulas, it is clear that *the last thing* the world needs now is another vitamin and mineral manufacturer.) Nor does the consumer need more formulas from marketers who try to create a big splash for the "latest and greatest" with flashy advertising that will "push" their products on the public. What is needed is something solid—supplements so nutritionally valuable that if the consumer were stranded on a deserted island, he or she could actually live off of them—supplements so thoroughly clinically validated that the results consumers and patients can expect are expertly detailed in published studies—supplements crafted from a modern day Garden of Eden and that are as Nature intended—free from pesticides, grown organically, unadulterated—yet, proven through rigorous science.

For us, the center of health is the gut—the body's gastrointestinal tract. And that's why our whole food concentrates are always targeted, in one respect or another, to aiding gastrointestinal health. One of our mottos surely is that, "you are not what you eat, but what you assimilate."

But the gut is more than the second brain; it is also the seat of the body's defenses, the center of immune function. In addition to the lymphoid tissue concentrated within the lymph nodes and spleen and immune cells circulating in our bloodstream, lymphoid tissue and immune cells are also found at other sites, most notably the gastrointestinal tract, respiratory tract and urogenital tract. Such lymphoid tissue is termed MALT or mucosal-associated lymphoid tissue. In the gastrointestinal tract, however, it's called the GALT or gut-associated lymphoid tissue. Our gut produces about 75 percent of our body's total immune system cells. So when we want to boost immunity, we must also look at improving gastrointestinal health.

Studies show that over 40 percent of patients visit their doctors for gastrointestinal problems, with complaints ranging from irritable bowel syndrome, abdominal bloating, and diarrhea to constipation. Often there are no answers to these problems because of a lack of diagnosed anatomical or chemical defects. Doctors tell patients that their gut problems are imaginary, emotional, or all in their heads, attributing their problems to brain malfunction. Needless to say, the quality of life for these patients will not be ideal until their problems are understood and a method to enhance the body's healing response is found. An understanding of the enteric nervous system and the importance of the gut to overall well-being should help to provide cures for many conditions well beyond those that center on the gastrointestinal tract. After all, the gut is the center of our own happiness and well-being.

There's a good reason why Primal Defense™ with Homeostatic Soil Organisms (HSOs) has become our flagship formula at Garden of Life. Every idea that we have put into action has come from the premise of this formula and the lessons it has spawned. A lot of diseases, we now realize, result from living too far removed from our microscopic allies, the beneficial bacteria in our environment.

Let's look more closely at these ancient soil organisms.* In the *Townsend Letter*, Dr. Morton Walker reports on their discovery and the implications of this discovery:[4]

There are relatively few areas of the world today whose natural ecology has been untainted by modern man. While hiking through a remote area on another continent in 1978, an American scientist discovered some mounds on the ground that he recognized as homeostatic soil organisms of an unusual nature. He brought a small quantity of the HSOs to the United States for use in experimentation. Because these bacteria are not regularly found on the North American continent, the scientist had to create a new culture for research purposes. Over the next three years his research team performed studies on the unknown homeostatic soil organisms. These researchers: (1) identified exactly what the various strains were; (2) determined toxicity or pathogenicity of the bacteria for humans or animals; (3) ascertained if the HSOs are beneficial for animals or humans and found they were useful to both. *In vivo* tests on rodents and other animals proved that nothing toxic came from the bacteria. Botany studies conducted indicated the HSOs were beneficial to plants and soil. Next, at U.S. and Mexican institutions, human beings—including the biochemist himself—underwent clinical tests with the bacteria by applying them topically to open wounds. Then the organisms were ingested. No toxicity reactions or side effects were observed; in fact, the HSOs offered no adverse responses in the test subjects even with greater amounts consumed....

Over time, the scientist and his co-workers perfected a process for selectively breeding superior strains of the microorganisms until they produced cultures that furnished good, positive body reac-

* We call them homeostatic soil organisms because science now shows us clearly that these organisms return the body to a state of dynamic homeostasis.

tions such as more normal bowel movements, improved sleep patterns, fewer colds and flu, and greater amounts of energy. During the breeding experiments, the scientist brought his HSOs to university laboratories in California for experiments. He collaborated with professors and utilized the universities' computer data banks.

Dr. Walker reported that neither the scientist nor his collaborators ever made any changes to the bacteria by mutation or other means. These homeostatic soil organisms appear to be as old as the Earth.

I mentioned that once my story became public through the *Townsend Letter* demand for these homeostatic soil organisms was incredible. I became the "hub" for anyone in the world with a gastrointestinal problem who couldn't get better and soon I began receiving thousands of phone calls. Eventually, I had to create a formula containing these organisms. I called the product Primal Defense, because I believed that what we were doing was original and primitive, closely approximating one of the truly important, beneficial influences upon our Earth's first inhabitants.

I chose a name for the company—Garden of Life—to exemplify my belief that our Creator gave us everything we need within His creation to have abundant and healthy lives.

Once I began Garden of Life, there were many things I wanted to accomplish. I went full speed ahead with my own medical education at the Peoples University of the Americas School of Natural Medicine and in so doing began to develop the concepts and ideas that would form the basis for the way we do things at Garden of Life. I also began studying the nutritional supplement industry to learn what companies were doing, both right and wrong. I found a lot more that was being done wrong than right.

Most companies start out trying to create a market. They ride that pony until it is all ridden out. Then, they go onto the next fresh horse and ride that one until it is broken down too. Their major source of research is all too frequently the Xerox copier. Borrowed science is the norm for the nutritional product industry. Few companies invest significant sums of money into research. Most copy products from their competitors. This is sad because one day, for most of these companies, their reliance on knock-off products will become the knock-out punch of their businesses and much of the nutritional product industry.

We were lucky. Garden of Life was created not to find a market, but by the force of a *huge* consumer demand. Believe me, people suffering from severe digestive disorders are not very patient—and there are a lot of such folks throughout the industrialized nations, especially in the United States where fast-food is king and almost everything is disinfected with powerful bacteriocides.

Among the most critical areas for the nutritional products industry are sourcing raw materials and their handling, all the way from soil to store shelf. You probably don't know this, but most herbs today are fumigated and irradiated in order to kill all microorganisms. Not very natural, if you ask me. We wanted all organic ingredients, if possible, which is very rare even in the natural products industry. To ensure potency and that our formulas embodied the physics of healing, we would employ low-temperature processing (see Chapter 7). We also found that vegetables and herbs are better absorbed when they are predigested through lactic acid fermentation, and that these herbs are more potent when grown in certain areas of the world. Thus, our unique Poten-Zyme™ fermentation process encourages populations of beneficial microorganisms that make our whole foods and herbs so much more available even to disease-weakened bodies. (To learn more about Poten-Zyme, see Chapter 4.) Our whole food and herbal ingredients are grown especially for Garden of Life in Australia, California, Arizona, Japan, France, Spain, and even regions of the former Soviet Union, and, of course, on our own certified organic farm, including a full-scale fermentation and drying facility located in southern Utah.

These were just some of the issues we met head-on here at Garden of Life. Also, we have invested almost one million dollars to date in primary research, including laboratory and clinical studies to scientifically validate not only our cornerstone formulations, Primal Defense, RM-10™ and FYI™ (For Your Inflammation™), but our new formulas.*

~~~~~

A sthma. *Allergies. Irritable bowel syndrome. Rheumatoid arthritis. Lupus. Crohn's disease. Chronic fatigue syndrome. Immune disorders. All are reaching epidemic proportions.*

To protect yourself from these disorders and insure long-term super health—as well as to aid your body's healing quest in the case of these and other related disorders—may I respectfully suggest you eat some dirt?

Do not be surprised by what I say. Dirt—or to be more specific, the Earth's soil—is one of your body's best friends.

Dirt or soil is so essential to health that if you or a loved one is suffering from any of the above conditions, this may be due to a lost connection with Earth.

When we were back in the era of primitive man, we got dirty. We were exposed to all sorts of microscopic bugs. Our food was dirty. But was this all bad? Not really, and it's a shame that today words like dirt or soil are such a negative concept.

Even today as children, we are meant to make mud pies, to play in the mud, to get dirty. It is as necessary to our long-term health as almost anything. Our immune systems need this kind of exposure to learn how to react later on in life to real or not so real threats to our health. You see, without early exposures to all sorts of organisms in the soil, later in life when our immune system is exposed to various benign intruders, it may overreact. Hence, we develop autoimmune diseases, some types of asthma, and allergies. And that's just one of the consequences of our lost connection to Earth. Our immune system may never truly reach its full zenith of defensive powers against disease-causing organisms or chemical toxins without re-establishing this lost connection to the Earth.

So while modern civilization proceeds full speed ahead with technology, we must not allow ourselves to become apart from Nature. It is in our best interest to maintain contact with the good Earth. Most of us don't.

* If you want to learn more about all of our Garden of Life formulas, see Appendix B.

Therefore one premise—one guiding light for Garden of Life—is that most of us will benefit by returning to our bodies these missing microorganisms.

I know what I'm saying may strike some readers as crazy, and they may wonder where I'm coming from. Yet, prestigious health experts at our most respected medical and scientific institutions worldwide have come to these same conclusions.

In fact, society's growing separation from dirt and germs may well be the cause of the growing incidence of a wide range of maladies, says epidemiologist David Strachan, who first advanced the over-cleanliness theory in 1989 when he was at Britain's London School of Hygiene and Tropical Medicine.[5]

At that time, Dr. Strachan noticed that children belonging to large families were much less likely to develop asthma, hay fever or eczema. Dr. Strachan theorized older children coming home dirty with all sorts of resident soil microorganisms were actually protecting their younger brothers and sisters.

We need dirt, says Dr. Strachan. He may be onto something.

Throughout the world, scientists are carrying spoons and sandwich bags no matter where they go, in search of ever-exotic sources of such soil organisms. They are seeking out new and unique soil organisms in bat caves, hot springs, undersea volcanoes, and even from mummies. Each exotic locale may yield a completely new discovery. Indeed, these vast resources have not even begun to be tapped. Even the National Cancer Institute is getting in on the action and funding research on soil organisms. It is thought by some of our leading government officials and scientists that in our soil we may find a treatment for AIDS, cancer, and other deadly diseases. Consider these discoveries:

- While vacationing in Norway, an employee at Sandoz Pharmaceutical took home a mold found in soil that later led to development of the anti-rejection transplant drug cyclosporin.
- A scientist scouring the soil of an Indonesian temple discovered microbes that can turn starch into sugar.
- In Japan, a scientist picked up a clump of soil from a golf course that is now used to cure parasitic infections plaguing livestock.
- Most current antibiotics come from microbes in the soil, including streptomycin, the first treatment for tuberculosis, and vancomycin, currently the drug of last resort for the toughest infections.[6]

And consider this: unknown organisms make up 99.9 percent of all the microbes in the soil. One gram of soil—the weight of a little packet of sugar—can contain as many as 10,000 species unknown to science, notes Jo Handelsman, a professor of plant pathology at the University of Wisconsin. As *Business Week* online notes, "Now, for the first time, she and her colleagues, along with several other research groups working independently, are learning to extract the DNA of these mysterious creatures and clone it. They are finding that the microbes differ so profoundly from known bacteria that they could represent entirely new kingdoms of life—as different from other bacteria as animals are from plants. That means that the proteins produced by these creatures could have properties unlike any other such substances known." Already, Handelsman says, several new antibiotics have been identified from such soil microbes.

But here's the clincher, from the same article on Business Week online—there is a great explanation as to why the HSOs helped turn around my health problems and why anyone with Crohn's or any other disease might well benefit from them:

> Even human intestines—an environment most people consider pretty familiar—are home to perhaps 10,000 kinds of microbes.... Indeed, one of the surprises in the decoding of the human genome was that it contains more than 200 genes that come from bacteria. Microbes not only keep us alive; in some small part, we are made of them.

> [Researchers are] now looking at how these largely unknown microbes might play a role in Crohn's disease, an inflammation of the small intestine. [They have] found that the makeup of the mixed "community" of microbes in the intestines changes in people with the disease. A similar thing might happen with tuberculosis…leading [researchers] to wonder whether some diseases might be caused not by a single dangerous microbe but by a change in the microbial community— an ecological imbalance inside the human body.

So there you have it. Our soil is home to countless numbers of microorganisms and our gut is also populated with far more microbes than we have ever known. Inside and out we are at one with the Earth. At least we should be. After all, the Bible says that man was made from the dust of the Earth. That is a bit of wisdom that we can't even yet begin to understand or comprehend.

HOW DIRT IMPROVES HEALTH

The idea that dirt is good for our health is paradoxically due to our exposure to both protective and infectious microorganisms found in soil. According to a recent report in the *New Scientist*, researchers have discovered the microorganisms found in dirt influence maturation of the immune system so that it is either functional or dysfunctional.[7] The organisms to which we are exposed "condition" our immune system so that it intuitively knows when to produce and activate T-helper (Th) cells.

Among the cells of the immature immune system are so-called non-differentiated T-helper cells (Th cells), which are primarily produced by the thymus gland. These Th cells control the initiation or suppression of the body's immune reactions and regulate many other immune cells. Among the TH cells are two types that develop as we mature: Th1 and Th2 helper cells.

The quality of an individual's immune system can be evaluated through the balance of cytokines it is producing. This increasingly popular classification method is referred to as the Th1/Th2 balance.

Interleukins and interferons are called "cytokines" which can be grouped into those secreted by Th1 type cells and those secreted by Th2 type cells. Th1 cells promote specialized cell-mediated immunity, while Th2 cells induce humoral immunity (this refers to immunity to infection created by proteins termed antibodies, specialized proteins secreted by "B" cells or B lymphocytes).

Th1 cells are the quintessential cop who does his job of defending your body very efficiently—with little wasted effort. The body's Th1 cells produce only as many germ-zapping antibodies as necessary to stop an invader. The message here is economy of action.

But on the other hand, Th2 cells are the armed forces of the body and when they go out to do battle it is like sending in the army, navy, marines and air force. The Th2 cells are "total response" defenders.

These two different methods by which the body fights infections exist side by side. While cellular immunity (Th1) directs natural killer T-cells and macrophages to attack abnormal cells and microorganisms at sites of infection inside the cells, humoral immunity (Th2) results in the production of antibodies used to neutralize foreign invaders and substances outside of the cells. Imagine the skies over Baghdad during the Gulf War and you get a sense of the mayhem created by Th2 cells when they are in overdrive, overproducing germ-zapping antibodies.

In many cases, an infection is fought with both arms of the immune system. At other times, predominantly one is needed to control an infection. A healthy immune system is both balanced and dynamic: it should be balanced between Th1 and Th2 activity, switching back and forth between the two as needed. This allows for a quick eradication of a threat and then a return to balance before responding to the next threat. The inability to respond adequately with a Th1 response can result in chronic infection, chronic fatigue syndrome and cancer; an overactive, yet paradoxically ineffective, Th2 response can contribute to allergies and various syndromes, and play a role in autoimmune disease.

A failure of the Th1 arm of the immune system and an overactive yet ineffective Th2 arm are implicated in a wide variety of chronic illnesses. These include AIDS, chronic fatigue syndrome, candidiasis, multiple allergies, multiple chemical sensitivities (MCS), viral hepatitis, Gulf War syndrome, cancer, lupus, and many other illnesses. If these two arms of the immune system could be balanced by stimulating Th1 cells and decreasing Th2 cells, then many of the symptoms associated with these chronic illnesses would diminish or disappear and we would have found the answer to immune restoration and balance, or come darn close to the equivalent of a cure.

ARE TODAY'S CHILDREN TOO CLEAN?

When we are children, if we are exposed to an adequate amount of viruses and bacteria and other microorganisms—if we are allowed to play in the dirt, put our fingers in our mouths and make mud pies—our Th cells will mature in the proper proportion into desirable Th1 cells. But without adequate internal exposure to soil microbes, our immune cells have a tendency towards overreactions and they are more likely to mature into Th2 cells. We have failed in our immune system's educational processes.

Too many children, today and in the last fifty years, have been denied this much-needed exposure to soil microorganisms. In other words, we're living in too clean an environment. The immune systems of children and even adults are no longer being properly educated.

Perhaps a sense of balance is required, and we have overemphasized elimination of microorganisms from our environment. This, coupled with the fact that most of the country has become so urbanized that kids are hardly ever found playing in the garden or walking on country roads, shows us that we have lost contact with our bacterially rich Earth.

Today, more than ever, we oversterilize everything. We have disinfectant dishwashing soap and disinfectant body lotions and skin bars with disinfectants like triclosan—and even disinfectant produce washes when, in fact, we need the beneficial organisms in our food supply.

We sterilize our agricultural soil with pesticides and herbicides, destroying beneficial and harmful bacteria alike, even harming plants' natural immune systems. Our food used to have loads of bacterial organisms which became part of the plant and which we consumed. Now, our soil is sterile; our foods are sterile; (and, in a sense, for too many, our own lives are sterile). Pesticides and herbicides do pretty much to the soil what overuse of medical antibiotics has done to the human gut—eliminate not only the bad but also the *good* guys. And that's not good.

Oh, sure, we are exposed to some of these microorganisms on a limited basis, but leading researchers say that on a daily basis, most people are no longer exposed to large enough quantities of microorganisms from our soil, dust, air, water and foods to achieve optimal health. With an overly sterile environment, our relationship to Earth has been severed. We live in air-conditioned offices and homes and pass from one to the other walking upon concrete or traveling in cars on polluted highways. Our foods are irradiated to further kill the microorganisms. We use antibacterial preservatives. The idea of fermented foods is almost foreign to Americans. With our modern, high-tech processing methods, food manufacturers remove and destroy many of our food's most important life-giving nutrients. Our children stay indoors watching TV and playing video games instead of playing outside. It is ironic that, even though our parents yelled at us for eating mud pies, perhaps it was the best thing we could have been doing for ourselves.

From thousands of years up to about half-a-century ago, the American agricultural system raised fruits and vegetables in soil exceedingly rich in bacteria and other organisms. After World War II, however, these homeostatic soil organisms were displaced as a result of chemical farming and pesticide usage by big agricultural business.

In their quest to reduce unwanted disease-causing pathogens, agribusiness groups sterilized the soil and water (chlorination), thereby eliminating the beneficial bacteria as well as the harmful ones. We now even give antibiotics, hormones, and other drugs to chickens and cattle—so much so that all of the European Common Market refuses to import livestock from American farms.

Even if we don't take antibiotics, we almost certainly consume them in animal products. Over 35 million pounds of antibiotics are produced in the U.S. each year, and animals are given the vast bulk of them. Cattle, pigs and poultry are routinely given big helpings of antibiotics to prevent infections from spreading in their stressful, crowded quarters. In Western Europe, giving antibiotics to cattle is outlawed, as is the importation of American beef; this is, in part, due to all the antibiotics fed to U.S. cattle. Researchers estimate that by consuming just one glass of commercial milk we are unknowingly ingesting the residues of up to 100 different antiobiotics. This constant exposure to low-dose antibiotics is leading to an increase in antibiotic resistant bacteria.

A healthy intestine in both children and adults contains billions of bacteria—including up to 10,000 different species. Optimally, the body's beneficial or benign bacteria should outnumber the cells of the body by approximately one-hundred fold! But this is no longer the case.

These friendly bacteria are our first line of immune defense. They displace and fight off *unfriendly* bacteria and internal fungi that can set the stage for both adult and childhood illness. They even increase the body's levels of interferon, a mighty immune-boosting chemical. They are as essential to health as water and food.

This is all very critical to our health. If harmful bacteria propagate and gain the upper hand, we will not only be prone to infectious disease but our bodies will produce toxic, carcinogenic substances. We will also suffer digestive problems including constipation and diarrhea.

But here's the problem that adults—and children especially—face as they grow up in a toxic world. Stress, medications and poor diet reduce friendly bacteria even further, leaving them even more vulnerable to disease. Antibiotics can be the biggest culprits in destroying our friendly bacteria. At high dosages, they wipe out *all* bacteria inside your child's body, the good along with the bad.

Once that happens, the race is on as to which microorganisms, the good guys or the bad guys, set up shop in that empty real estate inside your or your child's gut.

This is why we must be extra careful to replenish and stabilize friendly bacteria in the gastrointestinal tract. In essence, with the HSOs in Primal Defense, we have positioned on our side a massive army of health defenders in our intestines that is ever on guard to protect our health as well as maintain a balanced immune system, reacting only as needed, never over- or under-reacting.

We can support balanced immune function with soil organisms. These produce proteins that the body interprets as antigens (a protein from a foreign substance or microorganism that is capable of stimulating an immune response). The immune system reacts to these proteins. The way that HSOs stimulate the immune system's Th cells will also influence other immune cells, especially B lymphocytes that are manufactured in the bone marrow and produce nonspecific or un-programmed antibodies. These un-programmed antibodies have the ability to take a fresh, new look at newly introduced bodily invaders. They have not been preprogrammed to overreact and are freely available to travel where and when needed. It is as if we are sending our immune cells back to school to learn their jobs all over again so that they can perform them even better.

The beauty of it all is that this huge reservoir of extra antibodies is always on hand for the immune system to utilize as long as the individual is taking the HSOs regularly. Without them, this reservoir of extra antibodies is unavailable. Thus, by ingesting homeostatic soil organisms on a regular basis, the effectiveness of one's immune system becomes vastly enhanced.

The HSOs help to accomplish the educational process that was earlier disturbed when the link between beneficial soil organisms and the human body was broken. They help to educate the body's Th cells as they may never have been during childhood; the process might be more aptly called building immune "tolerance" or "maturation."

Through constant exposure to the lost HSOs, the body's Th cells become re-educated and "tolerant" and mount only necessary, not excessive, immune responses. In a sense, this formula gives the immune system the workout it missed when the patient was young, due to living in our modern, highly sanitized world. But that is only part of what HSOs do. Like any other great advance in healing, the science is there in abundance to back up the positive clinical outcomes complementary physicians are seeing with their patients.

In the natural environment, HSOs help plants to digest inorganic substances, protect root systems from parasites, yeast, and fungi, and provide growth factors and different hormones. They do the same for human health and the gastrointestinal tract. We are, after all, part of Nature. William C. Bryce, M.D., Ph.D., of Huntington Beach, California, notes: "Just as HSOs destroy molds, yeasts, fungi, and viruses in the soil of the organic garden, they perform the same function with pathological organisms present in the gut, which greatly enhances the body's immune system."

UNBALANCED GASTROINTESTINAL ECOLOGY

Scientists and doctors are prone to use fancy words that leave the average person wondering what the heck they're jabbering about. This imbalance, when pathogenic microorganisms outnumber beneficial bacterial species, is referred to as *dysbiosis*. Put simply, dysbiosis is one of those fancy words for a condition that occurs when the population of organisms residing within the gastrointestinal tract becomes imbalanced, often resulting in acute or chronic sickness.

Normally, populations of pathogenic organisms are kept in balance by competition from good bacteria and because of *symbiosis*, which is the mutually interdependent relationship among the hundreds of intestinal microbial species. According to Gershon, "One reason that the bacteria in the lumen of the colon do not break out and infect the body is that they are at war with one another. No one kind of germ gains ascendancy and takes uncontested possession of colonic turf. The constant competition between otherwise nasty germs helps to keep the bacterial population under control." The problem is that, after antibiotics have wiped out all or much of the entire gastrointestinal landscape, the bad bacteria have the upper hand because they love the types of foods that we typically consume in our diet, especially the carbohydrates found in bread, pasta, milk, candy, baked goods and soft drinks. So, when the balance of good and bad bacteria is disturbed by antibiotics, it's the bad bacteria that get the head start in repopulating the barren property within your gastrointestinal tract. And especially consider this: the kind of food people who are sick or have been sick love to eat is what we call comfort food—you know, milk shakes, breads, pastas, cookies, fries—the very kind of food that promotes the growth of disease-causing bacteria.

Dysbiosis results in abnormal fermentation in the small intestine.[8] In the large intestine, some fermentation is desirable because it produces butyrate and other short-chain fatty acids that nourish the cells of the intestinal wall.[9] In the small intestine, however, growth of yeast, fungi and/or fermenting pathogenic bacteria can result in damage to the gut lining, absorption of toxic by-products, and impaired absorption of nutrients.[10]

Repeated use of broad-spectrum antibiotics, oral contraceptives and steroid medications can set up conditions for opportunistic overgrowth of organisms that are not affected by the drugs or that are able to re-colonize rapidly once treatment has ended. This is particularly true of yeast and fungal organisms. Their metabolic products appearing in urine are the strongest physical evidence of intestinal overgrowth of these organisms. "As an internist, I can't tell you how often we have seen patients treated with antibiotics, especially our women patients, whose bodies are overrun by candida," notes Dr. Loes. "For men, such treatment often results in residual urinary tract bacteria, resulting in urinary tract infections and prostatitis (bacterial inflammation of the prostate gland)."

So, dysbiosis is a fancy word for the imbalance of microorganisms in your gastrointestinal tract. But what we need to keep in mind is that persistent dysbiosis can have serious health consequences.

It surely causes gastrointestinal problems, but it can also lead to a weakened immune system. As the body loses its ability to cope with the offending infections and pathogens, a host of chronic conditions appear that, on the surface, seem to have little to do with gastrointestinal disturbances.

This means that gastrointestinal health has far-reaching implications for general health, much more so than is commonly recognized. Indeed, doctors may have to do quite a bit of medical sleuthing to track down patients' complaints finally to attribute them to dysbiosis or an imbalance of their gastrointestinal bacteria. But once we do so and then take appropriate pathways to enhance the healing response, patients often respond far more favorably than anticipated.

When the friendly bacteria are decimated by antibiotics, other harmful bacteria, yeast and fungi already living in the body, which were held in strict check by the friendly bacteria, begin to multiply profusely. The overgrowth of one especially potent yeast-like fungus, *Candida albicans*, leads to a potentially serious condition called candidiasis. Depending on its locale of action, candidiasis can inflame the tongue, mouth or rectum. It can also cause vaginitis and may be instrumental in triggering a range of mental and emotional symptoms, including irritability, anxiety and even depression. Many allergies that manifest themselves as digestive disorders, such as bloating, heartburn, constipation and diarrhea also have been causally linked to candida yeast overgrowth.

Knowing how to use antibiotics in a safe and effective manner is critically important to doctors, pharmacists, and consumers alike. But it starts with our children. The American Academy of Pediatrics recently observed that 95 percent of children in the United States will have been treated with antibiotics for a middle ear infection by the age of five. Some children will be fine—but others won't be; their systems might become ravaged by the antibiotics, their populations of beneficial bacteria decimated.

Not surprisingly, dysbiosis or dysbacteriosis and its prevention or treatment are among the most topical and challenging problems doctors face today.[11] In dysbiosis—when protective friendly bacterial species are reduced in population—even organisms traditionally thought to have little ability to cause disease, including usually benign bacteria, yeasts, and some parasites, can induce illness by altering our nutritional status or immune response. The consequences of intestinal dysbiosis extend beyond the immediately obvious gastrointestinal distress. Studies have implicated intestinal bacterial imbalances as a basis for conditions ranging from recurrent infections and immune breakdown to chronic fatigue. In today's world, when we're looking to maximize our health, dysbiosis may leave us predisposed to a host of common ailments including diarrhea, constipation, irritable bowel syndrome, colon cancer, allergies, vaginitis, increased susceptibility to infection, food cravings, lack of mental clarity, hypoglycemia symptoms and many more conditions that doctors rarely connect to the bacterial populations of the gastrointestinal tract. Equally important, however, are the effects on tissues far from the intestinal site, such as the brain, joints and muscles, as well as on the immune system. Effects can be as diverse as headaches, learning disorders, insomnia, immune dysfunction, behavioral disorders, chronic fatigue, joint pain and nutritional deficiencies. More familiar to many patients are conditions such as irritable bowel syndrome, Crohn's disease, fibromyalgia, leaky gut syndrome, wasting disease, diverticulitis, hemorrhoids, and breast and colon cancer—all of which may have their genesis in an upset in the gastrointestinal tract's bacterial population. Abnormal bacterial populations which lead to dysfunctional gut fermentation have adverse effects on nutrient assimilation and production, especially the B vitamins, and absorption of calcium, magnesium and zinc.[12] These nutritional deficits explain how abnormal bacterial gut populations may cause many other significant adverse effects on health. As for breast cancer, who would've thought the bacteria in our gut are responsible for detoxification of potentially toxic metabolites of hormones such as estrogen?

COSTLY NATIONAL CONCERN

Today, we know that digestive diseases and other conditions related to unhealthy imbalances of intestinal flora have an enormous impact on our health. They are also extremely costly to the nation.

- Digestive diseases, which often are caused in part by or result in dysbiosis, cost nearly $107 billion in direct health care expenditures in 1992.[13] Digestive diseases result in nearly 200 million sick days, 50 million visits to physicians, 16.9 million days lost from school, 10 million hospitalizations, and nearly 200,000 deaths per year.
- The most costly digestive diseases are gastrointestinal disorders such as diarrheal infections ($4.7 billion); gallbladder disease ($4.5 billion); colorectal cancer ($4.5 billion); liver disease ($3.2 billion); and peptic ulcer disease ($2.5 billion).
- Cancers of the digestive tract, which includes the colon, the gallbladder, and the stomach, are responsible for 117,000 deaths yearly. Non-cancerous digestive diseases cause 74,000 deaths a year, with 36 percent caused by chronic liver disease and cirrhosis.
- Of the 440 million acute non-cancerous medical conditions reported in the United States annually, more than 22 million are for acute digestive conditions, with 11 million from gastroenteritis and 6 million from indigestion, nausea, and vomiting.

Digestive diseases have an enormous impact on the health care system in the United States. New technologies and new drugs have revolutionized the understanding and treatment of peptic ulcer disease and gastrointestinal esophageal reflux disease (GERD). Successful outcomes of future research will hopefully continue to reduce the economic and health care costs related to diagnosing and treating digestive diseases. But no matter what new medicines we come up with the bottom line remains: your body desperately requires healthy intestinal flora, while many environmental and dietary conditions threaten this balance. We should be handing out HSOs to everyone.

So where did it all start? Where did our fastidiousness become a case of widespread social germ phobia? As the practice of soil and water sterilization increased over the years, the beneficial bacteria in American's bodies decreased correspondingly. Normally, we should have a balance of 85 percent "good" bacteria to 15 percent "bad" bacteria in the intestinal tract. But today, most of us show the reverse ratio; therefore, it's no coincidence that the incidences of chronic and degenerative diseases have multiplied dramatically since World War II.

Sophisticated lifestyles among Western industrialized countries contribute greatly to critical gastrointestinal disruption among the populations. Antibiotic usage, excessive stress, consumption of excess sugar and alcohol, the regular drinking of carbonated beverages, and frequent consumption of over-the-counter drugs alter the acid/alkaline balance of the intestinal tract, creating the perfect environment for pathogenic microbial activity.

How Do You Know if You Have Dysbiosis?

The most common symptoms of intestinal dysbiosis are bloating, abdominal cramping, constipation and diarrhea. In other words, chronic indigestion is a surefire sign of dysbiosis. Lactose intolerance, increased gut permeability, food allergies and intolerances, fatigue and immune suppression frequently accompany intestinal dysbiosis.

Common Symptoms of Intestinal Imbalances

- Abdominal pain or cramps
- Colon cancer
- Constipation or diarrhea
- Distention/bloating
- Fatigue
- Fatigue after eating
- Flatulence
- Bad breath
- Body odor
- Food allergy
- Hypoglycemia
- Inability to lose weight
- Irregular bowel movements
- Irritable bowel syndrome
- Itchy anus
- Leaky gut syndrome
- Poor complexion
- Poor digestion
- Rheumatoid arthritis
- Spastic colon

Major Causes of Dysbiosis

- Decreased immune function
- Decreased intestinal motility (constipation)
- Drugs—especially antibiotics, oral contraceptives and cortisone-like medications
- Intestinal infection
- Maldigestion and malabsorption
- Poor diet—excessive carbohydrates, sugar and trans fats
- Stress—including long-term emotional stress

Nutritional researchers are now convinced that as much as 90 percent of known systemic diseases may be caused or exacerbated by gastrointestinal imbalances. My case of Crohn's disease is a severe example of what can occur from gut bacterial imbalances.

When toxins are dispersed through the bloodstream, a precondition of "intestinal toxemia" (i.e., poisoning by harmful gut bacteria) occurs. "It is now universally conceded that autointoxication is the underlying cause of an exceptionally large group of symptom complexes," said H.H. Boeker, D.C., as far back as 1928.

Take another case in point: our drinking water. Once, drinking water teemed with mycobacteria. Now, I'll be the first to tell you, some of these pathogens were deadly, and the fact that today our water supplies are disinfected and so much safer than a century ago is no doubt important to public health and reduced morbidity and mortality. On the other hand, I should also point out the fact that populations in countries with low rates of asthma still drink water with billions of mycobacteria per liter. The chlorination process used to disinfect water also disinfects the human body, again eliminating both good and bad microorganisms.

In order to restore health, many people need to restore their connection to the soil. While obviously not everyone can go out and start making mud pies, do a little gardening or hike in the mountains, there is another way of doing so: our HSOs seem to be the healing link between our soil and our bodies.

By reintroducing HSOs to the human body, persons in pain—and who are suffering from immune disorders including food allergies, irritable bowel syndrome, rheumatoid arthritis, lupus, and Crohn's disease, and many other conditions—finally have the missing link their bodies require to enhance the healing response.

Board-certified gastroenterologist Joseph Brasco, M.D., of Indianapolis, Indiana, and I met in 1999 when I attended a Designs for Health nutritional seminar. I was there both to speak and because I was researching more about the principles of the ancestral diet. Dr. Brasco was there too, investigating new options for his patients with gastrointestinal disorders. When it came time for my talk, Dr. Brasco was there in the front row. "Wow, so you're the guy whose miraculous recovery I read about in the *Townsend Letter*," he said after the talk.

We went to lunch and we've been close friends and colleagues ever since, though I have to admit that I was highly impressed by the fact that Dr. Brasco was willing to ask the advice of a brash 23-year-old (my age at the time).

"I'm intrigued," he told me at lunch. "All of this just makes great sense—your inclusion of kefir and other fermented foods, and the use of the Primal Defense. I've already been prescribing these supplements to patients. In my own practice, however, I'm taking things one step further. You see, my idea is that we can take the healing of patients through diet and universalize it not just to an individual but to a whole group of people—all our patients."

Eventually, our partnership resulted in *Restoring Your Digestive Health* (Kensington Health Books 2003).

Recently, when we spoke, Dr. Brasco told me why he is such a fan of HSOs when it comes to his patients' health problems and for maintaining their health. Again, our theme returns to our oversterilized environment. He is also very keen on the inclusion of fermented foods in our diet and the role they can play in the healing process. Indeed, HSOs and fermented foods—especially our Poten-Zyme process—naturally fit well together.

Keep in mind Dr. Brasco is a board-certified gastroenterologist. Here's what he says about the value of HSOs in his own practice and why he thinks they are so essential to our health and well-being:

Eating vegetables directly out of the soil as part of food was good for primitive man. The organisms living in that soil caused primal man to thrive. But today it's different! Given the paranoia that modern men and women in western society feel against ingesting soil of any kind, these ancient soil-based organisms no longer are part of our food supply. Yes, times do change! It used to be that a pioneering farmer working his fields, the so-called 'sod-buster,' who became hungry simply dug into the ground, pulled up some carrots, brushed off the dirt, and chomped away on vegetables containing the residual dirt and all. The farmer kept his gastrointestinal tract functioning well by ingesting these extracurricular homeostatic soil organisms. But that's not the way it is anymore. So fastidious are residents of Western industrialized nations that too much cleanliness has become somewhat detrimental to one's gastrointestinal tract. We have to eat dirt once in awhile.

But, in fact, the reestablishment of the HSO-body link yields far more benefits than simply aiding in cases of autoimmune disease. Overall bodily functions and immunity are greatly improved. Cholesterol levels are naturally reduced; energy levels are increased; and resistance to disease-causing organisms is enhanced. We have even seen increases in serum enzymes and normalization of serum albumin, indicating improved lymphatic flow and removal of lymphatic blockages.

With soil organisms, I was able to enhance my own body's healing response. Upon ingesting them, the soil organisms maintain a healthy balance of intestinal flora by also producing organic compounds such as lactic acid, hydrogen peroxide, and acetic acid, which increase the acidity of the intestine and inhibits the reproduction of massive amounts of harmful microorganisms. These soil organisms also produce substances called bacteriocins, which act as natural antibiotics to kill almost any kind of pathological bacteria and to fend off threats they themselves face from pathogenic microorganisms.

Two of the soil organisms in Primal Defense are *Bacillus subtilis* and *Bacillus lichenformis*. In studies conducted in Germany at the University of Berlin's Max-Volmer Institute, both were shown to inactivate human immunodeficiency, herpes simplex (HSV-1 and HSV-2), simian immunodeficiency, feline calicivirus, murine encephalomyocarditis, and other lipid envelope viruses—along with mycoplasmas, fungi and bacteria. They do so by producing a potent chemical called surfactin, a detergent-like substance that dissolves the lipid membranes of lipid envelope viruses, thereby rendering them completely inactivated.

The soil organisms provide even more important health benefits. They establish colonies in the entire digestive system, starting in the esophagus and ending in the colon, by attaching themselves to the walls of these organs. Burrowing behind the putrefaction, which lines the intestinal walls, they eat and destroy unfriendly microorganisms. The decay is then dislodged and flushed out of the body in the normal evacuation process. This aids in detoxification of the intestinal tract, increases the body's ability to absorb nutrients, and, again, makes the immune system super-strong by removing mucoid plaque that covers the gut-associated lymphoid tissues, especially aiding the body's ability to fight off infectious viruses and bacteria.

HSOs are extremely aggressive against all pathological molds, yeasts, fungi, and viruses and they help the body to efficiently eliminate such pathogens. Moreover, protozoa, worms, and other parasites are eliminated as well by the aggressive action of the HSOs, both within the intestines and throughout the other organs and tissues. *Candida albicans*, other yeasts, and molds are obliterated.

Among the health benefits we receive from ingestion of the soil organisms are the following:

- **HSOs Pool New RNA/DNA in the Cells** HSOs are rich sources of DNA and RNA, the naturally coded instructions for the cells to reactivate their own repair. Working in a symbiotic relationship with bodily tissues, HSOs create a pool of extra DNA/RNA raw materials that are immediately available when needed, accelerating healing of wounds and other tissue disturbances including burns, surgical incisions, and infections.

- **HSOs Quench Free Radicals by Creating SOD** HSOs produce the free radical-quencher, superoxide dismutase (SOD), a powerful antioxidant. Unless extinguished at once, free radicals attack any physiological molecule, causing cancers and other tissue damage. SOD, working enzymatically, is a first-line defense against free radicals before they can cause organ damage.

- **HSOs Stimulate Alpha Interferon Production** HSOs stimulate the production of a key immune system regulator, the polypeptide alpha interferon (a molecular protein). The scientific community has long known about the virus-fighting ability of alpha interferon and sought to enhance the body's production to aid the healing response when faced with certain health maladies. Research documents over 50 immune-regulating effects. Alpha interferon has been synthesized and used for a variety of illnesses, notably cancer, but the recombinantly derived version is extremely costly, inefficient, and has many adverse side effects. Researchers at the State Academy of Medicine in Apodaca, Mexico, report that the HSO formula, "when consumed at the recommended dosage, stimulates the body's endogenous alpha interferon production. The product itself does not contain any alpha interferon but comprises a singularly efficient set of nutrients that seem to increase specifically and most effectively the body's natural alpha interferon production." Working on human patients with various immune dysfunctions, the research team demonstrated the human body requires only small daily quantities of alpha interferon to maintain a lively and effective immune response. Scientists note that even small increases in the body's production of this therapeutic substance, produced by the immune system in reaction to soil organisms, can become an effective neutralizer of the toxic effects of pathogenic viruses that cause herpes, hepatitis B, hepatitis C, influenza, and other potentially life-threatening illnesses.

- **HSOs Stimulate the Production of Human Lactoferrin** Present in the homeostatic soil organisms themselves is a certain substance that stimulates the formation of human lactoferrin, a member of the family of iron-carrying proteins. Lactoferrin is found in the specific granules of neutrophils where it exerts antimicrobial activity by withholding iron from ingested pathogenic bacteria and fungi. For this reason, HSOs exhibit characteristics akin to fungicides, virucides, bactericides, and parasiticides. Iron carried by lactoferrin is extremely bioavailable—greater than 95 percent—yet it will not be delivered to noxious microbes.

So wide-ranging is the impact of our gut on human health that each of the following conditions may be caused by intestinal toxemia and can be aided by soil organisms:[14]

- **Allergies.** William Lintz, M.D., reported in 1939 in *Gastrointestinal Allergy, The Review of Gastroenterology* that he successfully treated 474 patients suffering allergies by elimination of pathogenic bacteria and their toxins.
- **Asthma.** Dr. Allan Eustis, an instructor at Tulane University of Medicine in the early twentieth century, noted that eliminating intestinal toxemia relieved 121 cases of bronchial asthma.
- **Arthritis.** Dr. Anthony Bassler treated some 344 arthritic patients by relieving intestinal toxemia.
- **Cardiac Arrhythmias.** Dr. D.J. Beary, a professor of physiology at Queens College, Cork, England, noted in 1916 that: "There seems to be little doubt that substances that have a deleterious action on the heart musculature and nerves are formed both in the small and large intestine, even under apparently normal circumstances."
- **Ear, Nose and Throat Problems.** J.A. Stucky, M.D., noted, "In several hundreds of cases of diseases of the nasal accessory sinuses, middle and internal ear…I have found unmistakable and marked evidence of toxemia of intestinal origin as evidenced by excessive indican in the urine, and when the condition causing this was removed there was marked amelioration or entire relief of the disease."
- **Eclampsia.** Dr. R.C. Brown, an obstetrical surgeon in England in 1930, linked intestinal toxemia with eclampsia.
- **Eye Problems.** C.W. Hawley, M.D., treated many causes of eyestrain and disease with success by relieving intestinal toxemia.
- **Thyroid Gland Disease.** W.S. Revano, M.D. theoretically linked goiter to "a toxic process in the intestinal tract."

The science of soil organisms is exploding, and what we are learning is essential to good health. The newly recognized ability of soil organisms to aid our quest for healing and maintaining good health is one of the most exciting breakthroughs in modern health. Of course, the irony is that we are talking about soil organisms as old as the Earth. I would urge anyone with intractable autoimmune conditions, allergies, low energy, inability to gain weight, fibromyalgia and chronic fatigue syndrome to take advantage of HSOs. Parents of children with chronic middle ear infections would do well by their child to get him or her on

HSOs. Even our beloved pets, who today are suffering from the same diseases as humans, can benefit from the inclusion of HSOs in their diet. Many veterinarians are currently using HSOs to treat animals with intractable digestive and immune system disorders.

"I believe that Primal Defense is applicable as a food supplement for everyone, whether a person is sick or not," notes Dr. Brasco. "The probiotic microorganisms found in this formula are proven to be helpful for the enhancement of health and prolongation of life. Such proof has been shown ever since mankind inhabited the Earth. Primitive man absorbed the product's soil-based organisms from the environment in different ways; for instance, he buried meat and other food in the ground as a form of preservation. Such meat would combine with soil-based bacteria and be eaten to become a part of the human physiology, thus changing into what science now identifies as body-based organisms. Such friendly microorganisms, having established themselves in the human gut, create an environment for optimizing human nutrition.

"Where Primal Defense kicks in is that its microorganisms are unlike other probiotics or beneficial gut bacteria. Rather, they are quite unique. Their homeostatic soil organisms maintain intrepid health for modern men and women the way primitive man experienced it. Where people specifically find advantage in using Primal Defense is in situations involving chronic disease of gut origin. Since my expertise lies in the area of gastrointestinal disorders, this product is a primary therapy that I utilize on a routine basis. Certainly with my seeing patients suffering from inflammatory bowel disease, it is one of the main tools I employ for treatment. I use this probiotic, which combines predigested plant nutrients from cereal grass juices and micro algaes in a formulation that is ever being improved, exactly as the manufacturer dictates. I give everyone a trial on Primal Defense. My standard procedure is to work up a patient to his or her optimal dosage and then maintain that dose as long as it's effective. So, I use it both preventively and therapeutically because the product's homeostatic soil organisms have definitely been part of the human diet for many thousands of years. Only, the HSOs have been lost as a result of our modern food processing methods. People with arthritis, chronic constipation, Crohn's disease, colitis, and other gut-linked systemic conditions improve by supplementing with the Primal Defense whole food ingredients.

"Allow me to offer an illustrating case history. About sixteen months ago, Marion Frome, an eighteen-year-old manicurist from a nearby Illinois town, consulted me for the treatment of Crohn's disease. She arrived after many forms of therapy had failed her. It was only after I prescribed Primal Defense that her diarrhea came under control, abdominal cramping stopped, malabsorption corrected itself, and fistulae around the anus healed. She had an exceedingly positive response, and my perception has been that this is standard procedure for Primal Defense. My medical associate has had similar experiences with the product, too."

"Based upon Dr. Brasco's excitement with Primal Defense, I became interested in the product approximately two years ago," confirms family medicine specialist Joseph M. Mercola, D.O., who worked with Dr. Brasco at the Optimal Wellness Center in Schaumburg, Illinois.* "Today, this probiotic has become the A-number-one nutritional supplement that we use in our Optimal Wellness Center. From its possessing at least fifteen different strains of beneficial bacteria efficacious for the gut, we are getting marvelous results with Primal Defense. I have literally put thousands of people on it, which is incorporated into a full detoxification program by me. The product is an incredibly potent and effective agent for the treatment of inflammatory bowel disease [IBD], and most especially for this condition's subset, Crohn's disease. I recommend all of my IBD patients to take it.

"If I see any reduction in results from a person's daily usage of Primal Defense, I switch my patient off the product and onto something else. I use only what is working for the individual. That has been my rule in this medical center during the entire length of its operation for the past fifteen years," says Dr. Mercola. "And successful case histories are easy to come by; for instance, a couple of years ago I was visited by Mrs. Sarah Haimes, a thirty-eight-year-old homemaker being treated with various steroids and antibiotics for the control of symptoms related to irritable bowel syndrome. She suffered with recurrent abdominal pain accompanied by spastic colon, functional diarrhea, a great deal of psychological stress, and emotional conflicts, all of which are characteristic of IBS. Mrs. Haimes was desirous of having a child, too, but the constant discomfort of her symptoms prevented conception.

"But then the situation changed for this patient. After she took Primal Defense for a period of six weeks, all of her health problems had become better. In fact, some months later Sarah reported that she had improved so much, she was able to become pregnant. Today, I'm happy to advise that mother and baby are doing very well."

In Lake Charles, Louisiana, John Moreno, Ph.D., conducts the successful multifaceted Lake Charles Advanced Medical Diagnostic Center, with two physician partners and other staff members. It is the largest practice of complementary and alternative medicine (CAM) in the state of Louisiana. In fact, Dr. Moreno is the only practitioner of CAM in Louisiana who has been granted hospital privileges.

"If a patient has any form of gastrointestinal problem, I start that person off with Primal Defense, because the product first stabilizes and then corrects GI problems," says Dr. Moreno. "It is the one therapeutic item that I make use of routinely. The first improvement I normally see is an increase in the patient's energy level, and that's good because this individual is then able to recognize how well the product is working. Furthermore, within the first few weeks both constipation and diarrhea clear up. They just correct themselves. So the patient observes himself or herself getting better. Such an experience is important for winning a person's confidence."

To illustrate the benefits of Primal Defense, a fifty-year-old Caucasian woman, Ms. Kate Robarts, the city's most popular church organist, consulted Dr. Moreno because of her constant feeling of fatigue, muscle pain, short-term memory difficulties, and a sense that, in her words, "I think I'm dying."

* Visit Dr. Mercola's excellent health website at www.mercola.com.

Although she did not exhibit any overt gastrointestinal problems, Dr. Moreno is a deep believer that intestinal toxemia may be the root cause of diverse human disease conditions. He started her on Primal Defense, which corrects intestinal toxemia—perhaps one of the most under appreciated chronic maladies in modern medicine. "Her improvement started with a vast elevation in energy," notes Dr. Moreno. "Songs she had seemingly forgotten on the organ keyboard came back to her mind, and the music she sent forth was reflected as sounds of great joy. Everyone hearing her play knew that Kate Robarts was feeling better.

"With her happiness restored, the lady has referred at least three dozen new patients to me," continues Dr. Moreno. "The music alone caused people to recognize that I had something going that was valuable treatment. Kate Robarts' case is the closest I've ever seen that could be described as a miracle response to a remedy I had prescribed."

Besides the Brasco, Mercola and Moreno reports, we have many such cases where HSOs have initiated powerful healing processes in sick persons. Having practiced chiropractic manipulation and nutritional therapy in Indiana, the late Phyllis Wilson Confer, D.C., revealed her experiences to Donald Boys, Ph.D., of Indianapolis, former member of the Indiana House of Representatives and columnist for *USA Today*. At the time of her interview, Dr. Confer told Dr. Boys she had 50 patients taking HSOs.

"One of my patients had exceedingly elevated blood triglycerides at 305 milligrams per deciliter (mg/dl)," she told Boys. "Six weeks later, after taking [soil organisms], her triglycerides dropped to a mere 151 mg/dl. I'm excited about the product. There are so many positive experiences associated with it.

"For instance, I had another patient with an enlarged prostate [benign prostatic hyperplasia] who was scheduled for surgery [transurethral resection of the prostate gland]," she continued. "Some weeks before his calendar date to undergo the operation, I put this man on those same [soil organisms] as an immune system booster so that he might heal faster. As a result of his taking the food supplement, his prostate gland shrank and the surgery was canceled. My patient had made no alteration in his usual lifestyle except to take capsules of the soil organisms as a food supplement."

Maxine Murray, N.D., C.N.H.P., M.A., treated patient Maria Strang, infected with Lyme disease, with soil organisms. After 10 days of taking 10 capsules per day of the soil organisms, she had her strength and vitality completely restored.

Murray also treated Manfred Rechsheim, a twenty-eight-year-old construction worker. He suffered from red-hot, open, bleeding sores all over his body and on his face. He felt emotionally depressed, had been fired from his job for absences caused by the skin lesions, and offered a long history of taking therapies. Operating on the theory that the skin is a reflection of the state of health of the gastrointestinal tract, she gave him soil organisms. "He took twenty capsules a day for six weeks until the skin lesions were entirely gone," says Dr. Murray. "They just disappeared. Frankly, I was amazed at the result. Today he takes five a day as a preventive measure, with his skin remaining smooth, clear, and flawless."

PUBLISHED STUDIES

Although they have been a part of the diet for centuries, product-specific studies on Primal Defense's soil organisms have only been recently conducted.

These studies have been accepted for publication in a special supplement of the peer-reviewed *Progress in Nutrition*.[15] Following are summaries of the studies from the journal.

In 1993, three single-blind, placebo-controlled studies on soil organisms were conducted at the Dispensario Medico, Partido de la Revolucion Democratica, a medical dispensary in Irapuato, Mexico. The researchers wanted to find out whether the soil organisms in Primal Defense could help people with high cholesterol and leukemia, as well as see if they made healthy test subjects feel more energetic and improved memory and concentration. Here are summaries of the results of the three studies:

- **High cholesterol:** Seventy patients with blood cholesterol counts higher than 300 milligrams per deciliter were given soil organisms or a placebo. Every subject given the soil organisms saw their total blood cholesterol count drop by 25 percent or more; the placebo subjects showed no change.

- **Energy levels, memory and concentration:** Seventy patients with no known pathologies were given soil organisms or a placebo. Of the 35 subjects given soil organisms, 33 reported feeling more energetic; vital hemoglobin (HGB) levels and red blood cell counts increased moderately in 33 subjects. In the placebo group, no subjects reported an increase in energy or vitality levels. Further, in the placebo group, only two subjects out of 33 (two subjects dropped out of the study) saw their HGB levels increase. In only one subject did the red blood cell count increase. Conspicuous increases in memory and concentration were seen in 28 out of 35 test patients, with only one patient improving in the placebo group.

- **Chronic Lymphocytic Leukemia stage II:** Thirty-five subjects with chronic lymphocytic leukemia were given soil organisms. The director of research reported that the soil organisms "attenuated the symptoms of approximately 80 percent of the treated patients." In 80 percent of subjects, white blood cell counts improved.

Here are results from additional studies:

- In a study conducted at Bio Inova Life Sciences Laboratories under the direction of Pierre Braquet, Ph.D., and Jean Michel Mencia-Juerta, Ph.D., researchers attempted to identify the antimicrobial properties of Primal Defense's soil organisms. The soil organisms were found to be effective in inhibiting various pathogenic microorganisms, including *Pseudomonas aeruginosa*, a rare but life-threatening infectious agent.[16]

- Another study conducted at Bio Inova Life Sciences Laboratories evaluated the effectiveness of soil organisms on the immune system. In this study, researchers looked at macrophage function and the production of cytokines, such as interleukins, and tumor necrosis factor. Macrophages are large white blood cells that also serve the immune system by killing foreign invaders. In the study, soil organisms were found to boost the immune system by enhancing macrophage function.[17]

- In another study at Bio Inova Life Sciences Laboratories, soil organisms were examined for inhibition of cancer cell lines. These were shown to inhibit the proliferation of cancer cell lines of the breast, liver and lung (see also Chapter 4 for our anticancer research).[18]
- Also at Bio Inova Life Sciences Laboratories, soil organisms were shown to enhance the production of healthy cells and tissue regeneration in the colon; this may positively affect those suffering from severe digestive disorders and oxidative stress.[19]

In an open-label, 120-day clinical pilot study conducted at the Diabetes Resource Center by Dr. Ernesto Perez, M.D., researchers determined whether the soil organisms could help control blood sugar levels and decrease the risk of cardiovascular disease in people with type 2 diabetes. Specifically, the researchers wanted to see if soil organisms could aid in controlling blood sugar levels and lowering cholesterol and triglyceride levels. The study showed that using soil organisms and following the diet and lifestyle recommendations of the American Diabetes Association lowers blood glucose levels, lowers HbA1C (a long-term indicator of blood sugar control), lowers total cholesterol, and decreases triglycerides. Overall, the subjects using soil organisms in the study lowered their risk of cardiovascular heart disease.

While the use of soil organisms did result in improved blood sugar balance, the real standout results were in the reduction of high cholesterol and triglyceride levels. The most dramatic results occurred among a subgroup of patients having the highest cholesterol and triglyceride levels.

These patients received two Primal Defense caplets, three times daily during week one; three caplets, three times daily, during week two; and four caplets, three times daily throughout the rest of the study. Here are some of the study highlights:

- One woman patient with a starting total cholesterol count of 356 mg/dl experienced a 56 percent drop to 224 mg/dl, while her triglycerides went from 1106 mg/dl to 205 mg/dl, an 81 percent drop. Her coronary heart disease risk factors dropped 44 percent from 10.7 to 6.0.
- In another case, a woman patient's total cholesterol went from 248 mg/dl to 181 mg/dl, a 27 percent drop, while her triglycerides went from 1,350 mg/dl to 167 mg/dl, an 88 percent drop. Her coronary heart disease risk factor rating also dropped 53 percent from 9.5 to 4.5.
- A male with cholesterol levels of 313 mg/dl experienced a 30 percent decline to 219 mg/dl, while his triglyceride levels went from 436 mg/dl to 253 mg/dl for a 42 percent decline. His coronary heart disease risk factor rating went down 16 percent (from 9.7 to 8.1).
- Another male with a cholesterol level of 179 mg/dl experienced a 12 percent decline to 157 mg/dl and a 20 percent decline in triglycerides from 172 mg/dl to 138 mg/dl. His coronary heart disease risk factor rating declined 14 percent from 4.2 to 3.6.
- Another male had a cholesterol reading of 199 mg/dl, which declined 27 percent to 145 mg/dl, while his triglycerides went down 44 percent (from 217 mg/dl to 121 mg/dl). His coronary heart disease risk factor rating went down 23 percent from 5.3 to 4.1.

- Finally, a woman with cholesterol levels of 194 mg/dl experienced a 10 percent decline to 174 mg/dl and an 11 percent decline in triglycerides from 413 mg/dl to 369 mg/dl. Her coronary heart disease risk factor rating declined 14 percent from 5.1 to 4.4

In an open-label, 120-day clinical pilot study conducted by Paul A. Goldberg, M.P.H, D.C., at the Goldberg Clinic in Marietta, Georgia, 17 individuals suffering from complex digestive and immune-system disorders were given Primal Defense HSOs for 120 days. The subjects' gastrointestinal and immune system disorders had been resistant to conventional and complimentary treatments. They had a variety of chronic diseases that were unresponsive to medical intervention for a minimum of three years. The subjects ranged in age from 20 to 65. No dietary or lifestyle changes were made. Of the 16 subjects, 15 reported clinical improvements in their overall health. They had partial to full relief from troublesome bowel problems, decreases in asthmatic symptoms, increases in energy levels, improvements in skin conditions, improvement in chronic sinus infection, and general improvement in overall well-being. No subjects reported a worsening of their symptoms.

Eight of eight subjects with elevated yeast levels as verified by stool and/or blood tests had a significant reduction in candida yeast growth. Three subjects with asthma had a 50 percent or greater reduction in usage of inhalant medications and asthma symptoms.

Moreover, three subjects who suffered from long-term chronic constipation and had laxative dependency were able to move their bowels daily without the use of laxatives.

Three subjects with chronic IBS showed between 25 and 100 percent improvement.

Four patients with chronic fatigue syndrome were completely free of symptoms by the end of the 120-day period. Before and after, blood tests and physical examinations showed that no subject experienced a worsening of conditions or exhibited any evidence of toxicity. Because this was not a placebo-controlled study, the results should be considered investigative and not scientific, but they deserve further research.

Let's look at the results for some individual patients:

Subject 1 A 53-year old male with a 27-year medical history of progressive psoriatic arthritis and ulcerative colitis experienced symptomatic improvement during the first three weeks with improvements in bowel function and arthritic pains followed by an exacerbation with increases in joint inflammation and bloody diarrhea. His Primal Defense dosage was reduced from 18 to two caplets, two times per day, with a reduction of symptoms. The patient increased his dosage over the next several days, returning to 18 caplets per day, completing the 120-day protocol. He reported that his bowel function improved 25 percent by the end of the study with occasional days of "near normal stools," which had not occurred for over five years. Improvements were also noted with less visible blood in his stool, better formed stools, and reduced incidence of cramping. There was no improvement in overall stiffness/joint discomforts. His sedimentation rate fluctuated, but, at the end of the study, remained close to what it had been at the start (55mm/hr). A follow up of the stool microbiology showed a significant reduction in the stool yeast count.

Results from Goldberg Study

Condition	Subjective Outcome	Candida Overgrowth (Bowel)*	Final Result	Elevated Candida (Blood)**	Final Result
Ulcerative Colitis	C	albicans 3+	No Yeast		
Ulcerative Colitis	C	tropicalis 3+	No Yeast		
Asthma	A			900 U/ml	438 U/ml
Chronic Sinusitis	A	albicans 4+, zeylanoides 2+	1+, 0		
Psoriasis	C				
Irritable Bowel Syndrome	C	albicans 2+	1+		
Irritable Bowel Syndrome	B	albicans 4+, lusitaniae 3+	No Yeast		
Irritable Bowel Syndrome	A				
Diverticulitis	D				
Chronic Constipation	A				
Chronic Constipation	A				
Chronic Constipation	A				
Rheumatoid Arthritis	A	albicans 1+, krusel 1+	No Yeast	1,688 U/ml	183 U/ml
Chronic Diarrhea	A				
Chronic Diarrhea	A				
Chronic Nausea	A	albicans 3+	No Yeast		
Asthma	B				

A=75% or greater subjective improvement
B=50% or greater subjective improvement
C=25% or greater subjective improvement
D=No improvement
E=Worsening of symptoms

*Bowel mycology testing was performed at Doctor's Data Diagnostic Laboratories, Illinois
**Candida serum antibody tests were performed at Great Smokies Diagnostic Laboratories, South Carolina

Subject 2 A 42-year-old female radiologist with a five-year history of chronic fungal infection of the lungs also had significant (approximately 25 percent loss of lung function. She had chronic chest pain upon breathing. Long-term use of the anti-fungal drug Sporonox® had not resolved the problem or allowed for any significant improvement. She also had chronic asthma and a significantly elevated serum yeast titer. At completion of the study, the subject reported feeling significant improvement. Her asthma symptomatology had improved by 70 percent, as rated by subject. She reported greater ease in breathing, improved bowel function, and more energy. She had a reduction in chest pain and significant improvement in spirometer testing by her medical pulmonologist in January 2002. Yeast serum antibody testing performed on this subject at the completion of the study showed a marked drop in the titer from 900 to 438 U/ml. Therefore, it would appear that her infectious state had greatly improved, leading to improved lung function.

Subject 3 A 36-year-old male with chronic psoriasis widespread over his scalp, elbows, face, torso and legs improved with approx. 25 percent of the psoriatic lesions clearing and a lightening of the remaining affected areas.

Subject 4 A 46-year-old male, with chronic irritable bowel syndrome since childhood that interfered with social and work activities, reported at end of the protocol a reduction in symptoms of cramping / diarrhea/ irritable bowel of approximately 25 to 30 percent.

Subject 5 A 35-year-old female, with chronic constipation of seven years duration and bowel movements that occurred once every three to four days, reported in the third week of the protocol that her constipation had abated entirely with bowel movements occurring every one to two days. She reported an enhanced sense of wellbeing.

Subject 6 A 43-year-old female, with chronic fatigue, constipation with laxative dependency, and depression, reported significant improvement in energy levels, reduction of depression, and complete relief from chronic constipation of five plus year's duration with her laxative dependency ended. *(Prior to protocol, this patient reported having a bowel movement once every three days. After the protocol, the patient reported a daily bowel movement without laxative usage.)*

A 90-day, 70-patient, blind placebo-controlled clinical study, also published in *Progress in Nutrition*, evaluated the effectiveness of Primal Defense HSOs as a primary treatment for chronic digestive disorder and malabsorption syndrome. Thirty-one patients in the study group and 14 patients in the placebo group completed the study. Some 52 percent of those taking Primal Defense achieved full remission of symptoms; 32 percent of the participants achieved greater than 60 percent; and the remaining 16 percent achieved a greater than 40 percent improvement of symptoms; no subjects had zero improvement or a worsening of symptoms.

According to the director of the study, Primal Defense's soil organisms qualify as an accomplished specific therapy with "significant efficacy" for treating chronic digestive disorders and malabsorption syndrome. "It is evident that the preparation triggers regulatory neuro-immune reactions, inducing healing processes of the herein indicated pathological conditions," note the researchers.

Additional studies conducted on Primal Defense showed the following results:

1) Individuals consuming Primal Defense had a marked increase in blood levels of several key enzymes:

Enzyme	Before HSOs	After HSOs	Change	Reference Range
Amylase	6.8 DU/mm	16.25	+139%	20-110 U/mm
Lipase	4.6 FCCLU/mm	20.0	+335%	7-60 U/mm
Protease 6.0	18.2 HUT/cu.mm	38.2	+110%	30-90 HUT/cu.mm
Protease 4.5	6.9 HUT/cu.mm	15.8	+129%	12-40 HUT/cu.mm
Protease 3.0	4.6 HUT/cu.mm	10.9	+137%	8-16 HUT/cu.mm

2) Individuals with low blood protein levels at the beginning of the study, after consuming Primal Defense, had an increase in blood protein levels. This signifies improved absorption and utilization of protein from the diet.

Marker	Before HSOs	After HSOs	Change	Reference Range
Total Protein (25)	3.86	7.03	+82%	6.4-8.4 g/dL

3) Individuals consuming Primal Defense had a marked improvement in symptoms of anemia and the use of the product seemed to have a "blood-building" effect.

Marker	Before HSOs	After HSOs	Change	Reference Range
RBC	3.5	1.1	+26%	4.5-5.6 Mios/cmm
Hemoglobin	9.3	12.9	+39%	12-16 G/dL

4) Individuals consuming Primal Defense had a marked improvement in blood levels of key minerals.

Marker	Before HSOs	After HSOs	Change	Reference Range
Iron	25.2	43.5	+73%	(40-80) ug/dL
Calcium	6.4	9.2	+44%	(8.5-10.6) mg/dL
Phosphorus	1.5	2.9	+93%	(2.5-4.6) mg/dL
Potassium	2.7	3.9	+44%	(3.5-5.3) mg/L

5) Individuals with abnormal immune markers showed a trend towards a modulation of the immune system as evidenced by a decrease in white blood cells; an increase in neutrophils; normalization of lymphocytes; and a decrease in elevated monocytes, eosinophils and basophils.

Marker	Before HSOs	After HSOs	Change	Reference Range
WBC (31)	11.2	8.6	-30%	4.5-9.5) Th/cmm
Low Neutrop (18)	45.3	55.3	+22%	(50-72) %
High Lymph (4)	44.75	33	-26%	(26-40) %
Low Lymph (16)	20	31	+55%	(26-40) %
High Monocytes (27)	13.4	6.9	-49%	(0-8) %
High Eos (6)	6.7	5.7	-15%	(0-4) %
High Bas (21)	10.3	2	-81%	(0-5) %

In addition, a significant number of beneficial observations were made in the course of the study which, due to the fact that they were beyond the scope of the established protocol, regrettably could not be incorporated in the official reports published in *Progress in Nutrition*. Thus these are presented here in an independent compilation:

• Fourteen patients (nine females, five males) reported remarkable increases in their energy levels beginning toward the end of the second month and continuing through the third month of treatment.

- Three female patients having suffered from chronic, recurrent migraine headaches, reported total remission from their headaches by the end of the respective studies.
- Six patients (five females, one male) having suffered from varied grades of chronic skin rash, reported total remission of these symptoms.
- Six patients (4 females, 2 males) reported significant vanishing of some of their facial wrinkles by the end of the study.

CASE REPORT #1
We Get Letters

Anthony C. was diagnosed with ulcerative colitis. Here is his HSO-healing story, in his own words in a letter to Garden of Life.

Dear Jordan,

I would sincerely like to take this opportunity and time to convey my personal experience with the usage of your product—Primal Defense HSO Immune Formula. To this date, words alone cannot express enough how immensely pleased and satisfied I am with achieving some positive benefits and significant improvements in my health.

In December of 1996, after complaints of finding traces of blood in my formed stools, I was diagnosed with proctitis, an inflammatory bowel disease primarily confined to the sigmoid of the lower rectum. Subsequently, as the year and months progressed my symptoms grew worse—left side bloating and pain of the left side, inflammation, rectal bleeding, blood mucus, uncontrollable bowel movements, up to five to seven times per day and weight loss. Obviously the condition had been deteriorating over time and the last colonoscopy had revealed that there was inflammation, sores, and ulceration now along the entire descending colon along the left side of the large intestine. The doctor's prognosis was ulcerative colitis.

In the course of the last four years I have seen no fewer than four gastroenterologist specialists and consulted with numerous alternative health care providers ranging from holistic doctors, Traditional Chinese doctors, homeopathic doctors, certified herbalists, naturopaths, Tibetan doctors and so forth. I had been prescribed and experimented with all known traditional herbs, supplements, and endless remedies documented to aid and/or alleviate and treat bowel diseases, but to no avail.

Then in late April of 2000 with hope dwindling, I came across one empathetic individual by the name of Jerry Zeifman. He encouraged me to try…Primal Defense…I was reluctant at first, but after reading some literature and one specific booklet called Beyond Probiotics, I resigned myself to giving it a go. I followed the protocol outlined in the booklet and after several weeks I started to notice some positive benefits in my condition. Going forward, the improvement gradually continued to a point where today I can report that I have no pain or discomfort on the left side, no bloating, no visible sign of blood or mucus from the rectum or in the stools, one to two formed bowel movements a day, and my weight has increased by seventeen pounds. I have to thank the Lord God Jesus for that encounter with Jerry who introduced me to…Primal Defense…or it was truly a blessing that has had a profound impact not only on my health but also on my life.

Yours truly, *Anthony C.*

CASE REPORT #2

Mike M. from Arlington, Texas, was suffering myriad symptoms: sinus headaches, severe vertigo, lethargy, irregular sleeping patterns, frequent colds and flu, food allergies, lactose intolerance, pain deep in the bowels, white fuzzy tongue, bloating and gas, blood and mucus in the stools, chronic diarrhea, inability to digest fruit and vegetables, and terrible low back pain. He was losing a pound a day on a 4,000 calorie daily diet.

Mike began taking one caplet per day of Primal Defense, increasing the dosage by one caplet every three days until he was taking eight per day.

After two weeks he began to cough up massive amounts of phlegm as his body began detoxifying. But by early April, he was feeling much more energetic.

"Although my gas and bloody stools continued, I knew Primal Defense was working," Mike writes. By late May, around day 80 of his use of the formula, his gas problems were history. Around day 90, his stools were no longer bloody.

"I would have never guessed back pain could be related to intestinal disease," Mike says. "But the pain slowly subsided and is now minimal. After 100 days of treatment with Primal Defense and Perfect Food, I have gained 15 pounds and feel tremendous renewal in my life. It is a terrible tragedy that millions of people today are suffering from digestive illnesses and other chronic problems due to intestinal toxemia [which may be a result of acidosis] simply because they are unaware of the solution."

If my experience can help one person, that's a blessing. Fortunately, as our files filled with letters indicate, many people have been able to overcome their own health challenges with the help of soil organisms combined with adherence to the Maker's Diet. And that makes what I went through worthwhile.

However, after getting well, I had to face another major health challenge. My grandmother Rose Menlowe, who was often my caretaker during my illness, was diagnosed with an aggressive cancer. I'll tell you about that next.

CHAPTER FOUR

Mankind's Most Powerful Immune Enhancer

The insurance industry is understandably dependent on statistics. Thus, both our average life span and the principal causes of premature death are continuously studied and monitored with greatest care. Nonetheless, I have yet to meet the first statistician who would have spelled out the paramount cause of death among the human population. The ultimate cause of untimely death is ignorance.

In the nineteenth century, the great French scientist Louis Pasteur offered the world the wisdom that most diseases were caused by harmful microbes. In the wake of his discoveries, more than a century ago, research and development in conventional medicine is focused on the theory that almost all pathology is brought on by germs, viruses, fungi and macroscopic parasites. Thus, to fight diseases, the onslaught of such invading germs must to be terminated. In order to destroy such microorganisms the pharmaceutical research was—and is—developing ever more potent medicines.

While these compounds have, indeed, succeeded in eliminating many forms of infections, their increasingly toxic effects revealed that the postulation of such theory has many irremediable deficiencies. In fact, it is my opinion that diseases are caused by a weak terrain in the body that becomes a prime target for infectious microorganisms. Even the great Pasteur himself as a dying man echoed the same sentiment. I've already mentioned the harm that indiscriminate antibiotic use poses to the gastrointestinal flora—the imbalance antibiotics can cause of populations of both beneficial and pathogenic bacterial species. Another problem worthy of mention is our population's growing resistance to these medical miracles.

During the past decades, we have witnessed the unequivocal repercussion and fiasco of antibiotics which, instead of delivering lasting solutions, turned into a veritable menace. In consequence to the aggression of ever more potent antibiotics, manifold strains of germs have mutated and acquired a resistance to the medications developed against them.

Antimicrobial resistance has been recognized since the introduction of penicillin nearly 50 years ago, when penicillin-resistant infections caused by *Staphylococcus aureus* rapidly appeared. Today, doctors and hospitals worldwide are facing unprecedented crises from the rapid emergence and dissemination of other microbes resistant to one or more antimicrobial agents.

In testimony, before the Senate Committee on Health, Education, Labor, and Pensions Subcommittee on Public Health and Safety on February 25, 1999, Anthony S. Fauci, M.D., director of the National Institute of Allergy and Infectious Diseases of the National Institutes of Health, presented his own disturbing views on the overuse of antibiotics:

> Many diseases are increasingly difficult to treat because of the emergence of drug-resistant organisms, including HIV and other viruses; bacteria such as staphylococci, enterococci, and E. coli which cause serious infections in hospitalized patients; bacteria that cause respiratory diseases such as pneumonia and tuberculosis; food-borne pathogens such as Salmonella and Campylobacter; sexually transmitted organisms such as Neisseria gonorrhoeae; Candida and other fungi; and parasites such as Plasmodium falciparum, the cause of malaria. According to the Institute of Medicine (IOM), the total cost of treating antimicrobial-resistant infections may be as high as $5 billion annually in the United States.

Consider the following facts:

- Strains of *Staphylococcus aureus* resistant to methicillin and other antibiotics are endemic in hospitals. Infection with methicillin-resistant *S. aureus* strains may also be increasing in non-hospital settings. A limited number of drugs remain effective against these infections. *S. aureus* strains with reduced susceptibility to vancomycin have emerged recently in Japan and the United States. The emergence of completely vancomycin-resistant strains would present a serious problem for physicians and patients.

- Increasing reliance on vancomycin has led to the emergence of vancomycin-resistant enterococci, bacteria that infect wounds, the urinary tract and other sites. Until 1989, such resistance had not been reported in U.S. hospitals. By 1993, however, more than 10 percent of hospital-acquired enterococci infections reported to the CDC were resistant.

- *Streptococcus pneumoniae* causes thousands of cases of meningitis and pneumonia, and seven million cases of ear infection in the United States each year. Currently, about 30 percent of *S. pneumoniae* isolates are resistant to penicillin, the primary drug used to treat this infection. Many penicillin-resistant strains are also resistant to other antimicrobial drugs.

- In sexually transmitted disease clinics that monitor outbreaks of drug-resistant infections, doctors have found that more than 30 percent of gonorrhea isolates are resistant to penicillin or tetracycline, or both.

- An estimated 300 to 500 million people worldwide are infected with the parasites that cause malaria. Resistance to chloroquine, once widely used and highly effective for preventing and treating malaria, has emerged in most parts of the world. Resistance to other antimalaria drugs is widespread and growing.

- Strains of multidrug-resistant tuberculosis (MDR-TB) have emerged over the last decade and pose a particular threat to people infected with HIV. Drug-resistant strains are as contagious as those that are susceptible to drugs. MDR-TB is more difficult and vastly more expensive to treat, and patients may remain infectious longer due to inadequate treatment.

- Diarrheal diseases cause almost three million deaths a year—mostly in developing countries, where resistant strains of highly pathogenic bacteria such as *Shigella dysenteriae*, *Vibrio cholerae*, *Escherichia coli*, campylobacter, and salmonella are emerging. Recent outbreaks of salmonella food poisoning have occurred in the United States. A potentially dangerous "superbug" known as *Salmonella typhimurium*, resistant to ampicillin, sulfa, streptomycin, tetracycline and chloramphenicol, has caused illness in Europe, Canada and the United States.

- Fungal pathogens account for a growing proportion of nosocomial (hospital) infections. Fungal diseases such as candidiasis and *Pneumocystis carinii* pneumonia are common among AIDS patients, and isolated outbreaks of other fungal diseases in people with normal immune systems have occurred recently in the United States. Scientists and clinicians are concerned that the increasing use of antifungal drugs will lead to drug-resistant fungi. In fact, recent studies have documented resistance of candida species to fluconazole, a drug used widely to treat patients with systemic fungal diseases.

- Recent years have seen the introduction of powerful new drugs and drug combinations against HIV. Although treatments that combine new protease inhibitor drugs with other anti-HIV medications often effectively suppress HIV production in infected individuals, results from recent clinical studies suggest that many treatment failures occur due to the development of resistance by the virus.

Consequently, many liberal-minded researchers are challenging the antibiotic theory of disease treatment and are seeking alternative solutions to the problems. Over time, two schools of therapeutic concepts have emerged. Orthodox medicine and its exponents have completely accepted the germ postulate. That is, germs, viruses, and fungi bring on most diseases, and somehow must to be obliterated. They assert that this goal can best be achieved through the use of potent antibiotics and specific chemicals.

Needless to say, the pharmaceutical industry enthusiastically endorses this theory and supports all research leading to the development of such preparations. Considering that there are factually billions of different harmful microorganisms, it is obvious that an endless stream of preparations must be developed in order to fight all of them. This, obviously, generates many billions of dollars in profits not only in manufacturing such products, but also in research and development of the same.

But, ultimately, we need to go beyond this theory because of the problem of emerging antibiotic-resistant pathogens. The second school of thought does, in fact, go beyond the use of ever more toxic drugs to destroy microbes and the assumption that these are the sole cause of disease. Our environment literally teems with billions of microorganisms, most of which are harmful. They thrive unchallenged in our air, water, and soil and even in our living tissues. Yet, thanks to the intricate and powerful design of our immune system, we are not only able to survive, but—judging by the global demographic explosion of our population—we are actually thriving amidst such a continuous onslaught. It is our proficient immune response that keeps us alive.

The immune system operating in a healthy human body is perfectly capable of annihilating injurious microorganisms, while leaving all benign and useful species undamaged. Thus, illness ensues when our immune system becomes defective and is unable to generate an appropriate immune response.

This also reveals why not everyone exposed to the assault of a given germ, virus or fungus succumbs to its harmful effects: their vigilant immune system is fully operational. Thus, the disciples of the second school of thought support the idea of continuously servicing and repairing the immune system by natural—that is, nontoxic—means that enhance our body's inborn self-healing abilities.

It is quite obvious—to say the least—that the pharmaceutical industry does not quite encourage the spreading of such ideas, since these generally must rely on the natural pharmacopoeia. Though likely to yield impressive health dividends, there is little profit to be generated by promoting natural means of health maintenance and repair and in teaching healthy lifestyles. Getting down to basics, this probably explains, at least in part, why the pharmaceutical industry and the medical establishment of conventional medicine frown on complementary and alternative therapeutic methods, purporting that they involve quackery.

Nonetheless, recent developments are proving them ever more wrong. Cancer incidence is irrepressibly increasing. In their important work *The Safe Shopper's Bible* (Hungry Minds 1995), David Steinman and Samuel S. Epstein, M.D., note that the National Cancer Institute (NCI) is responsible for directing the nation's "war" on cancer. Even so, from 1950 to 1989, the overall incidence of cancer in the United States (adjusted for the aging population) rose by approximately 44 percent, with lung cancer, due to smoking, accounting for less than a quarter of this increase.[21,22] Age-adjusted incidence rates for breast cancer and male colon cancer for the general U.S. population have increased by over 50 percent, whereas the rates for some less common cancers, such as melanoma, certain lymphomas, and male kidney cancer have increased by over 100 percent. Childhood cancer has also increased by about 20 percent, they note. Higher cancer rates still are seen for people living in highly urbanized and industrialized counties (in the vicinity of petrochemical, mining, smelting, and nuclear weapons plants), and for workers in these industries.[23] Today, more than one in three Americans will be stricken with cancer in their lifetime and more than one in four will die. Cancer has overtaken heart disease as the leading killer of middle-aged Americans,[24] and the baby boom generation is at far higher cancer risk than its grandparents' generation.[25]

Steinman and his co-author note that the NCI has taken a decidedly indifferent, if not hostile, view toward prevention despite the fact that the "war" on cancer is clearly being lost. For example, a recent Swedish study found that baby boomers face a higher risk of cancer than did their great-grandparents.[26] The study of nearly 840,000 cases in all groups reported to the Swedish government since 1958 revealed that the risk of developing cancer was almost three times higher in men born in the 1950s than in those born in the 1880s, and for women, the risk was twice as high. These differences held true even after accounting for smoking-related cancer. Despite growing evidence that cancer is caused by exposure to environmental carcinogens, NCI—which could direct millions of dollars into truly effective cancer-prevention programs that would focus on removing the environmental causes of this disease—continues its unsubstantiated claims that "victory" is only a "cure" away.

Meanwhile, AIDS researchers have finally admitted that flooding the organism with toxic medications does not offer solutions. The speed at which the several known AIDS viruses are able to mutate defies all attempts to develop a standard treatment against them. Furthermore, to heap insult over injury, the side effects of the hitherto proposed "cures" can prove even more lethal than the very virus.

Even today, we now know that our immune system is responsible in part for the prevention of heart disease, since infectious organisms account for increases in levels of inflammation, as measured by C-reactive protein. Inflammation levels, we now know, are quite adept at predicting risk of heart attack and stroke.

Thus, I truly believe that whichever pathology we are facing—except traumas, or other conditions, which clearly can only be assisted by surgery—the only obvious and feasible solutions are those that endeavor the revival, modulation, and regulation of the immune and self-repair systems.

Until quite recently, the very idea to find substances capable of achieving such goals evoked a storm of indignant and scornful objections from the medical establishment. However, fortunately times do change and nowadays this very notion is very much at the forefront of the interests of both conventional and naturopathic practitioners. The development of means for the enhancement of our immune responses has become a paramount priority—and, whether embraced by the medical establishment or not, health-conscious consumers intuitively and intellectually grasp the importance of immune health.

Regrettably, Americans are irrepressibly prone to follow fads. Most of these, I might add, do only conjure illusions. Yet, once in a while we learn about something that truly deserves our attention.

During my illness, my maternal grandmother, Rose Menlowe, took care of me whenever my condition became too much for my parents and they needed relief. Both times, when I was hospitalized, my grandmother slept in a chair next to the bed and was assuredly an angel who protected me and helped me to fight for my life.

You can imagine how devastating the news was when just a few years after my own recovery, I learned my grandmother had cancer.

In late spring 1999, when she was 77, my grandmother began experiencing excruciating stomach pain. She was throwing up constantly. But all of the laboratory tests kept coming back normal. My aunt and uncle asked Grandma to come stay with them. But, once with them in Atlanta, she began feeling even worse and had to be carried out of bed and helped out of the shower. She would rise in the middle of the night and throw up. The stomach pain was so unbearable, she asked my uncle (her son-in-law) to give her pills to help her end it all.

My uncle refused, of course. But Grandma's condition worsened. Soon after, the pain became so wretched that they rushed my grandmother to the emergency room in Atlanta where she immediately was put under for major exploratory surgery. When she awoke, the doctor told her she had multiple malignancies including a goblet cell carcinoid in her appendix and stage IV ovarian cancer that had spread to her lymph nodes and portions of her small and large intestines.

Stage IV, by the way, is the most advanced stage of ovarian cancer. Growth of the cancer involves one or both ovaries and distant metastases (spread of the cancer to organs located outside of the peritoneal cavity) have occurred. Finding ovarian cancer cells in her pleural fluid (from the cavity which surrounds the lungs) was also evidence of her stage IV disease.

The surgeon removed her ovaries, some of her lymph nodes, and portions of her small and large intestines, as they were cancerous as well. But the ovarian malignancy was extremely advanced and we already had evidence that the cancer had spread to other sites. Though the larger tumors were removed, the chance of recurrence was high. Because of her age and weakened state, her surgeon suggested we regularly monitor her situation rather than going with chemotherapy and radiation.

Grandma was born in Poland and lived on a farm in the country near Warsaw. As a child, her family consumed fruits and vegetables straight from the garden. The family had a mill where they pressed flax seed and poppy seed into oil. "I used to eat lignan cakes as snacks with black sourdough bread," she recalls. "Oh, the bread was as hard as a rock but so delicious. You cannot find that kind of bread anymore. We used to break off pieces from the flax cakes and dip them in fresh oil right from the press."

But by the time she was in her early teens, Europe was experiencing the devastating consequences of Nazism. "We were some of the last European Jews to arrive in America before the holocaust," she recalls. "I was 12 when we arrived—and, let me tell you, skinny, almost puny. In America, I fell in love with white bread and ate a lot of starchy things, cakes and doughnuts from the bakery …"

Immediately after surgery, Grandma became very depressed. She had the sense that she was going to die. She spoke of things in terms of having only limited time left. I was going to be married in September 1999. Her surgery was in June and all she hoped for was to live long enough to be at the wedding. "I was praying that I would live long enough to go to the wedding," she would confide to me later. It touches me now to recall her words. *"Jordan, you were my first grandchild. I want to do something so I might live to see you married. You must be able to come up with something."*

As any doctor will tell you, when a family member falls ill you would rather have them treated by anyone other than yourself. However, due to my grandmother's financial condition, I had no choice but to meet the challenge of her terminal illness.

In this case, I began studying the body's immune system components and natural methods of improving immune function, especially increasing the body's activity level of macrophages, natural killer cells, and cytokines (messenger chemicals). I had to somehow help strengthen Grandma's immune response to suppress her cancer cells and promote healthy cells.

My grandmother needed her white blood cells and cytokines to be not only at optimal population levels but also highly activated. Sometimes—as researchers now know—our immune cells are numerous in number but have been rendered inactive or ineffectual by various chemicals tumor cells secrete.

You see, a cancer cell wills itself to survive even if it causes the death of the host. To do so, it produces more and more of a growth factor called transforming growth factor-beta (TGF-β). As immune cells come nearer to extinguish this invader, the TGF-β causes the immune cells to become nonfunctional. TGF-β inhibits proliferation of T-cells, reduces the cancer cell-killing power of tumor necrosis factor, and inhibits the ability of macrophages, our immune system's first line of defense, to engage in phagocytosis. The body ends up thinking its forces are effectively attacking cancer cells. But they aren't any longer. The key was to activate them, to feed the hungry cells of her immune system.

That research led me to studying chains of complex sugars that today we call polysaccharides or glyconutrients (nutrients from sugar), or, more specifically, polysaccharide peptides or glycoproteins (polysaccharides that are bound to proteins)—and how they occur in Nature.

I learned that certain compounds, found in greatest abundance in edible fungi, enhance macrophage and natural killer cell production. This, in turn, enhances production of cytokines, which are immune cell secretions that facilitate cell-cell communications and fully optimize immune function. With glyconutrients we might even be able to overcome some of the deceptive practices of TGF-β. Do not confuse these sugar-based compounds with commonly consumed sugars such as fructose or starches. I call these highly complex compounds the *healing sugars*.

I also learned that our primitive diet used to contain a lot of these compounds, but now due to our modern refined diets our bodies are highly deficient in them. The richest source for these compounds is found in edible mushrooms, but, unfortunately, not the button mushrooms most of us buy at supermarkets.

Though our interest in edible fungi in America is limited, elsewhere in the world the healing powers of mushrooms have been known for more than 5,000 years. In the winter of 1991, hikers in the Italian Alps discovered the frozen remains of a man who had died some 5,300 years earlier. Found among the artifacts with which he was traveling, quite apart from his knapsack and flint ax, was a string of dried mushrooms called birch polypores (*Piptoporus betulinus*) and another as yet unidentified mushroom.

"The polypores can be used as tinder for starting fires and as medicine for treating wounds," writes fungi expert Paul Stamets, author of *Growing Gourmet & Medicinal Mushrooms* (Ten Speed Press 1993). "Further, a rich tea with immuno-enhancing properties can be prepared by boiling these mushrooms."

That mushrooms should possess significant healing powers, of course, is nothing new to Asian healing traditions. In the Orient, several types of mushrooms have been used for centuries to maintain health, preserve youth, and increase longevity. Although the healing aspects of mushrooms have been passed down through folklore, it has only been within the past 20 years that the scientific study of mushrooms and their healing properties has been initiated.[27]

In a 1996 article in Nutrition Reviews, R. Chang, of the Department of Medicine, Memorial Sloan-Kettering Cancer Center, New York, noted:

Edible mushrooms…may have important salutary effects on health or even in treating disease. A mushroom characteristically contains many different bioactive compounds with diverse biological activity…In order of decreasing cultivated tonnage, Lentinus (shiitake), Pleurotus (oyster), Auricularia (mu-er), Flammulina (enokitake), Tremella (yin-er), Hericium, and Grifola (maitake) mushrooms have various degrees of immunomodulatory, lipid lowering, antitumor, and other beneficial or therapeutic health effects without any significant toxicity.[28]

The complexity and variations in glyconutrients is truly mind-boggling. Each specific mushroom offers different combinations, involving far more complex and varied molecular structures than science has been able to identify or characterize. I also learned that various portions of the mushroom had different amounts of glyconutrients. For example, the mycelium of the mushroom, the seed of the mushroom so to speak (not the fruiting body which we see above ground), is a particularly rich source of protein-bound polysaccharides (glycoproteins).

The way mushrooms are cultivated, the various grains and seeds used, also influences mycelium glyconutrient content. Some mushrooms, like cordyceps, when found in the wild actually use caterpillars as a growth medium. And, of course, we now know that organic production truly enhances potency of all foods, including mushrooms, while minimizing exposure to pesticides and heavy metals.

Not only was I fascinated by the burgeoning amount of research being conducted into glyconutrients, apparently, so were pharmaceutical scientists. Some of the most potent anticancer drugs now in development are based on glyconutrients. These complex sugars are finding their way into other new applications such as wound and ulcer healing and cell transplantation (in diabetes). Another glyconutrient derivative is being heralded as a cure for influenza.

The commercial promise of glyconutrients eventually will lead to a new era of anti-inflammatory and anti-metastasic drugs. The future potential is enormous for the design of glyconutrient-based drugs.

No doubt, these drugs will be heralded as "new" breakthroughs. But are they really? After all, almost all synthetic drugs to be developed will be based on Nature's limitless molecular variations. I tapped into this mother load when I began working with medicinal mushrooms. Certainly, the same glyconutrients on which the pharmaceutical drugs are being based are already making their presence felt in the world of natural health.

THE MIRACLE OF POTEN-ZYME

But there was something more that I learned from my own illness. I realized people used to get much more reliable results from herbal medicines because their digestive tracts, at one time, were far more able to utilize foods and herbs than today. Today, for most of us, our digestive tracts are damaged to greater or lesser degrees due to our overuse of medications and poor dietary habits. Many herbs and other sources of natural healing agents, such as mushrooms, are fibrous and difficult for the body to break down. Some are as much as 60 percent fiber. Grandma's diet had changed so much since moving from Poland, she needed a delivery system that would enable her to utilize the herbs I wanted her to start using.

We took the fermentation process that helped heal me—what today we call the Poten-Zyme process, with more than 14 species of homeostatic soil organisms and other lactic-acid producing microorganisms—and used it to predigest the 10 mushrooms, aloe vera and cat's claw in the formula and thus "unlock" the active ingredients.

This is important. There are records of traditional herbalism from the Orient and other cultures in the Far East dating back 1,500 years ago, which talked about herbal remedies that were used to treat a variety of ailments. In the past, they provided very predictable, very effective, very potent results. Yet today, we are not getting the same kind of healing response from these herbs. The reason people today aren't being helped is not necessarily due to the lack of healing properties in the herbs themselves—it is the direct result of an ultimate breakdown in the human digestive tract. The nutrients and phytochemicals contained in herbs are not being broken down and utilized properly by the body, primarily because people's guts have been destroyed from the overuse of prescription medications—antibiotics, corticosteroids, and other immune suppressive drugs—as well as chlorinated and fluoridated water, ambient pollutants in our environment, and an overall poor diet coupled with a steady intake of junk foods. The application of the Poten-Zyme process is a way for the body to utilize all of the phytochemicals and phytonutrients available in these herbs, with very little stress on the digestive tract. This benefit is extremely important to those people undergoing chemotherapy and radiation, or those with AIDS or other immune disorders, who have very little digestive capability. This enzymatic "pre-digestion" process increases bioavailability and absorption of the medicinal compounds making them "body-ready" for everyone, even those with compromised digestion. In other words, the sickest persons, with the least ability to utilize fibrous herbs, receive a much greater boost from our nutritional formulas, thanks to the fermentation process that the whole food concentrates and herbs undergo, making their healing constituents far more available to the sickened person's body. Especially relevant to what I wanted to accomplish with my grandmother, some mushrooms are comprised of more than 80 percent carbohydrates and thus lend themselves well to fermentation, which unlocks their healing powers and makes them available to be assimilated by the body.

This ancient method of bio-fermentation incorporates beneficial microorganisms (probiotics) and their enzymes into the foods to gently break them down into their most basic elements. This is not something that any company could easily duplicate. Our fermentation, done in the U.S. Southwest and Australia, is not available anywhere else in the world. Our Poten-Zyme lactic acid fermentation process uses a "mother" culture that contains microorganisms resistant to many of the agents that kill more fragile probiotic species (such as acidophilus)—including stomach acid, heat, cold, chlorine, fluorine and ascorbic acid. We now have a rare, self-sustaining culture.

We take our young cereal grasses (from Australia and the Southwest United States), algae, seed, legumes or grains and cover these with our mother culture for three to six weeks (whereas typical fermentation lasts one to four days). The end result is a food that is nearly completely broken down and predigested with large amounts of probiotics, enzymes, B vitamins and proteins. But also created are several novel phytochemicals that the body craves, including the body's master antioxidant superoxide dismutase (SOD), as well as various immune-supportive beta-glucans, and many other antioxidants—all created from the "alchemy" involved in fermentation. Take our spirulina and grasses. We know spirulina and grasses are a rich source of beta-carotene and chlorophyll. However, when beta-carotene is taken into a human we are counting on the body to convert it to vitamin A or retinols; unfortunately, unhealthy persons cannot always make that conversion. Our spirulina is a dark blue-green at the beginning of fermentation, but a month or month-and-a-half later it is green with orange overtones because the carotenoids and chlorophyll have been liberated.

My grandmother began using the prototype medicinal mushroom and herbal formula immediately following her surgery.* "Not only did I gain weight; my energy level, physical appearance and general health improved to the point where they are now better than I can recall in the last 30 years," she recalls. "My digestion improved. But, most importantly, according my last CAT scan, I am cancer-free. Even the fatty liver that I developed (due most probably to metabolic imbalance) is gone now.

"Yes," she laughs, "I was able to see my first grandson marry his lovely bride!"

On Labor Day 2001, at the Cancer Control Society's 26th annual convention in Universal City, California, Grandma spoke before an audience of some 2,500 persons about her victorious battle with cancer.

"I told the people there that I used RM-10 continuously and do so even now. Today, more than three years after the discovery of my cancer, I told everyone, my CAT scans show no evidence of cancer. My energy levels are that of a 20-year-old. With help from my grandson, I hope to see my great-grandchildren grow up."

It was funny. On the way back from the conference site, we were walking along the CityWalk and all tired. We decided to take the tram to the hotel, which was a mile or two away. Grandma walked. She beat us there.

Stuart Zoll, O.M.D, L.Ac., director of the Centre for Preventive Medicine, Boca Raton, Florida, conducted one of the early pilot clinical studies to examine the clinical effectiveness of RM-10 when used for a wide range of immune-related maladies, including cancer, rheumatoid arthritis, bronchitis, and allergies.

Among Dr. Zoll's patients was a 14-year-old boy with brain cancer. He had been treated with an aggressive program of chemotherapy and his blood counts had dropped precipitously. But when Dr. Zoll added RM-10 to his treatment regimen, "the boy's blood counts stabilized" within months. With RM-10 as an adjuvant, his platelet count continued to improve, even as he completed his chemotherapy. In fact, while being treated with aggressive chemotherapy and taking RM-10 as an adjuvant, his blood work looked like that of a person *not* undergoing chemotherapy. But when the boy ran out of the product, within days his blood cell counts declined rapidly, once again indicative of someone on aggressive chemotherapy. Thus, the boy quickly resumed use of RM-10. The boy's oncologist also noted that his tumors had stopped growing and had begun to shrink, which was confirmed by magnetic resonance imaging.

"The boy's progress causes me to believe that, while RM-10 is not a solo treatment for cancer, it does have real value as a complementary therapy for anyone who is undergoing chemotherapy or radiation," says Dr. Zoll. "It may assist in stabilizing blood counts, especially for maintaining one's platelet levels. The product also seems to reduce symptoms of nausea, insomnia and fatigue."

---

* This formula eventually came to be known as RM-10™ (named for my Grandmother Rose Menlowe's initials and the fact that the formula contains glyconutrients from ten important medicinal mushrooms).

"There's been a paradigm shift in medicine and our revolutionary new vision of health requires a complete rethinking of the ways we treat disease today," says Garry Gordon, M.D., D.O., M.D. (H.), who also uses RM-10 extensively in his clinical practice. Dr. Gordon, who wrote the foreword for this book, currently is on the Board of Medical Examiners for Alternative and Homeopathic Medicine and is in charge of Peer Review in the state of Arizona for chelation therapy. He is the president of Gordon Research Institute, where his primary focus is research of natural products for every health problem, with particular emphasis on immune system support for heart disease and cancer.

"Let me tell you about my emerging views on cancer," he continues. "My main message is this: *treat yourself for cancer before you get cancer*. In other words, we all have cancer at every moment in our lives. But why are we waiting for the expression of cancer before we do anything?"

For many cancer patients, the clinically visible signs of cancer are the result of processes that might well have begun years or decades earlier, and that could have been stopped long before if we had only implemented a cancer treatment program before the cancer became clinically evident, says Dr. Gordon.

When Dr. Gordon speaks of treatment before the event, please understand he is not referring to chemotherapy, radiation or surgery. Rather, he refers to use of botanical and nutritional supplements and other natural healing pathways to be used long before the clinical signs of the disease emerge. This is when our natural pharmacy often works extremely well and gives us our best chance for delaying or completely eliminating expression of cancer in our lives.

"My entire program involves every aspect of your life—your diet, your exercise, your mind, your environment and judicious use of nutritional supplements," Dr. Gordon continues. "Now, I know that it is difficult for everyone to take as many different nutritional supplements as is optimal. So, if I were going to tell you about one formula for treating your cancer before you get cancer the formula I would recommend is RM-10 from Garden of Life.

"RM-10 has become a mainstay formula now as I work with patients and their doctors to implement a program of treating cancer before you exhibit its expression. I also use RM-10 extensively in treatment of cancer. In fact, I just had a wonderful success story, where I combined RM-10 with Wobenzym® N systemic oral enzymes for a breast cancer patient and we were able to reverse a metastatic ductal carcinoma when these formulas were used, in this case avoiding the need for surgery (other than biopsy).

"I have been a practicing physician since 1958, and actively involved in the study of immune support and trace element research for over 30 years. I have never seen an immune-support formula as universally applicable and multifaceted as we now have in RM-10. This formula not only captures but also unlocks the anticancer powers of ten different medicinal mushrooms, as well as properly sourced cat's claw and aloe vera.

"Let me explain. Mushrooms such as cordyceps, ganoderma, coriolus, maitake and shiitake, have tremendous anticancer potential. These are routinely prescribed by doctors worldwide to complement cancer treatments. *Cordyceps sinensis* (CS-4) inhibits the production of DNA and RNA synthesis in cancer cells and has displayed antitumor activity on bladder, kidney, colon, and lung carcinoma as well as fibroblastoma cell lines. *Ganoderma lucidum* (reishi) inhibits leukemia cell lines. Meanwhile, *Trametes versicolor* is the source of the highly potent immune-enhancing extract PSK, an immuno-modulator used primarily in conjunction with chemotherapy, radiation, and surgical treatments for cancer.

"But what Garden of Life has done is used their Poten-Zyme fermentation process to unlock all of the healing powers of these mushrooms and the cat's claw and aloe (all of which are organically grown)," asserts Dr. Gordon. "I assume now that none of my patients have adequate digestive processes and this is usually true. The Poten-Zyme fermentation creates a sort of 'alchemy,' wherein the phytochemicals in these medicinal herbs are unlocked and made more available than ever to be utilized by the body. I'm telling you, this is my patients' number one immune formula. If I had to recommend one immune formula to patients interested in the concept of treating themselves for cancer before they get cancer, RM-10 would clearly be my first choice."

Besides ten different medicinal mushrooms in the RM-10 formula, use of cat's claw is also exceedingly important. But not just any cat's claw…

Let's visit Peruvian traditional healing to learn why. According to the traditions of the Asháninka Indians of the Cutivireni region of Peru, one of the last refuges of the Asháninka tribe, only high-ranking healer-priests are able to guide the harvest of the cat's claw herb. That is because, as western scientists have learned, two distinct types of cat's claw grow in the wild, which are almost impossible to differentiate. Though they would not characterize these differences with the use of modern analytical chemistry terms, the high priests of the Asháninka tribe alone are able to discern which plants contain the correct chemotype.

The Asháninka healer-priests called the correct chemotype savéntaro (saveshi = plant, antearo = potent, or powerful plant) and regarded it as being inhabited by the good spirits of the forest.

That is because only those plants demonstrate the coveted immunomodulating properties assigned to cat's claw. The uncontrolled use of mixtures of the two distinctly different plants may lead to unexpected side effects. What's more, they can actually antagonize each other's effects, thus rendering the finished herb all but useless for medicinal purposes—and certainly unpredictable.

But when the proper cat's claw is harvested and processed, it possesses an uncanny ability to know when to stimulate or "down-regulate" immune activity. This, in turn, plays a role in the very positive observed clinical results for persons with autoimmune conditions, such as mixed connective tissue disease, rheumatoid arthritis and allergies, where the immune system is overstimulated and attacking the host's own tissues. In essence, the natural medicine is able to intuitively turn on or off the "switch" at the right time that has caused either an under or overactive immune state. RM-10 uses *only* cat's claw that would be chosen by the Asháninka tribe healer-priests.

With cat's claw alone, we have in RM-10 an ability to modulate disease states such as rheumatoid arthritis, lupus, inflammatory bowel disease and other inflammatory conditions caused by autoimmunity. We also have a powerful anticancer agent.

Two special notes should be attached to this discussion. First, the amount of active components found in the cat's claw contained in RM-10 is at least eight times greater than other formulas utilizing cat's claw. Second, cat's claw is a highly fibrous herb. The Poten-Zyme fermentation process does wonders for unlocking the powerful healing potential of the specific oxindole alkaloids and other phytochemicals present in the herb.

Finally, there is another little-known influence that these mushrooms have on the human physiological process. Perhaps in part because of their high glyconutrient content, these mushrooms have a tonifying effect. For example:

- Reishi (*Ganoderma lucidum*) alone has been shown to aid in blood sugar stabilization, normalization of blood pressure, and to offer neuroprotection.
- In Chinese medicine, cordyceps (*Cordyceps sinensis*) is utilized for circulatory, respiratory, immune, and sexual dysfunction, and other health problems. It is considered a tonic herb because of its ability to improve or normalize energy, stamina, appetite, endurance, and sleeping patterns.
- *Agaricus blazei's* glyconutrients (polysaccharides) activate interferon production to prevent viral infections.
- *Poria cocos* is used in Traditional Chinese Medicine with other herbs to promote blood flow and quell inflammation.
- Shiitake (*Lentinula edodes*) is the source of premiere anticancer agents used in Japanese medicine and is known for its cholesterol-normalizing benefits.

Thus, RM-10 is also a tonifying and longevity formula, in addition to the fact that it is immune-modulating.

RM-10—THE FORMULA

I created RM-10 by incorporating 12 different Chinese and Japanese mushrooms and herbs into a pre-fermented compound. The formula contains fermented:

Uncaria tomentosa (cat's claw)	*Trametes versicolor* (*Coriolus versicolor*)
Agaricus blazei	*Hericium erinaceus* (lion's mane)
Cordyceps sinensis (CS-4)	*Polyporus umbellatus*
Ganoderma lucidum (reishi)	*Tremelia fuciformis*
Grifola frondosa (maitake)	*Poria cocos*
Lentinula edodes (shiitake)	Aloe vera

Published Studies

Our RM-10 studies have been accepted for publication in a special supplement of the peer-reviewed *Progress in Nutrition*. Let's look at them in brief.

Our first study involved 20 "incurable" patients given only RM-10. The study was conducted by Missouri physician Lawrence Dorman, D.O., one of the founding members of the American Academy of Anti Aging Medicine (A4M) and graduate of the University of Health Sciences in Kansas City. Dr. Dorman has been practicing nutritional medicine for 30 years.

These non-responding patients had all but lost hope that they would ever find help for their ailments. Patients included in the Dorman study had been put on a standard detoxification diet but were classified as "nonresponders." Most doctors would have given up on them, and the patients would have gone from doctor to doctor and therapy to therapy in quest of the healing response.

The purpose of the Dorman study was to take patients with the most difficult-to-treat conditions that had not responded to either standard or complementary medicine and then to assess the efficacy of the RM-10 formula as a healing modality.

The patients maintained their standard detoxification diet (which consisted of removal of highly processed and other unhealthful foods) but they were removed from all other nutritional supplements and medications, unless removal of such medications would be considered life threatening. Dr. Dorman gave the patients nine caplets per day for 10 days followed by five caplets per day for 80 days as their sole therapy. This was an open-label study. The patients knew they were being given a nutritional formula. Thus, the study allowed for the rise and fall of a placebo effect. If only a placebo effect, it would have most likely waned prior to the two-month reporting date.

Dr. Dorman and I present these results on a case-by-case basis. They were compiled after only approximately two months of treatment:

1   A 51-year-old female, crippled with severe rheumatoid arthritis, suffered joint deformity and severe pain. She experienced a 50 percent decrease in pain and greater flexibility within one week of utilizing RM-10 in her nutritional program.

2   A 61-year-old female with polymyalgia rheumatica had worked with Dr. Dorman for eight months prior to inclusion in the study, showing little or no improvement. (Polymyalgia rheumatica causes stiffness and aching that begins in the neck, shoulder, and hip areas.) Her walking ease and distance improved by 80 percent and joint pain steadily diminished while on the protocol.

3   Another 51-year-old female with arthritis and irritable bowel syndrome experienced complete remission of her IBS and "gradual improvement" in her arthritis.

4   A 47-year-old female with loss of voice, thin vocal chords and hoarseness began using RM-10. Her symptoms began to disappear with use of nine caplets per day but returned when her dosage was reduced to five. She also experienced better sleep.

5   In the case of a 31-year-old female chronic fatigue syndrome patient, her life had been marked by chronic intermittent muscle pain and soreness, allergies, unremitting fatigue, fever, and sore throat. She could not accomplish anything with her life because every time she started feeling good, her condition knocked her down again, notes Dr. Dorman. Within eight weeks of placing RM-10 into her nutritional program, she was better. She has since remained better.

6 A 60-year-old female patient had angina and mixed connective tissue disease, the latter an autoimmune condition characterized by symptoms of scleroderma, myositis, systemic lupus erythematosus, rheumatoid arthritis and/or other autoimmune disease symptoms, all occurring together. She experienced complete cessation of her angina and marked improvement in her autoimmune condition after one month of use of RM-10. In a sense, rather than being stimulated, the formula down-regulated her immune system.

7 A 57-year-old female patient with adult-onset diabetes and chronic fatigue syndrome began using RM-10. Within one month, her chronic fatigue syndrome was "virtually gone" and her diabetes better controlled.

8 RM-10 was also beneficial to a 60-year-old male with elevated cholesterol and triglycerides, as well as psoriatic skin lesions. Within 10 days, his skin lesions improved by approximately 60 percent (see also our studies on Primal Defense for these conditions). His cholesterol dropped 15 percent and triglycerides by 20 percent within four weeks.

9 A 37-year-old female with colitis, gastritis and food allergies experienced "marked improvement" of her colitis and gastritis within one week of beginning use of RM-10. Her food allergies also improved significantly.

10 A 72-year-old female with cardiac arrhythmias experienced complete cessation within two weeks of using RM-10.

11 A 74-year-old male with indigestion and angina upon exertion began using RM-10. His indigestion disappeared completely within seven days. His angina improved significantly.

12 A 57-year-old obese female with bilateral knee pain and candidiasis experienced rapid improvement in her systemic yeast infection and modest improvement in knee pain.

13 A 46-year-old female patient with severe Crohn's disease improved dramatically (more than 90 percent) after two weeks of use of RM-10 with decreased pain, fewer bowel movements, and less mucous and blood in her stool.

14 A 51-year-old female's systemic yeast infection (chronic candidiasis) and allergies improved dramatically after four weeks of use of RM-10 (again, also see our Primal Defense studies).

15 A 19-year-old male with allergies since childhood and seizure disorder experienced a marked improvement in allergy symptoms within three days of use of RM-10. After two weeks, his allergies were virtually gone. He has experienced no additional seizures since.

16 An obese 81-year-old female with tendonitis and fluid retention began using RM-10. Her tendonitis was gone within four weeks and fluid retention was 90 percent improved. She lost a small amount of weight.

17 A 40-year-old male with a 10-year history of constipation and only one bowel movement per week increased his movements to three per week after four weeks of using RM-10. He reported feeling "much better."

18 A 47-year-old female with psoriasis experienced improvement after four weeks of use of RM-10.

19 A 76-year-old female with insomnia and a 30-year history of multiple treatment failures for neuropathy of her feet reported her insomnia to be gone within two weeks but did not experience improvement in her neuropathy.

20 A 38-year-old male with a four-year history of nausea and vomiting of an unknown etiology began using RM-10. His vomiting began to cease and his colon pain decreased and was less tender when palpated after six weeks of use.

"RM-10," says Dr. Dorman, "is one of the most phenomenal healing agents I have ever used. I had worked with some of these patients for years and never gotten results."

In addition to the Dorman study, work has been performed by Dr. Pierre Braquet, Ph.D., chief executive officer of Bio Inova Life Sciences Laboratories, Paris and Montreal. A noted researcher who studies both pharmaceutical and nutraceutical compounds, Dr. Braquet is credited for his discovery of some of the primary components of the herb *Ginkgo biloba*.

According to laboratory study results, RM-10:

• Performed notably well in its ability to enhance natural killer cell activity (critical to the body's healing response to cancer and infectious pathogens). Indeed, according to Dr. Braquet's associate researcher and board-certified immunologist Georges V. Halpern, M.D., Ph.D., Sc.D., "RM-10 increases NK cells better than anything else available, at minimal concentrations."

• Decreases proliferation of malignant cells and causes them to diminish in number.

• Significantly increases function of monocytes (large phagocytic white blood cells that eventually develop into the body's primary defenders, the macrophages).

• Increases interleukin-1 and interleukin-6 activity. These interleukins are anticancer cytokines that are secreted by activated macrophages. They are produced in response to infection and tissue injury. They stimulate production of antibodies and activate T-cells.

• Increases production of tumor necrosis factor. Tumor necrosis factor is an anti-angiogenic agent that prevents tumors from developing blood vessels for nourishing its growth. In particular, TNF-α (TNF-alpha) specifically initiates a cascade of cytokines that mediate the body's inflammatory response. It also regulates the expression of many genes in many cell types important for the host response to infection.

• Is safe to use by persons who suffer autoimmune conditions such as lupus, rheumatoid arthritis, and scleroderma and mediates the body's inflammatory response. Thus, RM-10 is not simply an immune stimulant but an immune modulator or normalizer.

• Demonstrates an anti-proliferation effect against K-562 cells. The presence of K-562 cells in the bloodstream predisposes persons to leukemia.

Another study conducted at Bio Inova Life Sciences Laboratories evaluated the effectiveness of RM-10 and 25 of the top-selling immune-enhancing products on the market for their ability to enhance immune system function. In this study, researchers looked at natural killer cell and macrophage function. Natural killer cells roam the bloodstream looking for and destroying foreign-invader cells. Macrophages are large white blood cells that also serve the immune system by killing foreign invaders and alerting other immune cells to invasions. In this study, RM-10 was found to boost the immune system by enhancing the function of natural killer cells and macrophages. The additional products included IP-6, transfer factor, colostrum, aloe isolate, yeast cell wall-derived beta glucans, carnivora, rice bran with arabinoxylane, ambrotose glyconutrient complex, arabinogalactan, sterols/sterolins, and many medicinal mushroom formulations including cloud mushroom extract, and PSP. *RM-10 outperformed every product tested in its ability to enhance the immune system and reduce the growth of certain cancers.*

In another study at Bio Inova Life Sciences Laboratories, RM-10 was shown to inhibit the proliferation of cancer cells in the breast, liver and lung.

In a 120-day, 70-patient, blind placebo-controlled clinical study conducted at the Peoples University of the Americas' School of Natural Medicine and directed by Jesus Garcia, M.D., researchers evaluated the effectiveness of RM-10 as a primary treatment for chronic fatigue immune deficiency syndrome (CFIDS). The end results of the study, in general, indicate that RM-10 qualifies as an excellent palliative and/or coadjuvant therapy for CFIDS, note researchers.

Considering that the target of the study is a pathology that resists all conventional therapeutic methods, it is noteworthy to underscore that approximately 30 percent of the participating test patients achieved full remission at the conclusion of the study. Moreover, each of the remaining participants attained varying yet considerable degrees of palliation. Each patient using the RM-10 formula improved by a minimum of 40 percent after only 120 days of treatment.

The placebo effects observed in the control group were completely negligible. Some 23 patients of the original 35 pertaining to the control group dropped out of the study because of disappointment, due to total lack of palliative results.

Additional Data from the RM-10 Study

1) Individuals consuming RM-10 with abnormal immune markers showed a trend towards a modulation of the immune system as evidenced by a decrease in white blood cells; increases in immunoglobulin G and neutrophils; normalization of lymphocytes and natural killer cells; and a decrease in elevated basophils.

Marker (number of patients)	Before RM-10	After RM-10	Change	Reference Range
Low WBC (4)	4.1	4.8	+17%	(4.5-9.5) Th/cm
Low Neutrop(11)	45.3	64	+41%	(50-72) %
High Lymph (16)	44.6	33.4	-25%	(26-40) %
Low Lymph (2)	18.5	29	+57%	(26-40) %
High Bas (18)	9.1	1.9	-79%	(0-5) %
Low IGg (33)	399.8	695.8	+74%	(572-1478) cu.mm
Low CD3/CD8(24)	142.5	415.6	+192%	(180-1170) cu.mm
Low Killer Cells(16)	763.4	1111.8	+46%	(1100-1200) cells/cu.mm
High Killer Cells(17)	1291.5	1147.6	-13%	(1100-1200) cells/cu.mm

2) Individuals with elevated uric acid showed a marked decrease. High levels of uric acid are characteristic of joint and muscle pain.

Marker	Before RM-10	After RM-10	Change	Reference Range
Uric Acid (23)	7.9	5.4	-32%	1.9-6.8 mg/dL

A significant number of additional observations were made in the course of the RM-10 Study:

- Three patients (two females, one male) suffered from sinus infections, which disappeared by the beginning of the third month of therapy with RM-10.
- Twelve patients (eight females, four males) reported remarkable increases in energy levels, beginning toward the end of the second month and continuing through the third month of treatment.
- Eleven patients (six females, five males) having suffered from chronic, recurrent migraine headaches, reported total remission from their headaches by the end of the respective studies.
- Five female patients reported significant vanishing of some of their facial wrinkles by the end of their respective studies.

Your risk for cancer and your ability to recover are not etched in stone. You should know that you can alter your cancer risk at any age.[29] This is a most positive and hopeful message. Cancer is not something we are born with and predestined to be stricken with; rather, it is often preventable. Personal risk can go up or down.[30]

We are so fortunate indeed, in our modern world where cancer is altogether too prevalent, to have powerful immune-boosting natural formulas. These include medicinal mushrooms, IP-6 with inositol, beta-glucans, MGN$_3$, and Mannapol. But, for the most part, these are only single-ingredient formulas. RM-10 was specifically created to be a multifaceted treatment approach for immune system disorders, especially cancer, and then subjected to experimental, laboratory and clinical studies that demonstrate its superiority to virtually all available commercial preparations.

CHAPTER FIVE

Attacking the Seven Causes of Inflammation

Al·che·my ('al-k&-mE): a power or process of
transforming something common into something special.
—*Merriam Webster's Collegiate Dictionary*

There is an alchemy that all of us are seeking in all aspects of life. Perhaps it will not be the discovery of a universal cure for disease or discovery of a means of indefinitely prolonging life or even transmutation of the base metals into gold; but, nevertheless, if we accept a more modest definition of this wonderful fourteenth century term, I believe that the best herbalists and formulators seek to achieve a certain alchemy.

I always try to study a problem thoroughly and then go about solving it in a comprehensive fashion. That's why I formulated FYI (*For Your Inflammation*) to attack the seven major causes of inflammation—and then took what amounted to a very great risk in putting the formula through extensive clinical trials.

I think if you answer the seven questions I've posed, you'll see why FYI can play such a key role in alleviating your inflammation, a condition we now recognize as being at the heart of many diseases—including arthritis, heart and circulatory problems, autoimmune conditions, and even some types of cancer.

Are old-fashioned soup stocks missing from your diet? Do you consume soup stocks regularly? Perhaps you should. Wonderful health benefits are to be derived from our traditional recipes. We are missing the gelatinous substances in stocks. "A lamentable outcome of our modern meat processing techniques and our hurry-up throwaway lifestyle has been a decline in the use of meat, chicken and fish stocks," say Sally Fallon and Mary G. Enig, Ph.D., in *Nourishing Traditions: The Cookbook that Challenges Politically Correct Nutrition and the Diet Dictocrats* (1999). "In days gone by, when the butcher sold meat on the bone rather than as individual filets and whole chickens rather than boneless breasts, our thrifty ancestors made use of every part of the animal by preparing stock, broth or bouillon from the bony portions." The authors add that stock "is also of great value because it supplies hydrophilic colloids to the diet. Raw food compounds are colloidal and tend to be hydrophilic, meaning that they attract liquids."

When cartilage deteriorates, we are left with bone against bone. But one of the beauties of traditional diets is that soup stocks made from whole chickens aid in rebuilding and maintaining cartilage by supplying high-quality gelatin and collagen, which are rich sources of glycosaminoglycans like chondroitin sulfate.

One thing collagen does is draw water to the joints, which, in turn, helps with cushioning. So do eat chicken and beef stock (organic whenever possible). The uniqueness of the Type II chicken collagen that we use in FYI is that it comes from the chicken's entire body, not just the sternum, as with many other types. In fact, I went to France to source our collagen because I wanted to work with farmers who don't farm chickens the way we typically do in America. (The chicken flocks that supply our collagen receive no antibiotics or mammalian remnants in their feed.)

Is your body overly acidic? Alkalize for joint health. Over-acidity is one of the major seven causes of inflammation. In fact, many experts consider over-acidity one of the major causes of inflammation, especially arthritic conditions. The body can only tolerate a small imbalance in blood pH and alkalizing the body can be important for arthritis (especially gout) sufferers.

A very interesting article came out in the October 2001 issue of the *European Journal of Nutrition*.[31] The message is that sodium chloride (NaCl) has been incorporated copiously into the contemporary diet, increasing the net systemic acid load imposed by the diet. The researchers note that their group "has shown that contemporary net acid-producing diets do indeed characteristically produce a low-grade systemic metabolic acidosis in otherwise healthy adult subjects, and that the degree of acidosis increases with age…" In a Russian-language journal, researchers studied changes in joint fluid acid-base balance in 65 rheumatoid arthritis patients.[32] They found increasing acidity to be correlated with the severity of joint damage and inflammation. It has also been determined that whole body potassium is significantly lower in older arthritics. The body can sink to almost half of normal in some cases. This again tells us that the body is in an overly acidic state.

That's why FYI is designed to aid correction of acidosis and ameliorate those conditions. I would argue that any level of acidosis may be unacceptable, and indeed, that a low-grade metabolic alkalosis may be the optimal acid-base state for humans. For this reason, I added fermented alfalfa grass juice to FYI. Alfalfa juice contains alkaline-forming minerals to help reduce acidity.* *Rhododendron caucasicum*, also in FYI, helps to reduce acidic deposits, particularly in gout. Rhododendron is used as an effective treatment for gout throughout the former Soviet Union.

Do you suffer from chronic low-grade infections? The arthritis-infection connection is now well established. Infections are clearly associated with the body's inflammatory levels, which can be measured with a high-sensitivity C-reactive protein test. But many infections do not manifest themselves as frank disease conditions such as the flu or common cold. They may simply cause minor symptoms like

---

*Such greens also oxygenate the body. Thus, users of grass juices may reduce their cancer risk. Otto Warburg, who won the Nobel Prize in the 1930s, demonstrated that cells with abnormal fermentation (in the absence of oxygen) are more likely to become cancerous. But cancer cannot develop in an oxygen-rich environment, which is often associated with healthy alkalinity.

skin eruptions or fatigue or the more serious conditions such as arthritis and even heart disease. FYI contains wild oregano concentrate and bayberry bark extract, both premiere infection-fighting herbs that aid the body's health against pathogens. In addition, FYI is processed using Poten-Zyme, which provides infection fighting probiotics, including bacteriocins.

Is your immune system overactive? FYI contains our specially harvested cat's claw because this herb, when harvested for its proper chemotype, has an almost intuitive ability to harmonize the body's immune system, helping to quell an overactive immune response, and to stimulate the underactive system. Many types of autoimmune arthritis or related inflammatory conditions (such as lupus) result from immune system dysfunction.

Are you taking arthritis drugs? We've all heard of celecoxib (Celebrex), refecocoxib (Vioxx) and other so-called COX-2-inhibiting drugs—the latest medical drugs to help people with arthritis. Unfortunately, the COX-2 drugs were promoted as safer alternatives to the stomach-harsh typical non-steroidal anti-inflammatory drugs (NSAIDs). But, as investigative reports and numerous legal torts demonstrate, the initial enthusiasm for these drugs by medical doctors might be unwarranted. The synthetic COX-2 inhibitors are not without their own side effects.

Natural COX-2 inhibitors, on the other hand, are safe. They also are effective. I've put several natural COX-2 inhibitors in FYI. Besides its infection-fighting properties, oregano contains rosmarinic acid, which has been reported in laboratory studies to have significant COX-2 inhibiting properties comparable to medical drugs such as ibuprofen, naproxen, and aspirin. Ginger and turmeric are also natural COX-2 inhibitors.

"In experimental studies, [ginger] has been shown to inhibit both the cyclooxygenase and lipoxygenase pathways and the production of prostaglandins, thromboxane, and leukotrienes, just as the NSAIDs do," says James B. LaValle, R.Ph., N.M.D., C.C.N, author of *The COX-2 Connection* (Healing Arts Press 2001). "Yet its clear advantage is that no significant side effects have been reported, unlike the NSAIDs, which can have quite serious side effects associated with their use."

Turmeric, closely related to ginger, is traditionally used to treat systemic inflammation. Researchers at New York Presbyterian Hospital and the Weill Medical College at Cornell University have shown that one of the major phytochemicals in turmeric has potent COX-2-inhibitory factors, notes LaValle. Additional research at Vanderbilt University and the University of Leicester in England has further confirmed the powerful COX-2-inhibiting capabilities of this ancient herb.

Because the herbs contained in FYI tend to be highly fibrous, we use our Poten-Zyme process to help to unlock their active constituents, making their phytonutrients even more bioavailable and easily assimilated.

Are you deficient in enzymes? Raw foods are an excellent source of enzymes and aid the body in maintaining the proper acid/alkaline balance, but most of us no longer consume adequate amounts of raw foods. Of course, only the overly brave would consume raw meats, due to the fear of bacterial contamination. The downside of this precautionary approach to eating raw meats is that we thereby miss out on some of the most potent proteases. Yet, enzymes can help to reduce circulating antibodies and have been shown to aid in all types of inflammatory processes. That's why FYI includes a wide array of inflammation-fighting enzymes, including proteases for protein digestion, lipase for fat digestion, amylase for carbohydrate digestion and cellulase for the digestion of plant fiber. FYI also contains appreciable amounts of the enzymes bromelain and papain. Bromelain, an enzyme found in the stalk of pineapples, is effective in reducing inflammation in living tissue. On the other hand, papain, the enzyme found in unripe papaya, is useful to reduce sites of inflammation where dead or diseased tissue has been lodged.

Are you suffering from oxidative stress? The use of antioxidants someday probably will be recognized as one of the most significant contributions to modern health practices. It's clear that you need basic vitamins and minerals as building blocks for structural support. However, antioxidants play an important role in fighting off the damaging effects of inflammation by quenching the devastating micro-cellular effects of free radicals that exert so much cumulative oxidative damage on joint tissues. *Rhododendron caucasicum* is high in polyphenolic antioxidants that are similar to those found in green tea, grape seed and pine bark extracts but is far more bioavailable. Turmeric and oregano are also powerful antioxidants that reduce oxidative stress. All will be found in the FYI formula.

PUBLISHED STUDIES ON FYI

The FYI studies have been accepted for publication in a special edition of the peer-reviewed *Progress in Nutrition*. Following are summaries of the studies:[33]

- A study conducted at Bio Inova Life Sciences Laboratories evaluated the effectiveness of FYI on the immune system. In this study, researchers looked at natural killer cells and macrophage function. FYI was found to boost the immune system by enhancing the function of natural killer cells and macrophages.
- In another study at Bio-Inova Life Sciences Laboratories, FYI was shown to inhibit the proliferation of cancer cells in the breast, liver and lung.
- In *in vivo* experimental studies by Michael Whitehouse, Ph.D., at the University of Queensland, Australia, FYI was found to reduce inflammation with continued use. These effects were seen to be comparable to common NSAIDs but without any gastrointestinal damage.

Taken as a whole, it should not be surprising that in a recent 90-day, 70-patient, blind, placebo-controlled clinical study directed by Jesus Garcia, M.D., 82 percent of the rheumatoid arthritis patients completing a study with FYI had a 60 percent or greater improvement in their condition, as measured by standard mobility evaluation tools and the commonly used RA latex test.[34] All patients experienced significant reductions in their C-reaction protein levels, indicating reduced inflammatory processes.

The placebo effects observed in the control group were completely negligible. Some 20 patients of the original 35 pertaining to the control group dropped out of the study because of disappointment due to total lack of benefit.

It was also shown that individuals consuming FYI with abnormal immune markers showed a trend towards a modulation of the immune system as evidenced by a decrease in white blood cells, an increase in neutrophils, normalization of lymphocytes and a decrease in elevated monocytes, eosinophils and basophils.

Marker	Before FYI	After FYI	Change	Reference Range
High WBC (15)	11.5	7.8	-32%	(4.5-9.5) Th/cmm
Low Neutrop (30)	42.7	60.3	+41%	(50-72) %
High Lymph (31)	51.6	36.3	-30%	(26-40) %
Low Lymph (2)	20.5	30	+46%	(26-40) %
High Monocytes (1)	8	0	NA	(0-8) %
High Eos (2)	6	1.5	-75%	(0-4) %
High Bas (9)	10.9	2.3	-79%	(0-5) %

Individuals with elevated inflammatory markers such as RA Latex and Uric Acid had a decrease in those markers with a corresponding improvement in symptoms.

Marker	Before FYI	After FYI	Change	Reference Range
RA Latex (33)	62.7	28.2	-55%	<30 IU/ml
High Uric Acid (26)	8.07	5.05	-37%	1.9-6.8 mg/dL

Patients in the study had the following additional improvements:
• Ten patients (seven females, three males), having suffered from chronic insomnia, reported total remission of this condition by the end of the study.
• Seven patients (four females, three males), having suffered from chronic, recurrent migraine headaches, reported total remission from their headaches by the end of the respective studies.
• Twelve patients (four females, eight males), having suffered from chronic digestive problems, reported significant improvement in their digestive deficit by the end of the study.
• Fifteen patients (ten females, five males), having suffered from chronic constipation, reported total remission of their condition by the end of the second month of their treatment.
• Three male patients, suffering from hearing deficit for several years, reported significant improvement in their hearing by the end of the study.
• Four patients (three females, one male), having suffered from varied grades of chronic skin rash, reported total remission of these symptoms.

Although we tend to think of inflammation almost solely in terms of arthritis, FYI is excellent for enhancing the body's healing response in cases of trauma and sports injuries, heart and circulatory disease, and virtually all other inflammatory conditions. By all means, I encourage you to take up the anti-inflammatory lifestyle.

CHAPTER SIX

You're Not What You Eat, But What You Digest

We can't really talk about gastrointestinal health without discussing the digestion of our foods. Digestion may be a most familiar household word. But far less commonly known is what a complex and manifold process is required to perform our digestion in order to extract the necessary nutrients from our food. To understand these mechanisms and put their potentials in proper perspective, we first have to become familiar with a few basic principles.

What is digestion? Digestion occurs without the need for central nervous system impulses. This, as mentioned, is the "law of the gut." Digestion entails the chemical breakdown of the ingested food, programmed and carried out with high precision. Thus, digestion is essentially a carefully executed decomposition process carried out by an independent enteric nervous system supported by an intricate array of interactive enzymes. The ingested food yields only a small proportion of substances that the body is able to assimilate. The rest is eliminated as waste. It is important to note that the body produces two fundamental kinds of waste: metabolic waste and digestive waste. Metabolic waste represents the cellular household waste and the breakdown of dead, discarded cells that are constantly being replaced in the body. Digestive waste comprises all the breakdown matter that is not absorbed. It is interesting to know that less than four percent of our metabolic waste exits the body with our stool. About 96 percent is eliminated through the kidneys.

Thus, to maintain its health and vitality, the human body requires a steady supply of many kinds of enzymes. Here again, before we continue, there are three basic tenets we'll have to become familiar with to understand why enzymes play a manifold role in our health:

- While there are thousands of different enzymes in Nature, they can be divided into two basic categories: lytic enzymes, which exclusively break down substances for which they were specifically designed— such as the legions of proteolytic enzymes in charge of breaking down proteins.

- The other category consists of enzymes responsible for the manifold processes of synthesis in the body. In other words, these induce the building of molecules and, eventually, tissues such as the telomerases.

• The human body is able to produce most of the enzymes it needs, but not all of these. Certain enzymes—such as cellulase, which is in charge of breaking down the fiber contained in plants—must be obtained from our food because the body has no mechanisms to produce them.

ENZYME DEFICIENCY CONSEQUENCES

According to the Surgeon General's report on nutrition and health, eight out of ten leading causes of death in the United States are diet-related. Digestive problems comprise the number one health problem in North America. Digestive complaints including everything from hemorrhoids to colon cancer result in more time lost at work, school, and play than any other health-related problem. Many of these digestive problems were rare or nonexistent less than a century ago.

Why is this? And how can we get back to the health of our ancestors?

Certainly, consuming enzyme-rich foods and "live" enzyme supplements is part of the answer.

It is easy to understand that a stable supply of all enzymes is necessary for the human body and is of paramount importance. Alas, our increasingly toxic eating habits and lifestyle not only deprives us of the enzymes we must import into our body, but also deteriorates the organs in charge of producing the body's own enzymes. The progressive, overall depletion of enzymes leads to a situation in which we can neither digest the food we eat, nor can our body synthesize the materials required for cell repair and maintenance.

Therefore, not only general but also a partial, specific enzyme deficit is unquestionably responsible for many of the diseases that escalate in the wake of our relentlessly deteriorating lifestyle.

Summing up the situation, the result of our increasingly worsening enzyme deficiencies is a progressive failure to digest proteins, fats, sugars, starches and other carbohydrates, which causes a great variety of diseases.

HOW ENZYME DEFICIENCY LEADS TO DISEASE STATES

It is the area of lymph gland blockage that should grab the attention of both health-conscious consumers and a wide range of health professionals. Incompletely digested protein and/or carbohydrate molecules trigger a domino effect in which the fragmentary breakdown compounds produce a secondary carbohydrate—*polysaccharides*. These then condense in the tissue fluids of the body and combine with excess proteins forming a substance known as *mucoproteins*, which are aggregates of undigested proteins that form long chains of polypeptides. These adhere to unassimilated carbohydrates in a process called glycation. Glycation then leads to overproduction of advanced glycation end products, which cause premature tissue aging. In a worst-case scenario, mucoproteins condense in blood plasma. The accumulation of such mucoproteins is the main cause of lymphatic congestion, which is the foremost trigger factor of a great variety of severe pathologies, blocking the lymphatic traffic in the interstitial tissues (i.e., the spaces between fine capillary vessels and cell structures).

This is important. And it's worth taking the time to explore the consequences of lymph gland blockage. The organs of the immune system, positioned throughout the body, are called lymphoid organs.

The word "lymph" in Greek means a pure, clear stream—an appropriate description considering lymph's appearance and purpose.

The lymphatic system defends the body from foreign invasion by disease-causing agents such as viruses, bacteria, or fungi. The lymph system contains a network of vessels that assists in circulating body fluids. Lymph bathes the tissues of the body, and the lymphatic vessels collect and move it eventually back into the blood circulation. Lymph nodes dot the network of lymphatic vessels and provide meeting grounds for the immune system cells that defend against invaders. The spleen, at the upper left of the abdomen, is also a staging ground and a place where immune system cells confront foreign microbes. Pockets of lymphoid tissue are in many other locations throughout the body, such as the bone marrow and thymus. Tonsils, adenoids, Peyer's patches, and the appendix are also lymphoid tissues.

Both immune cells and foreign molecules enter the lymph nodes via blood vessels or lymphatic vessels. All immune cells exit the lymphatic system and eventually return to the bloodstream. Once in the bloodstream, lymphocytes are transported to tissues throughout the body, where they act as sentries on the lookout for foreign antigens.

These vessels transport excess fluids away from interstitial spaces in body tissue and return it to the bloodstream for eventual elimination. Lymphatic vessels prevent the backflow of the lymph fluid. They have specialized bean-shaped organs called lymph nodes that filter out destroyed microorganisms. If your lymph system is malfunctioning, internal toxicity is quite likely.

This brings us to the next major problem resulting from enzyme deficiency: impaired immune function. GALT is an acronym for *gut-associated lymphoid tissue*. It is the responsibility of the GALT to discriminate between nutritious components present in the transiting stool and possible antigens, in which case it would alert the immune system to stage an appropriate immune response. Without a properly functioning GALT, our immune health is compromised and toxins can escape from the colon into the bloodstream. The outcome of such conditions can generate manifold illnesses that may involve any organ and even the entire body.

It is important to keep digestive waste freely moving through the intestines. However, if the in-transit food is isolated from the GALT by layers of gluey and hardened food (as a result of enzyme deficiency), no discriminatory action will ensue and no immune responses will be alerted; consequently, large amounts of toxic substances will be absorbed by the body.

Certainly one of the keys to improving our health, especially unblocking the lymph system and maintaining healthy immune function in the gut, is to insure an optimal amount of enzyme activity in the body. Enzymes are catalysts in the body, protein-like substances, which help maintain the tissues, orchestrate the many functions of the body, and digest food.

But they are so much more, notes Dr. Edward Howell, the groundbreaking physician who devoted his life to the study of enzymes and one of the great enzyme scientists of the twentieth century. Think of it this way: Enzymes are the "labor force" that builds your body, just like construction workers are the labor force that builds your house, he says. "You may have all the necessary building materials and lumber, but to build a house you need workers, which represent the vital life element. Catalysts are only inert substances. They possess none of the life energy we find in enzymes. For instance, enzymes give off a kind of radiation when they work (see also Chapter 7). This is not true of catalysts. In addition, although enzymes contain proteins—and some contain vitamins—the activity factor in enzymes has never been synthesized. Moreover, there is no combination of proteins or any combination of amino acids or any other substance which will give enzyme activity. There are proteins present in enzymes. However, they serve only as carriers of the enzyme activity factors. Therefore, we can say that enzymes consist of protein carriers charged with energy factors just as a battery consists of metallic plates charged with electrical energy."

Enzymes can be considered as important, if not more so, than perhaps any nutrient. Enzymes are responsible for nearly every facet of life and health. When we eat raw foods, we consume the enzymes in the foods. The foods are then digested easily by the body. When we eat cooked or processed foods, the body must provide the enzymes necessary to digest the cooked foods. Unfortunately, food enzymes are destroyed at temperatures above 118 degrees F. Thus, all cooked and processed foods are devoid of food enzymes. This constant need for enzymes depletes our store of enzymes, strains the body and causes the pancreas to enlarge. Without enzymes, we're as good as dead. Dr. Howell stated in his classic work, *Food Enzymes for Health and Longevity*, "After we have attained full mature growth, there is a slow and gradual decrease in the enzyme content of our bodies. When the enzyme content becomes so low that metabolism can't proceed at a proper level, death overtakes us."

Enzymes are not renewable resources. Once enzymes have completed their appointed task they are destroyed. For life to continue you must have a constant enzyme supply which requires continual replacement of enzymes. The best way to assure your body receives the adequate amount of enzymes every day is to consume a diet high in "live" raw and fermented foods and to consume a high-potency, broad-spectrum digestive enzyme supplement.

Thus, supplementation with a powerful and comprehensive enzyme formula is an ideal solution to both prevent and treat such conditions as digestive-related lymph gland blockage and impaired digestive enzyme activity.

GIVE DIGESTIVE ENZYMES A TRY

If you're at all skeptical about the effectiveness of these digestive enzymes, I challenge you to take two to four caplets or scoops of Omega-Zyme™ with each meal for about three to five days; then, stop taking them altogether for one to two days. You'll immediately notice the contrast as your body goes back to what you will now realize was your earlier sub-par state of poor digestion and low energy.

One of the true advantages of Omega-Zyme is its potency compared to other digestive enzyme formulas. This all-natural preparation is manufactured using a proprietary process of fermentation to pre-digest a synergistically combined array of nutrients, endowed also with a proprietary delivery system that ensures these effectively reach in unadulterated form the targeted organs and tissues. It is worthwhile mentioning that many digestive enzyme formulas have so little enzymatic activity, that they simply don't have the power to break down the amount of food you are eating at the time. For example, it takes approximately 1,000 ALUs of lactase to digest the lactose contained in eight ounces of milk in about 30 minutes. Each and every enzyme included in a formula needs to be provided in an effective dosage, but most products do not do this. We do, and we think this is why our formula is certainly among the best digestive enzyme formulations now available to consumers.

A CLOSER LOOK

A superior digestive enzyme formula, like Omega-Zyme, contains high amounts of the following digestive enzymes:

- **Protease Blend**—a blend of five proteolytic enzymes, including peptidase, which aid in the digestion and utilization of dietary proteins. Helps deliver the specific nutrients necessary for muscle and tissue repair, as well as for vibrant immune system function.
- **Amylase**—digests starch and carbohydrates. Acts in concert with proteases to stimulate immune system function. Acts in association with lipase to digest fragments of viruses and reduce inflammation and infections.
- **Lipase**—digests fats, thereby aiding in weight control, maintaining and enhancing cardiovascular health, and helping maintain proper liver and gall bladder function.
- Glucoamylase—breaks down carbohydrates, specifically polysaccharides.
- **Malt Diastase (Maltase)**—digests maltose, malt and grain sugars. May help relieve environmental sensitivities and allergies.
- **Invertase (Sucrase)**—digests sugars. Beneficial in helping prevent gastrointestinal problems and discomfort.
- **Alpha-Galactosidase**—aids in the digestion of difficult-to-digest foods such as beans, legumes and cruciferous vegetables such as cabbage, broccoli and cauliflower.
- **Lactase**—digests the milk sugar lactose. Extremely useful for individuals suffering from lactose intolerance. May be beneficial for those suffering from irritable bowel syndrome and other digestive disorders in which a high percentage are adversely affected by dairy products.
- **Cellulase**—digests fiber cellulose into smaller units, which include D-glucose. Helps remedy digestive problems such as malabsorption. Cellulase is a very important enzyme because the human body cannot produce it on its own.
- **Xylanase**—breaks down the sugar xylose.
- **Pectinase**—breaks down carbohydrates such as pectin (found in many fruits).
- **Hemicellulase**—breaks down carbohydrates called hemi-celluloses, which are found in plant foods.
- **Mannanase**—digest the sugar known as mannose.
- **Phytase**—breaks down carbohydrates, specifically phytates (phytic acid), present in many difficult-to-digest grains and beans. Especially useful for those suffering from serious bowel disorders which result

in an inability to handle phytates from soy and gluten from wheat, oats, rye and barley. Phytase may increase mineral absorption and the bioavailability of iron, zinc, calcium, and magnesium.

- **Beta-Glucanase**—breaks down polysaccharides and fibers known as beta glucans.
- **Arabinosidase**—digests the sugar arabinose.
- **Bromelain**—an enzyme from the stem of pineapples, breaks down protein and fights inflammation and reduces swelling. May speed the recovery of injuries and swelling resulting from athletics, childbirth and surgery.
- **Papain**—similar to the chymotrypsin, a protein-digesting enzyme produced by the body. Used to treat chronic diarrhea and celiac disease. Treats gastrointestinal discomfort due to intestinal parasites.
- **Poten-Zyme Ginger**—one of the most potent herbal digestive aids. Contains extremely potent protein-digesting enzymes. Frequently used to treat nausea and motion sickness.
- **Poten-Zyme Turmeric**—popular Indian spice that is commonly used to improve digestion and reduce stomach discomfort.
- **Poten-Zyme Barley Grass**—one of Nature's richest sources of alkaline-forming minerals and antioxidant enzymes. Provides the mineral co-factors necessary to enhance the functions of the enzymes.
- **Poten-Zyme Cat's Claw**—once called the "opener of the way" by a physician who treated hundreds of people suffering from digestive problems with this powerful herb. Cat's claw has been used for hundreds of years by native Peruvians as a treatment for digestive problems, urinary tract infections and arthritis.

These enzymes and other whole foods not only effectively aid digestion in general, but also help to remove accumulated, sticky waste adhered to the lining of the intestines and colon—what some health experts term "mucoid plaque"—that originates a whole array of digestion-contingent diseases.

Another reason Omega-Zyme is unquestionably the premier digestive enzyme formula now available to consumers is our Poten-Zyme process. By utilizing our unique HSOs, we are able to ferment our botanical blend of cat's claw, ginger, turmeric, and barley grass juice. Fermentation with Poten-Zyme produces a powerful array of beneficial enzymes, antioxidants, and other beneficial substances that also aid digestion.

In brief, Omega-Zyme participates in maintaining both the small and large intestinal environments and cleansing them of toxic residues and waste. This is an essential prerequisite for great health.

CHAPTER SEVEN

Capture the Power
of the Sun

Completely regardless of how improbable it may seem, light definitely does exist within our cells. In fact, light may be the basis of cell-cell communication. This is why at Garden of Life we do things the way we do—including drying our foods and herbs at the lowest possible temperature and employing temperature- and pressure-sensitive manufacturing techniques to preserve the vital living nutrients. This enables Garden of Life formulas to literally capture the photon powers of the sun.

Until quite recently, an unending universal confusion existed concerning the paradoxical discoveries revealed by the scientists dedicated to the exploration of the mechanisms that govern the immune response. The issue is this: How can so much information be processed so quickly throughout the body? Biochemical reactions alone are too slow. Perhaps the answer is *light*. Perhaps our body's communications themselves are carried out through biophotons at the speed of *light*.

In *The Whispering Pond: A Personal Guide to the Emerging Vision of Science* (HarperCollins UK 1997), author Ervin Laszlo gives a recent version of what turns out to be a fairly longstanding idea among scientists; that much of the physical world, and living Nature in particular, cannot be explained by current knowledge and that some form of unknown energy field is needed to explain it. This concept dates back to the 1920s when the famous Russian professor of medicine and biophysicist Alexander Gurwitsch empirically proved this surprising fact (in 1922) and postulated a morphogenetic field, a system-wide force field generated by the particular force fields of individual cells.[35] Laszlo calls this a fifth field (referring to the four accepted universal fields: the gravitational, the electromagnetic, the strong and the weak nuclear fields) and suggests that it might explain everything from the mysteries of the wave function in quantum mechanics, to the remarkable synchronicity found in Nature, even to psychic phenomena documented among people.

In fact, back in the 1920s, Gurwitsch had already established beyond any reasonable doubt that living cells and tissues generate an extremely weak, yet biologically active, form of electromagnetic radiation in the ultraviolet range; and that the presence of this radiation is somehow intimately connected with the nature of living processes themselves. Basically, Gurwitsch was able to show evidence of a weak but permanent photon emission of a few counts/(s.cm^2) in the optical range from biological systems, pointing out that it stimulates cell divisions. Gurwitsch was led to his experimental demonstration of what he called "mitogenetic radiation" in a lawful and rigorous way, as a by-product of his attempts to hypothesize a universal biophysical principle which (among other things) would encompass the paradoxical, but otherwise undeniable correlations between events of cell division (mitosis) and other events occurring in widely separated locations within a living organism.

After periods of neglect and even disregard, small groups in Russia, Australia, China, Italy, Japan, Germany, Poland, and the United States rediscovered ultraweak light emissions from living tissues by use of modern photomultiplier techniques, after the second World War. The researchers liken these force fields to the power of ultraviolet light. Since then, numerous scientists in several parts of the world unquestionably confirmed that in the core of living cells there is indeed perceptible light.

Eventually, after several decades of boisterous controversies, a team of German biophysicists irrefutably corroborated the postulate in 1975, under the direction of the professor Fritz-Albert Popp, conforming to the strictest requirements of the scientific method.*

In general terms, it is understood that the term *photon* refers to a "quantum of light." We know that a quantum constitutes the minutest and totally indivisible component of the Universe. Popp, who placed the prefix bio in front of photons, with the intention of suggesting that these may be emitted by living cells, coined the expression "*biophoton.*"

In 2002 in *Physics Letters*, Popp and co-researchers note that while there is now agreement about the universality of this effect for all living systems, no agreement has been achieved in the area of interpretation.[36] Meanwhile, a group of German physicists, starting in 1972 at the University Marburg, hypothesize that biophoton emissions as subject of quantum optics has to be assigned to a coherent photon field within the living system, responsible for intra- and inter-cellular communication and regulation of biological functions such as biochemical activities, cell growth and differentiation. In order to examine this hypothesis, consider that it has been shown that biophoton emission can be traced back to DNA as the most likely candidate for working as the (main) source, and that delayed luminescence (DL), which is the long-term afterglow of living systems after exposure to external light illumination, corresponds to excited states of the biophoton field. In addition, all the correlations between biophoton emission and biological functions such as cell growth, cell differentiation, biological rhythms, and cancer development, turned out to be consistent with the coherence hypothesis but could be only rather poorly explained in terms of free radical reactions.

Currently, there remain no doubts about the existence of such intra-cellular luminescence. (Not to be confused with the bioluminescence generated, for example, by glowworms.) Contemporary technology has developed powerful instruments capable of intensifying and measuring extremely minute

---

* Popp, born in 1938 in Frankfurt, West Germany, received a degree in experimental physics in 1966 at the University of Würzburg (where Röntgen discovered x-rays), received the Röntgen-Prize of the University of Würzburg, and received his Ph.D. in Theoretical Physics in 1969 at University of Mainz. He has supervised approximately 30 diploma works and dissertations in physics, biology and medicine, and written approximately 150 publications on basic questions of theoretical physics, biology, complementary medicine and biophotons.

light quantities, known as residual light, which prove unquestionably the existence of the biophotons.

It was also established that that this biophysical force does not only pulsate in intensity, but also in frequency. This explains quite satisfactorily the dynamics of its inherent mechanisms of interactions, which unfold among the different organs.

The question that remained to be answered was why do our cells emit light? Popp explains "our organism must replace nearly ten million cells each minute." It is obvious that the information required to achieve such a feat can only be processed at the speed of light. Apparently, such an overwhelming amount of signal traffic of data transference and processing within any living organism—be that human, animal, vegetal or of insects—is achieved through biophotons with high precision. These minutest coherent rays of light are responsible for the maintenance and operation of the network of information linking all living cells in an organism, and likewise allow the continuous, unobstructed and intelligent updating of data.

These advancements in quantum physics definitely influence the way we do things at Garden of Life. Strange as it may seem, every time we consume some natural and fresh food, or their carefully preserved components, we indeed also ingest light that—in one way or another—triggers certain activities in our system.

In other words, when we ingest fresh food, once assimilated, their individual components emit luminous signals that inescapably participate in the development and management of certain biochemical endogenous processes. That is, the greater the capacity of light storage is in our nourishment, the more powerful will be their beneficial influence on our cells.

Modern men and women seemed to have lost touch with the powerful resonance within their own being whose source is linked to the photon-power of the sun. Then, in the 1960s, came *Sonnenenergie und der Mensch als Antenne (Solar Energy and Man as Antenna)* and a series of lectures, both by seven-time Nobel Prize nominee Dr. Johanna Budwig.

Dr. Budwig first earned fame as an analytical chemist who developed key analytical techniques required for identifying types of fats. At one time, science was unable to identify key distinct fats in foods such as omega-3s (found in wild coldwater fish and flaxseed) from omega-6s (found in grains, certain seeds and corn oil) and omega-9s (found in olive oil and avocado). Thus, the work of Dr. Budwig must be considered seminal in the advancement of nutritional science, particularly that of lipids.

However, Budwig's firmly grounded scientific work led her to intuit—and, then, later clinically validate—much greater truths so profound that they bring together modern physics, biology and even modern humanity's overall health.

"Sun rays reach the earth as an inexhaustible source of energy," she observed. "The sources of power in mineral oil, coal, green plant-foods and fruits are based on the energy supplied by the sun's radiation."

Indeed, today we know that the energy from the sun is in the form of photons, the fastest moving, smallest units of elementary energy known. This concentration of the sun's energy is accomplished by ocean and land plants into the compounds that comprise their cells and tissues. The energy is transferred into biophotons.

Our own health may be improved when we eat foods which, rich in electrons, have themselves captured the power of the sun. A high amount of these electrons, which are on the wavelength of the sun's energy, are to be found in seed oils, observed Budwig.

"Scientifically," she explained, "the oils are even known as electron-rich essentially highly unsaturated fats."*

The great leap Budwig makes, however, is the insight that modern men and women lack the proper foods to capture this elementary power of the sun for their vital health. It is intriguing that the most protective organ system in the human body, the central nervous system, requires the most unsaturated fatty acids, especially omega-3 fatty acids, for its cell membranes to function optimally. It is also interesting that Nature provides fatty acids in the cis form that bends fatty acids into the shape of a fish hook, rather than the trans form that would stretch the molecules into a more linear shape. The cis form intrinsically has more molecular electromagnetic tension than the trans form. Could it be that the cis configuration is a way of storing within each molecule a special storage form of the sun's energy?

OUR ELECTRON-DEPLETED MODERN DIET

It has long been known that, unless heroic preservation measures are taken, once seed grains are crushed they soon turn rancid. Because of the high vulnerability of their electrons to oxidation, these precious oils, much like fruits or vegetables, are highly perishable.

The husks and germ of grains first began to be removed in the mid-1700s in Great Britain, extending shelf life but removing their vital contents, thereby precipitating overt B-vitamin deficiency diseases such as pellagra and beriberi. The vital powers of these photon-rich foods were lost.

In the early 1900s much of our wheat and other grain products were made into white flour by removing the bran and germ and along with them most of the nutrients.

Along came the corn oil craze in the 1950s. The producers of the commodity launched a massive public misinformation campaign, taking out full-page advertisements in the nation's medical journals. This campaign convinced medical doctors that corn oil, so overloaded with omega-6 fatty acids, could prevent heart disease.

Another wrong turn occurred with the advent of hydrogenation, a process that turns vegetable oils into semi-solid fats.

* I also believe that when one consumes certain foods rich in saturated fats such as meat and dairy products from animals that feed on greens and herbs we are getting a pre-packaged rich source of these electrons. These fat soluble activators, as they are often called, have been transformed by the animals' digestive tracts into highly usable health-promoting compounds.

Fats and oils treated to preserve them longer have their electronic structure changed—otherwise oxygen would try to grasp vulnerable electrons in the molecules. But this modified form is not the form useful to the body and may, in fact, be detrimental. The irony of modern society is that electron-rich foods, particularly the good fats such as those found in fish, grass-fed animal foods and to some extent flaxseed, have become so rare. No wonder we have much higher rates of heart disease, cancer, multiple sclerosis and arthritis than primitive peoples!

When people began to process fats to make them keep longer on the supermarket shelves and when people began consuming refined polyunsaturated fats to such a great extent, no one stopped to consider the consequences to long-term health. These vitally important electrons in the double bonds found in seed oils and healthy animal fats, with their continual movement and wonderful ability to capture the elementary power of the sun, were destroyed!

Electron-rich foods, electron-rich seeds, healthy animal foods, herbs and spices, and vegetables and fruits which are rich in aroma and natural pigments from the color of the sunlight's photons—these all help the absorption, storage and utilization of the sun's energy.

The body's capacity to activate vital life functions is thus dramatically enhanced, resulting in extraordinary healing and rejuvenation.

Here it is important to note that these same principles begin to act—in fact, even more powerfully—when we administer food supplements that contain naturopathic factors that originate from biotechnological sources such as virgin plants, particularly seeds and sprouts, or even animal products and organs processed by special technical means that permit the preservation of their light-storing capacity, and their ability to induce coherent biological light in their intracellular environments.

The physicist Popp declared that, "The human organism is not only a carnivorous, or vegetarian being, but also a consumer of light. In fact, it behaves like a luminivorous creature."

This is why our formulas are rich in fermented grasses, herbs, sprouts and seeds harvested at the point of optimal nutritional value. At the time, I did not understand all of the science behind what we were doing, but I insisted that our Poten-Zyme medium be rich in seeds and chlorophyll-rich superfoods—spirulina, chlorella, dunaliella; young rye, wheat, barley, oat, and alfalfa grass; flax, sesame, sunflower, pumpkin seeds. In Perfect Food™, our super green drink formula, we go even further and apply Poten-Zyme to brown rice, flax, pumpkin, sesame, sunflower, and chia seeds, as well as garbanzo, red lentil, soy, kidney, and azuki beans, and young shoots of oats, barley, rye, millet, maize and buckwheat—all organically grown. Most of our formulas are rich in greens, sprouts, seeds and other sunlight-rich foods.

But we go further. I wish you could come with me to southern Utah. It's a beautiful little farm town. This is where our superfoods and cereal grasses are grown, fermented and dried you would see for yourself that the growing and processing temperatures are so low it is akin to a moderately warm summer day—certainly not the drying inferno that has become standard practice in processing herbal extracts that include using autoclave and other high heat and pressure sterilization techniques.

The fermentation process is an artisanal craft and not an industrial process. Our fermentation process takes place at a temperature of approximately 98.6 degrees and lasts between three and six weeks. These conditions make our end products what I like to call "body ready." Our fermentation process can be likened to the aging of a fine wine. Over the weeks of fermentation, wonderful flavors and aromas develop, not to mention the many health-enhancing compounds that the process generates. Once fermentation is finished, the material is dried at extremely low temperatures very quickly. You will never see artificial heat sources, solvents or other extraction materials because we don't use them.

You see, the heat and solvents destroy the biophotonic energies of our foods and herbs. We don't want heat. We don't use irradiation, either, another common practice in sterilizing herbs used in the natural products industry. This is all wrong and a violation of the principles of natural healing, one of the dirty little secrets the natural products industry doesn't particularly want health-conscious consumers to know about. We do want you to know the facts and truths, though, because at Garden of Life we do things differently. We avoid irradiation, our foods are grown purely organically, and, when they are dried, it is at low temperatures never exceeding 90 degrees Fahrenheit with the express intent of preserving their electron-rich nature, their biophotons—their force fields to which modern physics and natural health must certainly now ascribe a portion of the healing power of whole foods and herbs.

Our steller super green food Perfect Food is a prime example of biophoton nutrition at its best. I'll tell you about that next.

CHAPTER EIGHT

The Healing Power of Green Foods

I know by now you know to expect the unexpected from me.

You should eat grass.

You'll be a lot healthier.

Once, we recognized the value of grass.

We no longer do.

We don't even really know what grass is. We should. Did you know that we eat the fruits of grass all of the time? No? Well, did you know that the fruit of grass is grain? Or that wheat, rye, corn, rice, oats, barley, sorghum, millet, spelt, kamut, and even bamboo and sugarcane are grasses? Or that grasses offer their greatest nutritive value at a specific point of physical growth, long before the bearing of their fruits?

Walt Whitman, the great American poet, wrote a series of beautiful poems that he called *Leaves of Grass*. Most of us today are too busy to read Whitman or even contemplate the grass beneath our feet that softens the Earth and makes it so much more of a beautiful habitat. Perhaps no popular writer today writes as knowledgeably about grass as Steve Meyerowitz who observes, "We step on it, sit on it, lay on it, jog on it, picnic on it, walk the dog on it, mow it, water it, in fact, we do most everything on it, for it, or with it except eat it! Wherever there is sun, water and earth, there is grass. From the outback down under to the one inch Arctic tundra of Greenland…to the hundred food tropical bamboo, grass is the most fundamental form of vegetation on the planet."

WHAT PROGRESS LEFT BEHIND—ANCIENT WISDOM FORGOTTEN?

In their ancient wisdom, our bodies crave grass. Though vitamin, mineral, and herbal supplements can be beneficial to our health, none of these match the nutritive value found in grasses. It is interesting to note that in 1936 cereal grass tablets were considered the first multi-nutrient in this country. Cereal grasses are the only foods in the vegetable kingdom that, even if consumed alone, enable animals to continually maintain weight, strength and optimal health. Grasses are considered to be at or near the base of the terrestrial food chain. The powers of the sun that are trapped in its blades produce rich amounts of chlorophyll and other green photosynthetic pigments. Once, even the prestigious American Medical

Association recognized the value of grass. In 1939, the *Journal of the American Medical Association* Council on Foods announced that Cerophyl, a whole food concentrate made with young rapidly growing leaves of wheat, oats and barley, would be "listed in the book of accepted foods." But then, following World War II, the concept of "better living through chemistry" took hold of the nation. Most of us forgot our ancient wisdom. Vitamins could be synthesized, minerals isolated.

Yet, in spite of these wonderful technological advancements, the ancient wisdom of the grasses could not be duplicated within the test tube.

NUTRIENT-DENSE GRASS

Why do we crave green foods? Cereal grasses—known today as green superfoods—supply many nutritional factors that even today scientists cannot duplicate. Is it the chlorophyll—the trapped sunlight—that is the basis for life? Or is it the grass juice factor or enzymes in these plants that are thought to be found nowhere else? We can't deny this fact: cereal grass is perhaps the most nutritious food on this green Earth.

Based on data from the U.S. Department of Agriculture Nutrient Data Laboratory, grasses are richer than spinach, broccoli, eggs and chicken in virtually every nutrient category: protein, calcium, iron, magnesium, phosphorous, potassium, zinc, copper, manganese, vitamin C, thiamin, riboflavin, niacin, vitamin B_6, folate, vitamin B_{12}, carotenoids and vitamin E.

THRIVE ON GRASS

In the 1930s and 1940s, America's leading scientists, led by biochemist George Kohler, worked on grass research at the University College of Agriculture, University of Wisconsin, Madison. The Kohler team was remarkable. They made the discovery of niacin (vitamin B3), as well as the grass juice factor, a nutritive compound in grass that still can't be duplicated by vitamins or minerals.

In an experimental study, published in the *Journal of Nutrition*, Dr. Kohler and his team compared the growth of animals fed either dried grass powder, lettuce, cabbage, or spinach. For eight weeks, young guinea pigs received only the combination of lettuce, cabbage, spinach, or dried grass powder.[38] The animals receiving the lettuce or cabbage lost weight. With spinach, the animals barely sustained their weight. But with cereal grass, the animals thrived and gained much weight. The researchers noted, "the growth stimulating factor of grass was distinct from all the known vitamins." This study was confirmed in subsequent studies, published in the same journal or presented at the Cornell Nutrition Conference.[39,40,41]

MORE ANCIENT WISDOM

Better yet, you should eat fermented grass. Most of us have never known the power of fermentation. We often think the superior way to consume veggies and fruit is raw. But this isn't always so. Sometimes proper food preparation methods release important compounds that would otherwise pass undigested and unused through our systems. Fermentation is Nature's method of preparing foods for easy assimilation in the human body. But most of us don't even know that lactic acid fermentation is driven by beneficial microorganisms, producing enzymes that break down foods into useable compounds. Farmers know. In fact, cattle ranchers produce something called silage, which is fermented grass or hay, to feed to their cattle. This predigested grass allows the cows to get more nutrition from less grass. Farmers know that even cows with their multiple stomachs and strong digestive power can use a little help from our little probiotic friends.

Every long-lived culture in the world has consumed fermented foods with their meals—fermented vegetables, dairy, meat. The Inuits or Eskimos bury their walrus meat or fish and then pull these out, consuming this "rotten" meat to inoculate themselves against pathogenic organisms. The aboriginal peoples of Australia buried sweet potatoes in the soil for months, removed them, and then consumed the sweet potato loaded with living microorganisms as a means of stimulating health. Even in this country, our favorite condiments had their origins in lacto-fermented foods. Mayonnaise, mustard, ketchup, salsa, relish, guacamole, and jams all once were fermented foods replete with enzymes and living bacterial cultures that aided our digestion and nutrient assimilation, and protected us from pathogenic organisms.

"It may seem strange to us that, in earlier times, people knew how to preserve vegetables for long periods without the use of refrigerators, freezers or canning machines," note Fallon and Enig. "This was done through the process of lacto-fermentation. Lactic acid is a natural preservative that inhibits putrefying bacteria. Starches and sugars in vegetables and fruits are converted into lactic acid by the many species of lactic-acid-producing bacteria. These *lactobacilli* are ubiquitous, present on the surface of all living things and especially numerous on leaves and roots of plants growing in or near the ground.

"The ancient Greeks understood that important chemical changes took place during this type of fermentation. Their name for this change was 'alchemy.' Like the fermentation of dairy products, preservation of vegetables and fruits by the process of lacto-fermentation has numerous advantages beyond those of simple preservation. The proliferation of *lactobacilli* in fermented vegetables enhances their digestibility and increases vitamin levels. These beneficial organisms produce numerous helpful enzymes as well as antibiotic and anticarcinogenic substances. Their main by-product, lactic acid, not only keeps vegetables and fruits in a state of perfect preservation but also promotes the growth of healthy flora throughout the intestine. Other alchemical by-products include hydrogen peroxide and small amounts of benzoic acid.

"A partial list of lacto-fermented vegetables from around the world is sufficient to prove the universality of this practice. In Europe the principle lacto-fermented food is sauerkraut. Described in Roman texts, it was prized for both for its delicious taste as well as its medicinal properties. Cucumbers, beets and turnips are also traditional foods for lacto-fermentation. Less well known are ancient recipes for pickled herbs, sorrel leaves and grape leaves. In Russia and Poland one finds pickled green tomatoes, peppers and lettuces. Lacto-fermented foods form part of Asian cuisines as well. The peoples of Japan, China and Korea make pickled preparations of cabbage, turnip, eggplant, cucumber, onion, squash and carrot. Korean *kimchi*, for example, is a lacto-fermented condiment of cabbage with other vegetables and seasonings that is eaten on a daily basis and no Japanese meal is complete without a portion of pickled vegetable. American tradition includes many types of relishes—corn relish, cucumber relish, watermelon rind—all of which were no doubt originally lacto-fermented products. The pickling of fruit is less well known but, nevertheless, found in many traditional cultures. The Japanese prize pickled *umeboshi* plums, and the peoples of India traditionally fermented fruit with spices to make chutneys."

Lacto-fermentation, as I mentioned, is an artisanal craft that does not lend itself to industrialization. Results are not always predictable. "For this reason, when the pickling process became industrialized, many changes were made that rendered the final product more uniform and more saleable but not necessarily more nutritious. Chief among these was the use of vinegar for the brine, resulting in a product that is more acidic and not necessarily beneficial when eaten in large quantities; and of subjecting the final product to pasteurization, thereby effectively killing all the lactic-acid-producing bacteria and robbing consumers of their beneficial effect on the digestion."

Predigestion of the nutrient-rich superfoods contained in Perfect Food is accomplished by use of the proprietary Poten-Zyme process. This ancient method of bio-fermentation incorporates beneficial microorganisms (probiotics) and their enzymes into the foods to gently break them down into their most basic elements. This is not something that any company could easily duplicate.

The end result is a food that is nearly completely broken down and predigested with large amounts of probiotics, enzymes, B vitamins and proteins. But also created are several novel phytochemicals that the body craves, including the body's master antioxidant SOD, as well as various immune-supportive beta-glucans, and many other antioxidants—all created from the 'alchemy' involved in fermentation.

Perfect Food's blend of grasses, legumes, seeds and key vegetables provides the highest concentration of greens of any combination green food product today, including five key nutrient treasures: chlorophyll, which aids in the elimination of harmful bacteria, promotes skin repair, transports oxygen and deodorizes the intestinal tract; polypeptide vegetable proteins that enhance growth and immune function; an abundance of bioavailable minerals and their cofactors gathered by the grasses' deep traveling roots; unique enzymes for digestion and nutrient assimilation; and grass juice factor—the X factor of green foods, especially prevalent in barley greens, which is anti-inflammatory and promotes the growth of healthy tissue.

Many consumers often wonder whether, since they are taking a multiple vitamin/mineral formula, they should also consume green foods. The enzyme-rich "live foods" in Perfect Food provide vitamins and minerals as Nature intended, with all of the naturally occurring co-factors and synergistic compounds intact. These whole foods contain hundreds and possibly thousands of yet to be discovered nutrients that cannot be isolated and put into a vitamin/mineral supplement.

In December 2000, Iris Roswell, a 51-year-old unmarried social worker, visited the office of Terry Morse-Stupka, N.D., who is married to Mark Stupka, N.D. The team of Stupka and Stupka practice together as naturopathic doctors at their Center for Natural Healing in Baton Rouge, Louisiana.

Roswell was suffering from many health troubles, among which were severe indigestion of fats, excessive weight, sinusitis, unclear thinking, confusion, insomnia, perimenopausal difficulties, and massive amounts of body congestion.

Roswell's circulatory, lymphatic, and elimination systems were dysfunctional. Her spleen and thymus were ineffective in their operation. She showed definite signs of yeast and bacterial infections, and there was some compromise in the woman's bone structure. Also, this patient's pH was too alkaline.

"A hair test sample that we took of Ms. Roswell was evaluated by the Analytical Research Laboratory of Phoenix, Arizona, and it indicated that her sodium-potassium (Na-K) ratio remained out of balance at 1.56," notes Terry Morse-Stupka. "A normal reading would have been 2.5 in favor of sodium for expediting the Na-K pump effect at the human cellular level. The patient's disproportionate Na-K ratio occurred from chronic and long term stressors affecting her body. Her adrenal glands were operating 43 times faster than normal, and her thyroid was functioning at only 3 percent of what it was supposed to be. From reading her laboratory tests and observing the clinical symptoms she displayed, it became obvious that Ms. Roswell was in true physiological distress.

"Before treatment, this patient was a very fast metabolizer so that her metabolism was out of control, in a catabolic state which resulted in consumption of her own tissues. She was going downhill too fast. My husband and I considered nutritional restoration to be vital for the woman so we dispensed Perfect Food to her, and it worked beautifully."

Roswell gained immense amounts of energy, lost ten pounds quickly (she declared, "I feel lighter"), found fat digestion improving, experienced brain clarity, and her metabolism normalized as did the woman's many laboratory tests.

"Two months after our patient underwent her initial hair mineral analysis, when we first started her onto Perfect Food, a new hair test was administered," notes the doctor. "It showed that the green product was improving her laboratory numbers and bringing them back to normal levels. We saw an increase in her calcium and magnesium, and these are the two calming minerals which are bringing down Ms. Roswell's metabolism from functioning overly fast to much lower readings. Three trace minerals, cobalt, selenium, and lithium, had been exceedingly low for her, but they are now raised considerably. In contrast, the toxic metal nickel, which was poisoning Ms. Roswell by being much too high at 0.58, is now reduced to near-normal at 0.11. The most homeostatic reading for nickel should be 0.10. Our patient is very close to that norm."

Something else happened to Ms. Roswell from taking Perfect Food. Her metabolism of simple and complex carbohydrates increased greatly. "The normal sugar metabolism ratio for such carbohydrates is 6.67, but her ratio had been elevated at 11.33; now it's fallen to 9.25," the doctor points out. "And this woman's hormones are more balanced today. While earlier she was too low with a hormone ratio at 5.58, currently Ms. Roswell's hormones stand at 7.33. The correct hormone ratio for any woman to maintain balance is 8.0. Finally, our patient's sodium-potassium level has increased from 1.56 to 1.71; her cellular metabolism has enhanced significantly by the regular daily intake of Perfect Food.

"Mark and I are happy with our patient's physiological improvements, and she is happy too. Invariably when Iris comes into our office now she is singing, laughing, joking, and declaring that she feels on top of the world. The two of us attribute this woman's new love of life to her regularly supplementing with the green, powdered Perfect Food.

But, they add, "Iris Roswell is just one example of what we've found with dispensing this super green food. From our experience, Mark and I know that using it tends to eliminate the need for individual supplemental vitamins and minerals. At some point during their treatment programs we get all of our patients consuming Perfect Food. There is no question that every person requires more fruits and vegetables in their diets, and this product is so far above any other marketed green supplement that nothing else sold is able to compete with its quality and quantity of nutrition what with the excellent enzymes, probiotics, and live foods that it contains. There isn't anything else on the market like Perfect Food. My husband and I would not allow our patients to take any other green food supplement except this one."

"I have been recommending the daily drinking of Perfect Food to my patients for over two-and-a-half years," says Peter Cloete, M.D., Ph.D., who practices family medicine at the Center for Biomolecular Medicine in George, a town located in western South Africa.

"Although the patient's clinical picture determines my treatment, I do use this green food product on almost every person," says Dr. Cloete. "It's just good nutritional medicine, especially for relieving any type of gut pathology such as poor absorption or irritable bowel. Perfect Food works wonders for almost all of those kinds of gastrointestinal tract problems. If a patient has gut absorption trouble, it just makes sense to give him or her the finest available food to eat and assimilate. This product does not demand a well-functioning digestive system to support the body because the super green drink is absorbed so readily and well. By its usage, the patient's digestion will improve."

Dr. Cloete finds Perfect Food works especially well on younger children—babies and toddlers—who are affected by antibiotics often prescribed for otitis media and other childhood diseases. By adding the drinking of Perfect Food to the patients' diets, the doctor will see a massive pickup in their well-being.

"I can describe the medical history of one baby who at two-and-a-half years old was chronically ill from birth and appeared white or sallow-colored all the time. She had no energy, acted lethargic, cried constantly, suffered from otitis media, had chronic bronchitis, spiked fevers that came on for no apparent reason, and required the need for pediatrician attention every week. Infections permeated her body, and antibiotics had become an integral part of the child's daily routine." When Dr. Cloete took over this baby's care, Perfect Food was among the first and most important prescriptions for her. "I reduced the abundant amount of carbohydrates the baby was being fed and got Perfect Food into her on a daily basis. That one action did the trick in just a couple of weeks. Now, after six months on the super green drink, she has not required medical attention more than once. About three months ago, I was called upon when the mother brought her baby into me for a general checkup and progress report. Today that baby is fine.

"Patients who feel miserable from Crohn's disease and colitis respond exceedingly well to Perfect Food," says Dr. Cloete. "I treat an awful lot of people with bowel disorders, and the green drink is the specific medicine for them. Treatment for such gut troubles falls to me after the patients have been butchered with bad drug medicine and/or surgery. Good management using the super green food's certified organic ingredients offers complete relief for the individual suffering with digestive disturbances."

POSTPARTUM FATIGUE & OTHER COMPLAINTS

Noelle Nielsen, M.D., of Saratoga Springs, New York, is an ob/gyn who has prescribed Perfect Food for women requiring improved nutrition after childbirth. "For one of my patients, a registered nurse age twenty-five, the recommendation to drink this super green food was mandatory for her six-months postpartum breast feeding. Because she was suffering from excessive weight gain during her pregnancy along with chronic fatigue, the new mother needed this extra boost to her menu plan. Positive effects for her kicked in by the end of a week. She found more energy, and a twenty-five-pound weight loss occurred over a couple of months. The woman returned to her pre-pregnancy weight, and generally felt restored. Both my patient and I attribute this excellent effect to her taking of Perfect Food. While as a nurse she knew how to take care of herself, this green drink is what the nurse ascribed as her source of improvement.

"I drink Perfect Food myself as do my two sons, and we make taking it a routine part of our daily nutrition intake," adds Dr. Nielsen. "Just recently it was revealed to me that Perfect Food mixes well with the high protein goat's milk drink, Goatein™ (also from Garden of Life), so now I combine them as a more complete nutritional beverage."

GREEN SUPERFOOD ALONG WITH DETOXIFICATION

Colon hydrotherapist Carmen Howard of Lake Ann, Michigan, is knowledgeable about Perfect Food. She takes it as her means of preventive maintenance. Howard is an athlete who runs 35 miles a week, and she supports her personal physical effort with the best in whole food eating. This colon hydrotherapist actively engages in good health practices and advocates the same for those clients who consult her for colonic health.

In addition to administering colonic irrigation, Howard offers clients nutritional supplements as a means of preparation for bowel cleansing. "As part of my client services, I dispense the most nutritious super green food existing on our planet and people thrive on it," she says. "I eat this perfect food myself every day, as does my family. When taken as a supplement to one's regular menu plan, two tablespoonsful of my super green food do offer the equivalent of up to 10 servings of vegetables, including certified organic greens, grains and seeds plus enzyme-active live foods, more than 90 antioxidants, and over 100 minerals and vitamins. It provides the omega-3, -6, -9, and -18 essential fatty acids.

"The super green food complex that I recommend is brandnamed Perfect Food by its United States manufacturer/distributor, Garden of Life, Inc. of Palm Beach Gardens, Florida," advises the colon hydrotherapist. "And my observation is that Perfect Food in powder form shaken with water or mixed into a smoothie is superb as a drinkable antidote for almost any form of intestinal malabsorption. I advise putting two tablespoons of the green powder into 6 ounces of fresh-made carrot juice and drinking this for optimal nutrition. In fact, if someone needs to be more economical, just one tablespoonful of the green supplement will provide that person with the equivalent of five servings of vegetables and one serving of brown rice," states Howard. "I know that this type of excellent nourishment helps to repair the body by giving it whole food that's readily available for absorption.

"By a client ingesting Perfect Food regularly, my job as a colon hydrotherapist becomes easier because less preparation time is required to get that person's bowel ready to receive colonic treatment. I consider Perfect Food to be the finest possible fast-food for ongoing health maintenance. It behaves adjunctively to what people usually eat by causing bowel function to be easier and more regular," affirms Howard. "From such good functioning, skin troubles such as psoriasis, acne, dermatitis…all get better.

"I am an animal lover and choose to feed my German shepherds Perfect Food for the nutritional excellence of its formulation. My dogs are happy, healthy, and beautiful show animals as a result. I declare that Perfect Food is the perfect food for pets exactly as it is for humans.

"I've analyzed the cost breakdown of Perfect Food as a nutritional agent and have figured out that a heaping tablespoonful costs less than the price of a small bag of corn chips and a can of soda pop per day—somewhat less than 89 cents—and for this small expenditure of money, each consumer does get the perfect food."

"I have been dispensing Perfect Food for over three years, and I can't keep it in stock" says Ronald Wedemeyer, D.C., of Bakersfield, California. "Containers of this green-powdered superfood are snapped up and carried off by my patients as soon as shipments arrive. They love its nutritional content and what drinking the stuff does for them. It's the most popular nutritional supplement that I dispense from my office. It sells quickly because the people no longer need to swallow fractionated nutrient pills. All the nutrients are at hand in one serving of Perfect Food. I personally take a double dose of it every day as does my family.

"My patient, a thirty-five-year-old single mother named Simone Mauser who supported herself as a public school teacher, consulted me because of four particular health problems. Simone was overly skinny and could not gain weight; she experienced severe digestive imbalances from diverticulitis; she was troubled by allergies; and she had been trying to nurse her new baby but milk would not come. I started this woman on Perfect Food two years ago," explains Dr. Wedemeyer, "and since then weight came back aplenty; allergies left her; she produced abundant breast milk and still feeds her baby with it; and she has remained in remarkably good health—not even coming down with a cold. Simone Mauser has become one of my most active spokespersons for Perfect Food.

"I have purchasers of the green powder whom I don't ever see. They buy it by mail order. I love Perfect Food because it simplifies the patients' nutrient programs. They don't ever need multiple bottles of pills but only this single container of this true super food."

PERFECT FOOD IS FOR THE BIRDS, SAY LIZ AND BOB JOHNSON

I thought this story might amuse but also demonstrate how pure this food is. Liz and Bob Johnson of South Florida, administrators of the Shyne Foundation, a nonprofit organization which devotes itself to the health preservation and safety of parrots, cockatoos, macaws, and other tropical birds, feed their birds Perfect Food as the most nutritious nourishment available. (The Johnsons refuse to have their exact location identified because of dangers they face from bird thieves.) The Shyne Foundation is a quarter-acre, 16-foot-high, screened in section of rain forest. It offers a free-flight natural habitat sanctuary for numbers of neglected, abused, damaged, or handicapped parrots, some of which are quite valuable.

"There are thirty-two species of parrots, and we hold them in sanctuary here to heal, be safe, and enjoy life. The birds do not need to perform, and we avoid selling or breeding them," says Liz Johnson. "Bob and I agree that Perfect Food works wonders for our birds."

"Perfect Food is definitely for the birds, but we also take it ourselves every day. We feed the birds many nutritional supplements: homeopathics, herbs, nutrients, phytochemicals, and most especially this nutrition-packed, green superfood. We believe in employing a shotgun approach for attaining optimal nourishment," states certified nutritionist Bob Johnson, M.Ed. "Usually, I add the green superfood to the birds' water, sprinkle it on moist food morsels for purposes of improved digestion, and actually feed it into the mouths of young birds with a syringe.

"Although they prefer to eat bananas and crackers, greens are an exceedingly important part of the parrots' diet. Like children, however, some birds avoid eating greens so that Perfect Food fills their need as an agent adhered to cut-up fruits and vegetables" adds Bob Johnson. "A few of our 160 parrots eat directly from the Perfect Food container."

"Feathers that are missing on damaged or denuded birds are stimulated to grow in faster when they eat Perfect Food , and it gives their feathers a greater glossiness with brighter colors. Also it elevates the energy of droopy birds," says Liz Johnson. "They show more vigor, increased sexual activity, and become highly energetic from eating it."

"A parrot's metabolism is much more efficient than a human's so that when it is given optimal nutrition as with Perfect Food, it shows very quick healing and truly fast improvement in its physical abilities. We see results from feeding them the green superfood rather quickly," conclude the two conservationists.

Perfect Food is the only "predigested" green superfood on the market. This is a pure survival food. Perfect Food is truly a smart choice. Once you consume powdered green foods, your body tells you immediately, "Hey, I like this. I feel better." It is instinctual. That is why, we must warn you, once you start having a green food power drink in the morning, you won't be able to give up the habit. Why should you give up such a healthy habit? The perfect combination of grass therapy and fermentation has been combined in the powdered (or caplet) super green food.

Be sure to mix one to two level tablespoons in eight ounces of juice or water one or more times per day. Perfect Food may be taken with or without food. Children may take one-fourth to one-half the adult serving if desired.

Perfect Food Ingredients

Green Superfoods: Wheat Grass Juice*, Barley Grass Juice*, Rye Grass Juice*, Oat Grass Juice*, Alfalfa Grass Juice*; Spirulina, Chlorella, Dunaliella, Kelp, Dulse and other sea vegetables. Green Superfoods are a rich source of vitamins, minerals, enzymes, amino acids, chlorophyll and antioxidants. (The product is gluten-free.)

Vegetables: Carrot Juice*, Beet Juice*, Tomato Juice*, Sweet Potato*, Broccoli*, Kale*, Cabbage*, Cauliflower, Brussels Sprouts, Parsley*, Spinach*, Asparagus*, Celery*, Cucumber, Green Seeds*, Chia Seeds*, Garbanzo Beans*, Red Lentils*, Soy Beans*, Kidney Beans*, Azuki Beans*, Millet*, Brown Rice*, Maize* and Buckwheat* (gluten- and phytate-free). These predigested grains, seeds and legumes, provide vitamins such as B complex and vitamin E, isoflavones, fiber, and essential fatty acids including, Omega-3 and -6 fatty acids. Pepper*, Garlic, Ginger* and Onion. Vegetables are Nature's richest source of phytochemicals including lycopene, sulforaphane, allicin and bioflavonoids.

Grains and Seeds: Flax Seeds*, Sesame Seeds*, Sunflower Seeds*, Pumpkin

Acerola cherry: Nature's richest source of vitamin C. Vitamin C is crucial as a premier antioxidant and is important for the overall health of the immune system.

*Organically or biodynamically grown (free from pesticides and grown according to the Maker's intent).

Part III–
The Garden of Life Healing Program

CHAPTER NINE

Return to the Maker's Diet

You would think if anyone would have developed lifelong-health eating habits, it would have to be me. After all, my father is a trained naturopath and chiropractor. He is well versed in the Hippocratic philosophy that food shall be thy medicine. So naturally you would think my family's diet should have been great.

We ate what we considered to be the healthiest foods. Although I slathered my bagels with cow's milk cream cheese, at least they were *whole-wheat* bagels. I ate turkey cold cuts instead of pork. Hold the sodium nitrite, please. I even had yogurt occasionally, albeit frozen. I ate vegetables and whole grains instead of polished white rice or enriched flour. I had an apple, if not every day, every few days. We avoided the use of sugar and preservatives. I thought my diet was pretty good.

And, truthfully, compared to most Americans' eating habits, mine were probably better than average. But then again perhaps there's a good reason why jaded nutritionists have coined *SAD* as the acromym for the *Standard American Diet*. I may have been eating a diet that made me a little nutritionally smarter than the average bear. But that isn't saying a whole lot. For most Americans, our diets are truly *SAD*.

When I was sick, awake in bed and unable to do much of anything, I read a lot of books—especially about diets—from *Dr. Atkins' New Diet Revolution* to *The Zone*. I also spoke to a lot of nutritional experts by phone or visited their clinics. One thing I learned from my own struggle is that our dietary habits are the key to our good health. But, unfortunately, I've also seen that so much of what we've learned about what constitutes a good diet is wrong—plain wrong—even from the so-called nutrition experts and from our highest paid health officials. Healthy eating has become politicized and commercialized—and we've really made far too many compromises that victimize our health. It's a pity, too, that so many of us must suffer. Our life habits must change in so many ways in order for us to reach the full potential of our health. Our eating habits are in desperate need of a complete overhaul.

Most Americans simply do not eat the nutritious diets that our own ancestors ate to remain healthy and live long, disease-free lives.

Instead, we have strayed from the foods of our Creator, foods that at one time nourished the world's healthiest peoples. We have altered the Maker's intent, and we have allowed food to become our idol.

We are becoming fat, sick and sedentary. I know it's harsh. I also know it's true, and what all of us need now is a lot more truth and a lot less fluff. The kind of things that pass for food today—what we choose for table fare—are pathetic!

Consider this: diseases of civilization—including arthritis, cancer, diabetes, heart attack, high blood pressure and stroke—are the top ten causes of death past the age of forty-five. These same diseases of civilization are becoming ever more widespread as civilization progressively becomes more industrialized. Certainly, our diets are a major factor in their spread. These were not common diseases—even among the oldest primitive persons—when we were maintaining a Biblical diet that was in keeping with the intent of our Creator.

I'm not about to tell you to toss off your clothes, put on a loin cloth, grab a long sharp stick and start to spear some fish in the nearest body of water for your lunch this afternoon—even if that is one of the ways our ancestors gathered their own food. The great 20th century novelist Thomas Wolfe once said you can never go back home again. We can't go back to the old ways completely. But we can learn from the old ways and improve our modern lives. The old ways—the primitive ways and heeding the word of our Maker—can help us to overcome modern diseases of civilization and help to provide the nourishment that will make us strong and disease-resistant.

Many cutting-edge researchers from both major academic institutions as well as "alternative" medicine now believe that a more primitive diet is superior in virtually all ways to the modern diet. But I want you to go further. I want you also to participate in the ultimate wisdom of the Maker's or Biblical diet.

Let me put it to you this way. Technology has advanced at far greater speed than our digestive tracts. We can process and preserve food now to make it last for decades. You can have an irradiated ten-year-old burger if you're so inclined. We can splice the gene of one species into another. If you want a peanut with the genes of a salmon, it's yours, baby. We can bioengineer foods with their own pesticides. If you want *Bt* with your potatoes, no problem.

We may be in the twenty-first century when it comes to cyberspace and our technological advancements. But our bodies are still back in primitive times, six thousand years ago. Our bodies will do better if we eat more like our primitive ancestors. I also believe we should be eating foods as detailed in the Bible. I know this may sound outrageous to some readers. However, whether you believe that the Bible is the inspired word of God or not, there is no denying that the Old Testament (or Tenach or scriptures, as the Jews refer to it) describes in great detail the dietary habits of a group of people who were healthier than all of their neighbors. All I'm saying is that there is wisdom in the Bible that goes far beyond the spiritual —especially when it comes to dietary considerations.

Let's look a little more closely at an overview of the Maker's Diet. In Genesis 1:29, God tells us, "I give you every seed-bearing plant on the face of the whole earth and every tree that has fruit with seed in it. They will be yours for food." Unlike our modern diet, the Maker's Diet provides a far greater amount of vitamins, minerals, protein and healthy fats, as well as substances in plants that are neither vitamins nor minerals, known as phytochemicals. The Maker is telling us that seed-bearing foods are healthy.

Fruits, vegetables, herbs, lentils, properly prepared whole grains—these are pretty much all good as long as we don't get fancy and impose too much modern technology on them. Rex Russell, M.D., author of *What the Bible Says About Healthy Living*, admonishes us, "Don't alter God's design."

On the other hand, the Maker's Diet contains no refined or processed carbohydrates and only a very small amount of healthy sweeteners. This is the opposite of our modern diet, which strays from God's design and delivers us techno-foods, rich in calories, filled with refined carbohydrates, and of inadequate nutritional value. The Maker's Diet fills us with foods from the Creator—unprocessed—replete with every healing miracle put on God's Green Earth. The modern diet perverts the design of the Creator, strays from the wisdom of our ancestors, and overloads our bodies with adulterated fats and refined, simple sugars—like those found in candy, baked goods and refined grains.

Our bodies do better with the old ways—with wild game instead of artificially fattened, estrogenized slabs of beef; fermented raw dairy instead of antibiotic- bovine growth hormone- and pesticide-contaminated pasteurized dairy; wild fish with fins and scales instead of farm-raised antibiotic-laden fish; nutritious fermented or sprouted whole grain bread instead of Wonder white; fermented relishes and condiments instead of sugary sauce substitutes.

The cure for modern disease—arthritis, cancer, diabetes, heart attack, high blood pressure and stroke—is found in the simple truths of living healthfully—in short, by following the Maker's Diet.

BRUTISH, SAVAGE & DUMB—THE MYTH OF PRIMITIVE MAN

It's hard to believe what I'm about to tell you, but it's largely true: our ancestors had some neat nutritional things going for them. So, let's drop the loutish, brutish, savage dumb stereotyping of our ancient predecessors here. There's a lot we can learn from them.

The biggest failing of our ancestors was simply that they did not have access to all of the technology that we have today—no neonatal units, ICU, antibiotics—and as a result many died during infancy or quite young. In fact, infant mortality was 20 to 30 percent, which isn't good; in fact, it was 10 to 100 times greater than it is today. However, if someone survived the first two years of life, their likelihood of living past 80 in good health was probably many, many times greater than today.

Talk to anyone today and the most common perception of our ancestors' more primitive lifestyle is that they were an undernourished, brutish group of filthy semi-human beings plagued by illness and their own stupidity. Think again. Our ancestors experienced robust health often until death. Our great, great-grandparents had no words for retirement or nursing home. They lived a lifestyle and consumed a diet that was suited to their bodies and it kept them strong and healthy well into the eighties and beyond.

THE PRIMITIVE AMONG US

We can learn more about the health of our ancestors by studying people who even to this day continue to consume a primitive diet and lead primitive lifestyles. We can also examine the records of anthropologists, explorers, and others who came into contact with primitive people during the nineteenth and twentieth centuries.

While it is true that some primitive people did not live long enough to acquire cardiovascular diseases or cancer, two of the major causes of death in the United States and Europe today, we know that the ones who did live long acquired these diseases infrequently.

We know this, in part, because cancer and heart disease are rare among people alive today who eat a more primitive, ancestral diet. Researchers made a survey on cardiovascular disease incidence and related risk factors among 2,300 subsistence horticulturists in the tropical island of Kitava, Trobriand Islands, Papua New Guinea.[42] Their most important findings so far published are that sudden cardiac death, stroke and exertion-related chest pain were nonexistent or extremely rare in Kitavans. (Infections, accidents, complications of pregnancy and senescence were the most common causes of death.) All adults had low diastolic blood pressure (all below 90 mm Hg) and were very lean (weight decreased after age 30). Tubers, fruit, fish and coconut were dietary staples in Kitava. The intake of western food and alcohol was negligible. Salt intake was far lower, too. Eighty per cent of both sexes were daily smokers, supporting the concept that smoking alone is not sufficient to cause cardiovascular disease. (The only available migrant was a 44-year-old urbanized businessman who had grown up on Kitava and who came for a visit during the survey. He differed markedly from all other adults regardless of sex: he had the highest diastolic blood pressure, the highest body mass index, and the highest waist to hip ratio, indicating that Kitavans are not genetically protected from hypertension or abdominal obesity.)

Michael Murray, N.D., one of our leading natural healing experts today, has also written extensively about the absence of modern disease from primitive cultures. He notes that among those aboriginal, primitive societies in Australia, Africa, and South America that survived into the twentieth century, the rates of cancer, rheumatoid arthritis, obesity, diabetes, osteoporosis, heart disease and other conditions were remarkably low until they switched to modern diets.[43]

Tragically, encroachment of modern civilization throughout the globe has led to the infiltration by modern culture of once-isolated societies. Today, few societies remain that have continued to consume the more primitive, simple diet of their ancestors. It would seem that canned food, refined sugar, and white flour are consumed nearly everywhere on Earth. Almost every society has made the transition from the primitive diet to the modern diet. But there is an historic record that tells what we need to know about the virtues of the primitive diet. In 1913, Nobel Prize winner, medical doctor and missionary Dr. Albert Schweitzer visited Gabon, Africa. "I was astonished to encounter no cases of cancer," he observed. "I saw none among the natives two hundred miles from the coast…. I cannot, of course, say positively that there was no cancer at all, but, like other frontier doctors, I can only say that, if any cases existed they must have been quite rare. This absence of cancer seemed to be due to the difference in nutrition of the natives compared to the Europeans."

Explorer and anthropologist Vilhjalmur Stefansson kept meticulous diaries of his adventures in the Arctic. In *Cancer: Disease of Civilization*, Stefansson told readers he searched in vain for cases of cancer among the Inuit peoples. He even cited the findings of a whaling ship doctor, George B. Leavitt, who found only a single cancer case in 49 years among the Inuit of Alaska and Canada. But by the 1970s, after the Inuit began consuming a modern diet, breast cancer was a frequent form of malignancy. Today, we know that toxic chemicals from our modern foods and industries have contributed to this condition.[44] Also, changes from the traditional way of life tend to increase the likelihood of Inuit developing the risk factors associated with heart disease and diabetes, according to a February 2000 report from Health Canada.

Once rare cases of diabetes in Australia among native Aborigines are now tenfold greater than among European arrivals, again due to dietary changes, notes Kerin O'Dea, a professor at Monash University. Interestingly, the Aborigines were once known for prodigious consumption of fermented sweet potatoes, a natural source of probiotics and soluble fiber that fed the good bacteria of the gastrointestinal tract and is thought to markedly reduce risk of blood sugar imbalances.

THE FINDINGS OF DR. WESTON PRICE

Dr. Weston A. Price, a Harvard-trained dentist, has been called the "Charles Darwin of Nutrition." Alarmed by the number of cavities, the crooked teeth, and the deformed dental arches he saw in his young patients, Dr. Price wondered if these abnormalities were caused by nutritional deficiencies. Price believed, and rightfully so, that dental health is a good indicator of physical health. Deformed dental arches, crooked teeth, and cavities are signs of physical degeneration and a vulnerability to diseases such as heart attacks and cancer, we now know based on scientific evidence. In his search for the causes of dental decay and physical degeneration that he observed in his dental practice, he turned from test tubes and microscopes to unstudied evidence among human beings.

With his wife Florence, he left his home in Ohio and embarked on a six-year journey that took him to primitive societies on five continents. Wherever Dr. Price went, he photographed and studied the inhabitants' teeth. He made detailed notes about primitive people's diet, the state of their health, and their way of life. Dr. Price chose an opportune time to undertake his study.

In the 1930s, the last remaining societies in the world where people ate a primitive diet were making the transformation to the modern diet. Dr. Price had a chance to compare people, sometimes in the same family or household, who had grown up with the primitive and the modern diet.

Price traveled the world over in order to study isolated human groups, including sequestered villages in Switzerland, Gaelic communities in the Outer Hebrides, Eskimos and Indians of North America, Melanesian and Polynesian South Sea Islanders, African tribes, Australian Aborigines, New Zealand Maori and the Indians of South America. Wherever he went, Dr. Price found that beautiful straight teeth, freedom from decay, stalwart bodies, resistance to disease and integrity of character were typical of primitives on their traditional diets, rich in essential food factors.

Dr. Price sought the factors responsible for fine teeth among the people who had them—the isolated "primitives." The world became his laboratory. As he traveled, his findings led him to the belief that dental caries and deformed dental arches resulting in crowded, crooked teeth and unattractive appearance were merely a sign of physical degeneration, resulting from what he had suspected—nutritional deficiencies.

Dr. Price reported his findings in an extraordinary book called *Nutritional and Physical Degeneration*. He found that primitive people who were cut off from the modern diet had very little tooth decay and perfectly formed teeth and jaws. The photographs in the book are astonishing. The narrow faces, misshapen jaws, and crooked teeth of people who ate the modern diet are shown in stark contrast to the wide faces, perfect teeth, and perfectly formed dental arches of their fathers, mothers, sisters, and brothers who ate a primitive diet. What accounted for primitive people's good physical health? Their diet, Dr. Price concluded. Wherever he went, he noticed that people who ate the modern diet suffered from physical degeneration. Dr. Price suggested, moreover, that dietary deficiencies may cause poor brain development and lead to social disorders such as juvenile delinquency and high crime rates.

In a period of history when primitive people were disparaged and sneered at, Dr. Price made the startling suggestion that modern humans could learn from primitives. He advocated returning to the primitive diet that had made our ancestors so healthy. He said we could learn much from some of their practices as well, especially those pertaining to child rearing and child development.

Dr. Price wrote:

No era in the long journey of mankind reveals in the skeletal remains such a terrible degeneration of teeth and bones as this brief modern period records. Must Nature reject our vaunted culture and call back the more obedient primitives?

When Dr. Price analyzed the foods used by isolated primitive peoples he found that they provided at least four times the water-soluble vitamins, calcium and other minerals, and at least ten times the fat-soluble vitamins from animal foods such as butter, fatty fish, wild game and organ meats.

The importance of good nutrition for mothers during pregnancy has long been recognized, but Dr. Price's investigation showed that primitives understood and practiced preconception nutritional programs for both parents. Many tribes required a period of premarital nutrition, and children were spaced to permit the mother to maintain her full health and strength, thus assuring subsequent offspring of physical excellence. Special foods were often given to pregnant and lactating women, as well as to the maturing boys and girls in preparation for future parenthood. Dr. Price found these foods to be very rich in fat-soluble vitamins A and D, *nutrients found only in animal fats*.

These primitives with their fine bodies, homogeneous reproduction, emotional stability and freedom from degenerative ills stand forth in sharp contrast to those subsisting on the impoverished foods of civilization—sugar, white flour, pasteurized milk and convenience foods filled with shelf-life extenders and additives.

Dr. Price performed a nutritional intake comparison between those primitive groups which demonstrated resistance to dental caries and freedom from degenerative processes with the diets of modernized groups who had forsaken their native diets for the foods of commerce, consisting largely of white flour products, sugar, polished rice, jams, canned goods and vegetable oils (resulting in loss of this immunity to dental caries and in loss of freedom from degenerative processes). (Figures given below show the number of times the amount of minerals and vitamins which are found in primitive diets compared with modernized diets.)

Group	Minerals[1]						Vitamins[2]	
	Ca	P	Fe	Mg	Cu	I	Fat Soluble	Water Soluble
Native Eskimos	5.4	5.0	1.5	7.9	1.8	49.0	10 plus	large increase
Indians-far North of Canada	5.8	5.8	2.7	4.3	1.5	8.8	10 plus	large increase
Swiss	3.7	2.2	3.1	2.5	*	*	10 plus	large increase
Gaelic- Outer Hebrides	2.1	2.3	1.0	1.3	*	*	10 plus	large increase
Aborigines of Australia	4.6	6.2	50.6	17.0	*	*	10 plus	large increase
New Zealand Maori	6.2	6.9	58.3	23.4	*	*	10 plus	large increase
Melanesians	5.7	6.4	22.4	26.4	*	*	10 plus	large increase
Polynesians	5.6	7.2	18.6	28.5	*	*	10 plus	large increase
Coastal Indians of Peru	6.6	5.5	5.1	13.6	*	*	10 plus	large increase
Andean Mountain Indians of Peru	5.0	5.5	29.3	13.3	*	*	10 plus	large increase
Cattle Tribes of Interior Africa	7.5	8.2	16.6	19.1	*	*	10 plus	large increase
Agricultural Tribes of Central Africa	3.5	4.1	16.6	5.4	*	*	10 plus	large increase

*Not given
1. Minerals: Ca=Calcium, P=Phosphorus , Fe=Iron, Mg=Magnesium, Cu=Copper, I=Iodine
2. Fat-soluble vitamins include A, D, E, K. Water-soluble vitamins include the B vitamins (folate, pantothenic acid, thiamin, riboflavin, niacin, B6, B12) and vitamin C

Here are some observations from his book *Nutrition and Physical Degeneration* (published in 1939):
• Switzerland: "The isolated groups dependent on locally produced natural foods have nearly complete natural immunity to dental caries, and the substitution of modern dietaries for these primitive natural foods destroys this immunity…"
• Outer Hebrides Islands: "I was advised that in the last fifty years the average height of Scotch men in some parts decreased four inches, and that this had been coincident with the general change from

Percentages of Teeth Attacked By Dental Caries in Primitive and Modernized Groups		
Group	Primitive	Modern
Swiss	4.60	29.8
Gaelics	1.20	30.0
Eskimos	0.09	13.0
Northern Indians	0.16	21.5
Seminole Indians	4.00	40.0
Melanesians	0.38	29.0
Polynesians	0.32	21.9

high immunity to dental caries to a loss of immunity in a great part of this general district. A study of the market places revealed that a large part of the nutrition was shipped into the district in the form of refined flours and canned goods and sugar."

- Alaska: "We neither saw nor heard of a case (of arthritis) in the isolated groups. However, at the point of contact with the foods of modern civilization many cases were found including ten bed-ridden cripples in a series of about twenty Indian homes. Some other afflictions made their appearance there, particularly tuberculosis which is taking a very severe toll on the children who had been born at the center."

- Tongan Islands: "Following the war (World War I), the price of copra [aged dried coconut meat] went from $40.00 per ton to $400.00, which brought trading ships with white flour and sugar to exchange for the copra. The effect of this is shown clearly in the teeth. The incidence of dental caries among the isolated groups living on native foods was 0.6 percent, while for those around the port living in part on trade foods, it was 33.4 percent. Now the trader ships no longer call and this forced isolation is very clearly a blessing in disguise. Dental caries have largely ceased to be active since imported foods became scarce, for the price of copra fell to $4.00 a ton."

- Ethiopia: "In one of the most efficiently organized mission schools that we found in Africa, the principal asked me to help them solve a serious problem. He said there was no single question asked them so often by the native boys in their school as why it is that those families that have grown up in the mission or government schools were physically not so strong as those families who had never been in contact with the mission or government schools."

- New Zealand: "Whereas the original primitive Maori had reportedly the finest teeth in the world, the whites now in New Zealand are claimed to have the poorest teeth in the world."

- Australia: "The rapid degeneration of the Australian Aborigines after the adoption of the government's modern foods provides a demonstration that should be infinitely more convincing than animal experimentation. It should be a matter not only of concern but deep alarm that human beings can degenerate physically so rapidly by the use of a certain type of nutrition, particularly the dietary products used so generally by modern civilization."

At times, Dr. Price writes rhapsodically about primitive people, their endurance, their stamina, their physical strength, and their natural beauty. They did not suffer from obesity, heart disease, digestive problems or cancer at the rates we do. Thanks in large part to their diet, they enjoyed a vibrant health that has been lost to modern civilization. But some folks have called Price's work biased. So let's go to the anthropologists and archaeologists to see what we can glean from their scientific work. I think you will find their body of evidence supports entirely the work of the late great Dr. Price.

We can study the skeletons and teeth of primitive people for evidence of vitamin and mineral deficiencies. And here's what we learn: The evidence suggests that humans before the advent of modern agriculture were stronger, bigger, and healthier. Generally speaking, whenever our primitive ancestors took to agriculture as their primary food supply, their health declined.

The Illinois Valley is one of the few sites in the United States containing an intact mortuary record dating back to when humans first populated the area.[45] In addition to skeletal remains, a large amount of archaeological dietary evidence has also been recovered. This enables us to draw conclusions on health and disease as it relates to subsistence during the various cultural components. One site, the Dickson Mounds in Illinois, provides ample data to show a correlation between increasing primary food production and overall health level.[46] The three components represented by sufficient data are the Late Woodland period (950-1100 AD), the Mississippian Acculturated/Late Woodland period (1100-1200 AD), and the Middle Mississippian period (1200-1300 AD).

The Late Woodland component is associated with a generalized hunting and gathering economy. From the appearance of the first people at the Dickson Mounds, there is a general increase in the reliance on maize as the primary food crop. The number of skeletons with non-specific skeletal infections greatly increases as the maize dependence increases. By the Middle Mississippian period, the infection rate more than doubled. Decreased host immunity resulting from severe iron-deficiency anemia due to the maize-based monodiet probably is responsible for the great increase in infection rates. Iron-deficiency anemia greatly inhibits the ability of the body's immune system to stave off infection because iron plays a key role in the function of the immune system.

Similar findings have been reported from ancient cultures elsewhere in the Americas. In East Georgia, maize cultivation occurs only after 1150 AD. After this time there is a progressive increase in habitation site density and distribution. There is an increase in overall bone infections for the agricultural-based people. The decrease in bone size, robusticity, and stature for the agriculturists is also evident. The fact that people became smaller can be attributed to the change in subsistence practices. When people became sedentary it greatly decreased their physical stress. As a result, their size and stature decreased. Another equal factor in this reduced size is nutritional- and disease-related stress.

Before the advent of widespread modern agriculture, the human diet consisted mostly of fruits, vegetables, wild grain and seeds, fish, and meat from wild animals. No matter how far we have progressed socially and technologically, our bodies crave the foods of our ancestors. Our genetic constitutions and nutritional requirements were established during our past. Those people were optimally adapted to the types of foods that they could gather, and there's no evidence to suggest that modern humans are any different. We are literally designed to eat the same foods in the same proportions as thousands of years ago. Our physiology and biochemistry cry out for a primitive diet with its plentiful amounts of healthy meat, fish, fruit, vegetables and nuts. We have departed so far from the wisdom of our forefathers that fully 55 percent of the American diet is "new food" not eaten by our ancestors.

So how do you do it? How do you move from the modern diet to the Maker's Diet? Let's look in detail at some of the components of the Maker's Diet.

Fruits and vegetables. Primitive humans ate three times more of a wide variety of fruits and vegetables than we do. Fruits and vegetables (along with legumes and nuts) provided a startling 50-65 percent of daily calories and up to 100 grams of fiber a day—five times today's level. Vitamins, minerals and antioxidants were supplied in amounts people now get only through supplements. Modern research clearly shows that heavy consumers of fruits and vegetables have less cancer, heart disease, diabetes, high blood pressure and other chronic ills.

Grass-fed meat. Our not-so-distant ancestors consumed 35 percent of their calories in protein. The difference: their protein came from pasture-fed animals, wild game and fish, which also supply highly beneficial omega-3 fatty acids that protect against modern diseases like cancer, diabetes, and heart problems.

Our ancestors ate less of the following:

Grains, cereals, pasta, bread. The over-consumption of grain products is a huge problem in our world today. Grains contain nutrient inhibitors that prevent us from utilizing many minerals. Grains also contain disaccharides, sugars which are difficult to digest and can lead to the growth of undesirable microorganisms in the gut. The over-consumption of carbohydrate foods, particularly grains, can lead to the overproduction of insulin, which may be a major cause of many metabolic disorders and other illnesses. Most grains today are improperly prepared or refined and no longer supply important vitamins, minerals and phytochemicals. Some research has linked grains, notably wheat, to arthritis, gastrointestinal problems, headaches and depression, perhaps indicating subtle allergic food reactions.

Refined sugar. Rather than honey and fruit, today's main sweet is 120 pounds of refined sugar a year per person. Evidence shows sugar drives up blood levels of insulin, glucose and triglycerides, known factors in diabetes and heart disease.

Processed oils. Modern processing techniques have led to a dramatic change in the types and kinds of oils we now consume. Today, we consume highly refined, nutrient-poor vegetable oils and shortening. These cause our bodies to become overloaded with polyunsaturated fats and artificially created hydrogenated and trans fats that promote cancer, inflammation, abnormal types of cholesterol and heart disease.

Did You Know? Primitive Diet & Potassium

Our primitive ancestors got 7,000 mg potassium and only 600 mg sodium daily, compared with our 2,500 mg potassium and 4,000 mg sodium. We are the only free-living mammals that eat more sodium than potassium. Studies link high-sodium, low-potassium diets to high blood pressure, strokes and heart disease.

WATCH OUT FOR REFINED CARBOHYDRATES

The simple, refined carbohydrates we commonly call sugar are the primary modern fuel for the body. Anyone who has gone through a bout of three p.m. sugar cravings and found himself munching on a candy bar knows how intimately sugar governs alertness, mood, and all of our mental powers. Every cell of your body needs sugar. Your need for sugar is instinctual and genetic. After all, in primitive times our bodies knew that when we tasted something sweet it was coming from a ripened fruit or vegetable, replete with all of its nutritional bounty. But today, modern food processors have learned how to trick our bodies and exploit these ancient instincts. Hence, the lure of the candy bar or after-dinner dessert when we are feeling lethargic or to top off a meal is irresistible. But we are being nutritionally deceived. Instead of receiving the nutritional bounty of God's fruits and sweeteners, our body is simply receiving the empty calories of a Snicker's bar.

Refined carbohydrates like those found in candy, baked goods and other processed foods, are preferred by the pathogenic bacteria in our gastrointestinal tract. So eating too much of them can cause imbalances in the ratio of pathogenic to friendly microorganisms. They can also cause abnormal fermentation, which interferes with digestion. In addition, refined foods are almost identical to table sugar. They cause blood sugar levels to spike and then go down rapidly, exacerbating diabetic and pre-diabetic conditions.

Foods rich in refined carbohydrates are also nutritionally depleted and are substituted in our diet instead of more nutritious wholesome fare.

In addition, refined carbohydrates lead to hormonal imbalances. As most everyone knows, hormones are messenger proteins that regulate bodily functions, ranging from sexual maturation to tissue growth and sleep patterns. When you eat large amounts of carbohydrates, your body produces too much insulin. Not all of us with glucose/insulin problems suffer from overt diabetes. Most of us even with such imbalances would not be considered diabetic. However, according to experts, a lot more people are on the borderline of blood sugar disorders than are typically clinically diagnosed. Many such persons suffer from Syndrome X and have relatively serious blood sugar problems—though not diabetes. Fortunately, blood sugar imbalances can be positively influenced by the Maker's Diet (see Chapter 12).

Pure, organic fruits, vegetables, and a small amount of soaked, fermented or sprouted whole grains, nuts and seeds—grown and processed minimally as our Maker intended—should be our source of carbohydrates, not candies, bread, pasta, baked goods and table sugar. As in the Bible, our primitive ancestors did not eat sugar, either. Their source of sugary sweetness was the rare find of raw wild honey. And even honey, notes the Bible, should be consumed as a treat and not a staple. This is nothing to take away from honey, which, when unheated, raw and unprocessed, is a wonderful source of trace minerals, vitamins, and many other nutrients—especially amylases, enzymes that aid in the digestion of carbohydrates. Nevertheless, we are told in Proverbs 25:27, "It is not good to eat too much honey."

Another insidious form of refined carbohydrates comes from our processing of grains. I know what I'm telling you is probably difficult for some to digest (no pun intended). After all, the cultivation of grain is one of the hallmarks of the agrarian society—of the dawn of modern civilization. Indeed, the tillage of grains—especially wheat and corn—is at the heart of almost every civilization's agricultural practices. The use of the millstone—consisting of two circular stones used for grinding grain—is heralded as one of the great agricultural advancements of early humans.

Many anthropologists believe that our ancestors first stockpiled grains as a storable food source. Interestingly, when their grains got wet, they sprouted. People found that if the grain was planted it yielded yet more seeds.

Perhaps our primitive ancestors realized intuitively that when they sprouted, germinated or fermented grains, their phytonutrients became far more bioavailable. We now know sprouting grains and seeds unlocks their vitamin content, especially the B vitamins, and increases enzyme activity by eight-fold. Another advantage of sprouting and fermenting is that phytic acid and other enzyme inhibitors in grains are neutralized. Phytic acid is the great nutritional robber. It is found in the bran of all grains. If ingested in high amounts, it can rob the body of important minerals such as iron, calcium, and magnesium and prevent their absorption. Soaking and fermenting grains also limits enzyme inhibitors that interfere with the body's digestive enzymes, as well as breaking down the difficult-to-digest disaccharides found in the starch of the grain.

Once again, the Bible provides us with the wisdom our bodies require for the proper assimilation of grains. Take for example the word *pulse*. In Daniel 1:12, Daniel tells Beltashazar, "Prove thy servants, I beseech thee, ten days; and let them give us pulse to eat, and water to drink." In Daniel 1:15, we are further told, "And at the end of ten days their countenances appeared fairer and fatter in flesh than all the children which did eat the portion of the king's meat." We have two definitions of pulse. In the first, we think that pulse is a sprout. In the second we believe that pulse refers to rye grain. Perhaps in Biblical *pulse* we have sprouted rye. This makes sense.

Through much of history, a person's social station could be discerned by the color of bread they consumed. The darker the bread, the lower the social station. This was because whiter flours were more expensive and harder for millers to adulterate with other products and, because they were most expensive, were most coveted by the wealthy members of ancient society. Today, we have seen a reversal of this trend when darker breads are more expensive and highly prized for their taste as well as their nutritional value. Today we nutritionists have our own saying: "The whiter the bread, the sooner you're dead."

Go easy on, or better yet eliminate, pastas and regular breads. I know they seem like they are pretty innocuous foods. But they aren't. Most are highly refined grains and in keeping neither with the primitive diet nor the Maker's wisdom. I truly believe your health will improve tremendously, if you are careful to prefer sprouted or properly prepared sourdough bread from whole organic grains. In the health food store, a typical healthful bread contains organic sprouted wheat, sprouted barley, sprouted millet, sprouted lentils, sprouted soybeans, sprouted spelt. Not surprisingly, our Maker tells Ezekiel (4:9): "Take thou also unto thee wheat, and barley, and beans, and lentils, and millet, and fitches, and put them in one vessel, and make thee bread thereof…"

Today in natural food markets there are several sprouted breads baked by following the recipe found in Ezekiel 4:9.

PROTEIN POWER

Researchers estimate that 20 to 40 percent of our ancestors' diet was made up of protein-rich food, whereas today the percentage of our diet made up of protein is generally only about 15 percent. That's quite a difference, and I think that is why, in some respects, our nation's people are getting so fat. We eat way too many carbohydrates, not enough protein.

Consider that protein along with fat is an essential macronutrient. Believe it or not, the body can live without carbohydrates. If no carbohydrates are consumed, the body can covert proteins and fats into carbohydrates. Proteins are actually made up of long strings of amino acids. We ingest proteins from plant and animal foods and the enzymes in our digestive tract split these into smaller molecules, such as peptides and individual amino acids. These are then used or combined by other enzymes to form important messenger substances in the body (such as hormones, growth factors, cytokines and antibodies) that play key roles in muscle building and tissue repair, as well as immune function. You can see that protein is essential to life.

The body can produce certain amino acids. But others—the essential amino acids—must be obtained exclusively from our diet. Although vegetables and fruits provide proteins, they are incomplete sources of proteins because they lack one or more of the essential amino acids. Beef, chicken, fish, eggs and dairy are complete protein sources, providing all essential amino acids.

Unfortunately, most of what passes for meat today is pathetic. Farm animals are often too crowded and raised inhumanely, fattened on growth stimulants, given sub-therapeutic levels of antibiotics and even fed remnants of other warm-blooded creatures.

In these stifling, politically correct times, I have a different take on protein than a lot of other people. Although I am a complete believer in the humane treatment of all creatures, I don't ascribe to a vegetarian diet. I know People for the Ethical Treatment of Animals and other vegetarian groups oppose consumption of animal foods. Some groups even claim that a true Biblical diet shouldn't contain any animal products. However, two entire chapters in the Bible, Leviticus 11 and Deuteronomy 14 are devoted solely to the consumption of animal foods,which to eat and which to avoid. Jesus consumed and provided flesh foods to his disciples. In Matthew 15:36, we learn, "Then He took the seven loaves and the fish, and when He had given thanks, he broke them and gave them to His disciples, and they in turn to the people."

And in Luke 24:42, upon Jesus' resurrection, we are told that his disciples, "gave him a piece of a broiled fish, and some honeycomb."

As for the supposed dangers of consuming animal foods, our primitive ancestors received most of their protein from meat, fish, eggs, and cultured dairy products but rarely experienced heart disease. I know this may be confusing to some readers because after all we have been taught that meat—especially beef—is the cause of many major illnesses including colon cancer and heart disease. We have even been told that the saturated fat in meat causes clogged arteries and is implicated in heart attacks and stroke.

This couldn't be further from the truth. In fact, the preferred fuel source for the heart is saturated fatty acids. In primitive times, as well as containing healthy saturated fats, our meats were an important source of heart-protective omega-3 fatty acids and even conjugated linoleic acid. They provided the kinds of fats that kept our blood flowing smoothly, fought the ravages of cancer and aided our metabolism so we didn't get rolls of abdominal fat. That is because in the old days, animals grazed on grasses and they bio-accumulated these important fatty acids. Today, animals are kept in pens or otherwise confined and fed foods that are deficient in omega-3 fatty acids and abundant in omega-6 fatty acids (more on that later). As for dairy, it was usually from cows, goats or sheep that were strictly free-range and grass-fed (although goat's eat leaves, herbs and bark as well), raw, cultured and rich in beneficial bacteria, enzymes and other important substances. Our fish was unpolluted, not factory farmed or contaminated with mercury.

Wild meats eaten by our ancestors contained healthier fats than modern farmed cattle, claims Loren Cordain of Colorado State University. He and his colleagues have shown that meat from buffalo, wild elk, deer and antelope contain more beneficial types of fat than meat from today's grain-fed cattle.

Cordain and his team compared the muscle, brain, bone marrow and fat of wild animals with those of cattle. A wild steak has two percent total fat, as opposed to the ten to fifteen percent in commercially available lean beef. Wild meat also contains more omega-3 fatty acids, which are present in oily fish and have been linked to a reduced risk of heart disease and cancer. Meat from pasture-grazed cattle resembles wild meat more closely than meat from cows fed corn and sorghum. Cordain says, "We should try and raise our meat so it emulates wild meat."

Try to purchase only grass-fed beef, buffalo, lamb and venison and free-range or pastured chicken and poultry. Free-range chickens have a natural diet of grass, seeds, and insects. The meat from these chickens as well as their eggs are far more rich sources of all-important omega-3 fatty acids including docosahexaenois acid, an omega-3 fatty acid critical to brain development.

Also, be sure to avoid toxic meat sources. In Leviticus 11:3, God says, "You may eat any animal that has a split hoof completely divided and that chews the cud." In 11:9, we are told, "Of all the creatures living in the water of the seas and the streams, you may eat any that have fins and scales." And in the next verse, we learn, "You must distinguish between the holy and the common, between the unclean and the clean."

Scientists have confirmed the wisdom of distinguishing between the clean and unclean flesh foods. In 1953, Dr. David Macht of Johns Hopkins University conducted a study in which he took all of the clean and unclean foods in the Maker's Diet and compared them for toxicity. He did so by taking a growth culture and adding the flesh to it. If the flesh substance reduced the culture's growth rate below 75 percent it was considered to be toxic. Above 75 percent was considered nontoxic. In all cases, the flesh of the Biblically clean animals tested nontoxic and the flesh of the unclean toxic. The blood of all animals was more toxic than the flesh. We find similar results with clean fowl such as goose, chicken, coot, duck, pigeon, quail, swan and turkey when compared to the unclean, including cormorant, crow, eagle, falcon, hawk, heron, ibis, and raven. The findings are pretty remarkable. Clean animals such as calf, venison, goat, ox, buffalo and lamb were all rated 82 percent or higher. Unclean animals such as swine (pork), bear, camel, cat, guinea pig, dog, fox, groundhog, hamster, horse, opossum, rabbit, rat, rhinoceros, and squirrel rated from 39 to 62 percent. So remember, next time you are tempted to have a rhinoceros burger with cheese, I suggest you pass.

In Leviticus 11:4-8, we are told by our Maker:

Nevertheless among those that chew the cud or part the hoof, you shall not eat these: The camel, because it chews the cud but does not part the hoof, is unclean to you. And the rock badger, because it chews the cud but does not part the hoof, is unclean to you. And the hare, because it chews the cud but does not part the hoof, is unclean to you. And the swine (pig), because it parts the hoof and is cloven-footed but does not chew the cud, is unclean to you. Of their flesh you shall not eat, and their carcasses you shall not touch; they are unclean to you.

Perhaps no dietary commandment is as widely flaunted as that which cautions against consumption of pork. But, again, even in these modern times, there is good reason to heed our Maker's wisdom. In the June 2001 issue of Parasite, researchers from the Department of Animal Hygiene and Prophylaxis, Agricultural University of Szczecin, Poland, note that, "Pork and its products are still the main cause of human trichinellosis in Poland." Furthermore, "epidemics caused by eating wild boar meat suggested that this way of the transmission of Trichinella sp. larvae to humans might be of considerable importance."[47] This is a report from the year 2001 when the most stringent meat inspection procedures are in place in many nations. Imagine what perils our ancestors must have faced.

Many cases of trichinellosis remain undetected. The rate of Trichinella spiralis infection in swine through-out Bolivia is considered to be very high.[48] Although few cases of trichinellosis are reported among swine or humans, a high percentage of people have tested positive for exposure to this parasite. Many people also report various symptoms of trichinellosis, such as headaches, fever, and swelling in the extremities. Clearly, many people are made ill from this parasite, though it remains underdiagnosed.

The Maker warned against consumption of creatures of the sea without fins or scales. Why would we be warned against shellfish consumption? Again, these foods are likely to carry dangerous pathogens. A friend of mine who served on the seafood safety committee of the National Academy of Sciences tells me that committee members considered the odds to be about one in 300 that anyone eating raw or cooked shellfish in American today will become seriously ill with infectious disease. That's a very high rate of potential for serious illness. Shellfish are a source of cholera as well as diseases involving paralysis. Shellfish are filter or bottom feeders. They help to purify their environment but they themselves accumulate pathogens and other contaminants. Many caretakers of ponds and other bodies of water know the best way to purify a freshwater pond or lake is to throw loads of scallops in and wait a few days. The lake will be purified and the scallops will float to the top. The same can be said of other scavengers such as oysters, clams, shrimp, and lobster.

The scavengers that the Maker warned us against play a critical role in our environment. But, remember, our Maker told us to eat only certain flesh foods with cloven hooves and that chew the cud and certain fowl. As for the rest, this question is posed in Job 14:4: "Who can bring a clean thing out of an unclean? Not one."

THE SEARCH FOR A HEALTHY PROTEIN POWDER

There is no question of the importance of protein in our diet. But when I began my search for the ultimate protein with which to supplement our diet it was a more difficult task than first thought. Nearly every producer of protein powder in the industry provided product from non-organic, highly processed cow's milk or soy. Due to the fact that I consider both sources inadequate at best, I began to search for alternatives. Then it happened, and I found what I consider to be the world's finest protein powder ever offered—one suited for infants, the elderly and even professional athletes.

Goat's milk is the most widely consumed dairy beverage in the world. Fully 65 percent of the world's population drinks goat's milk. Goat's milk has been a staple in much of the world since Biblical times. For people with intestinal disorders, goat's milk and goat's milk products have the potential to heal. Whereas cow's milk requires up to three hours to be absorbed, goat's milk requires only twenty minutes. At half the size of those in cow's milk, the protein molecules in goat's milk have thinner, more fragile membranes. For that reason, they are easier to absorb through the wall of the small intestine. Here are some of the other advantages of drinking goat's milk:

- It is less allergic than cow's milk because it doesn't contain the protein complexes in cow's milk that stimulate allergic reactions. Children who have allergic reactions to cow's milk have seen their allergies improve after switching to goat's milk.
- It doesn't as readily produce gas or bloating. Because goat's milk is digested quickly, it doesn't remain in the small intestine and ferment. It contains seven percent less lactose than cow's milk.
- It is high in the medium-chain fatty acids that inhibit candida.
- It is not mucus forming.

- It is a rich source of selenium. This mineral is believed to be an immuno-regulator. It quickens a sluggish immune system but quiets an overactive one. In this way, selenium keeps the immune system in tune and well balanced.
- It doesn't contain the *Mycobacterium avium subspecies paratuberculosis* (MAP) microorganism.

As quoted by world-famous clinical nutritionist and chiropractic physician Bernard Jensen, Ph.D., D.C., of Escondido, California, the *Journal of the American Medical Association* (*JAMA*), under its heading of Dietetics and Hygiene, states: "The goat is the healthiest domestic animal known. Goat milk is superior in every way to cow's milk. Goat milk is the ideal food for babies, convalescents and invalids, especially those with weakened digestive powers. Goat milk is the purest, most healthful and most complete food known."[49]

Goatein, the first and only protein powder made from goat's milk, is a highly concentrated powdered protein rich in amino acids in both their peptide and free forms. Among the goat products' components are the biologically active amino acids cystine, glycine, and glutamic acid. These three are precursors to glutathione formation by the body. As is generally known, glutathione functions as a principal antioxidant, scavenging free radicals and environmental toxins such as lipid peroxides that often damage and destroy healthy cells. Anyone suffering from oxidative stress, with its resultant nervous system, immune system, and endocrine system dysfunctions accompanied by fatigue, undergoes marked loss of physiological glutathione.

Goatein also provides immunoproteins such as albumin, lactalbumin, and lactoferin, which have been proven to stimulate immune response. Additionally, it's a balanced combination of whey protein and milk proteins that offers a favorable ratio of amino acids.

The amino acids vital for health maintenance present in one serving of Goatein are shown in the table (*below*). Goat's milk furnishes the growth materials each person requires for tissue repair, energy, the production of hormones, enzymes, antibodies, cellular components, amino acids, immunoglobulins, and every other part of the human physiology. As an animal source, it contains complete protein unlike any vegetable protein such as soy; and goat's milk is much less allergenic than cow's milk.

"The fat particles in goat's cream are five times smaller than those in cow's milk and much less hard on the liver," says Dr. Jensen. He adds, "Goat's milk is sometimes superior to mother's milk, because goat's milk contains food elements that mother's milk does not contain."[50]

Dr. Gloria Gilbère Counteracts Her Patients' Multiple Chemical Sensitivities with Goatein

Being aware of the statement from *JAMA* about the nutritional superiority of goat's milk, the practicing naturopath, homeopath, and ergonomist Gloria Gilbère, N.D., D.A.Hom., Ph.D., states: "Goat protein (in the form of Goatein) has been special in my practice because almost exclusively I put my

The Amino Acid Profile of Goatein

Alanine......................2.8%	Isoleucine*................4.8%	Threonine.................4.8%
Arginine 2.9%	Leucine*....................9.4%	Tryptophan*..............1.0%
Apaftic Acid 6.0%	Lysine*......................6.4%	Tyrosine.....................3.9%
Cystine/Cysteine........0.5%	Methionine*..............2.9%	Valine* 7.1%
Glutamic Acid 21.2%	Phenylalanine*..........4.4%	*Essential Amino Acid
Glycine.....................1.4%	Proline....................12.5%	
Histidine 2.6%	Serine*......................5.4%	

attention on chemically induced immune disorders and leaky gut syndrome. Most of the patients who consult me for treatment are so chemically sensitive that most of the time they're unable to assimilate any kind of food except perhaps vegetable juices and wild rice. This same circumstance happened to me too from my being affected by multiple chemical sensitivity. That's why I moved to this out-of-the-way but pristine environment, Bonners Ferry in northern Idaho. Along with avoiding chemicals of all types, eating a purely natural and nontoxic diet, and taking various nutritional supplements containing no binders, my personal treatment involves drinking copious quantities of goat's milk in the form of Goatein powder ingested in smoothies, shakes, cooked oatmeal, muffins and other ways."

As its medical director, Dr. Gloria Gilbère administers to patients attending her Naturopathic Health and Research Center. The tiny town of Bonners Ferry is located 90 miles south of the Canadian border, sandwiched between Montana and Washington State. This natural health doctor tells her inspiring tale of immunological restoration from multiple chemical sensitivities in a book she published last year under the title, *I Was Poisoned By My Body*, with a short excerpt reprinted in the *Townsend Letter for Doctors & Patients*:[51]

"People who are nutritionally deprived or those who suffer from livers overburdened with immune system breakdown due to their excessive use of prescription drugs, street drugs, overindulgence of alcohol, environmental toxins, eating overly processed diets, or just engaging in bad lifestyle choices, do reach a point where protein can't be handled any more. By ingesting Goatein the way I do in a smoothie, shake, or in cooked but cooled cereal, concentrated protein becomes available to them so that their bodies can use all of it. That way they avoid anaphylactic shock and still receive excellent nourishment," Dr. Gilbère affirms. "This goat's milk protein becomes bioavailable, is easy on the digestive system, and brings on absolutely no disturbance to serious gastrointestinal disorders such as Crohn's disease, irritable bowel syndrome, leaky gut, and other conditions which lock people into acute states of chemical sensitivity. Remember, in my practice I deal strictly with people who are highly sensitive to almost anything. Items such as nightshade foods, soy, cow's milk, wheat, and gluten set them off. They are predisposed to respond adversely with serious symptoms such as skin rashes, gastrointestinal refluxes, anaphylaxis or some other negative reactions," explains Dr. Gilbère. "When I recommend that they use Goatein and they do, I never need to worry about negative reactions because in this goat's milk product there are no pesticides, hormones, antibiotics, steroids, or any other chemicals to which such sensitive people can react. I dispense Goatein to my patients with peace of mind.

About 14 months ago, one such patient, a surgical nurse, age 54, moved into a recently constructed hospital facility and became chemically sensitive almost overnight from all of the outgassings of new building materials," explains Dr. Gilbere. "The overriding symptom was her inability to eat anything—no appetite at all. Within a couple of months her body weight dropped by over 35% to just 92 pounds. She became a shadow of her former self. Her weakness prevented the performance of any meaningful activity—certainly she could not work in surgical nursing or do her housekeeping chores.

"Immediately I began my patient on a detoxification program because she failed to eliminate her body wastes. She was experiencing just one bowel movement per week," states Dr. Gilbère, "and that was accomplished only with much concentration. She would spend large amounts of time in the bathroom trying to eliminate and often without result. But the goat's milk protein along with other components of my program changed all that.

"After finding that the nurse could not tolerate even the blandest vegetable juices, I introduced her to Goatein combined with rice milk as a smoothie drink. She took to this protein drink well and relied on it as almost the only thing ingested; it helped her put on 12 pounds in five weeks without any gastrointestinal cramping," Dr. Gilbère says. "Her bowels became more normal with a movement occurring every second day. It's now a year later, and my patient experiences two bowel movements daily.

"She currently supplements any form of protein she ingests with Goatein because even today, this surgical nurse is unable to eat any other animal-derived products—no yogurt, cow's milk, eggs, fish, shellfish, meat, or poultry. Moreover the patient is highly lactose-intolerant, but she finds Goatein to be quite digestible as the mainstay of her diet. It is a minimally processed product that does not cause excitation to a lactose intolerant bowel. Truly, I am an enthusiastic advocate of using Goatein for any chemically sensitive patients," affirms Dr. Gilbère.

The Nutritional Science Behind Goatein

Biologically active proteins make up much but not all the nutrient components in Goatein. As mentioned, this product furnishes the only available protein powder that comes from organically raised goat's milk. All other milk products consumed in North America are manufactured from bovine sources or from vegetables such as rice. Goatein is minimally processed. Most other milk protein powders are made from cow's milk and, even though cow's milk manufacturers claim that their product is "minimally processed," they may use several invasive processing steps, including heating at high temperatures. These methods denature many important amino acids and destroy enzymes and beneficial bacteria. Research suggests that processing whey with heat and acid (i.e. ion-exchange) results in the loss of several key amino acids including 73 to 77 percent of cysteine, 35 to 45 percent of threonine, 18 to 30 percent of serine, and 19 to 20 percent of lysine. Because Goatein is processed without the use of acid or excessive heat, the amino acids, enzymes, and beneficial bacteria remain in their natural form.

Nanny goats produce milk which almost duplicates human breast milk. The nanny's natural function is to feed her kid (a baby goat) weighing between seven and nine pounds, which is the size of a human baby. In contrast, the cow's newborn calf weighs as high as 90 pounds so that bovine milk's chemicals, including its fat and protein, are tailored to fit the needs of a baby animal quite different in size than a newborn human. Molecules of the cow's milk protein are overly large for digestion and absorption by human infants, and for this reason, among others, cow's milk frequently incites allergic responses in a child.

By being injected with bovine growth hormone (BGH), a dairy cow can produce 12 gallons of milk daily as opposed to the goat which can produce only up to 2 gallons a day. The BGH stimulates a cow's mammary glands to secrete excessively, but the hormone is absorbed in the animal's dairy product. There is risk associated with endocrine imbalance caused by cow's milk. In contrast, Goatein is free of hormones, antibiotics, and pesticides. The goats graze on pasture and are fed chemical-free feed.

Since it goes through the most minimal processing of any protein product on the market today, the very low heat drying process for Goatein leaves its nutritional values intact. The product is highly concentrated. It takes four gallons of goat's milk to produce one container of Goatein. Moreover, as I will discuss below, highly beneficial microorganisms or probiotics are contained in Goatein.

The English word protein comes from the Latin proteus, which means of primary importance. The vast number of amino acids in Goatein protein are essential for normal growth. They give rise to all connective tissues, enzymes, hormones, antibodies, muscles, skin, bones, hair, nails, heart, teeth, blood, brain, biochemical activities, and the entire nervous system. Protein deficiency is responsible for the lowering of immune function and for much of the immune system suppression diseases that the medical community is currently confronting.

This product is ideal for those who prefer not to eat meat because of its hormonal content. Athletes who must maintain an anabolic state (the building of tissue) certainly wish to avoid residues of hormones in meat. But most cattle is fed or injected with female hormones for purposes of producing greater amounts of meat. Unless they are labeled growth hormone-free, every protein powder marketed today is most likely produced by cows treated with hormones. Goatein is not; it is growth hormone-free. No goat which could be medicated in any way is allowed to be milked for this food powder's production.

Added to these attributes, Goatein contains super-potent proprietary strains of probiotics. These super-strains of probiotics are grown in goat's milk protein creating biologically active lactic acid and increasing the absorption and utilization of Goatein. Thus, energy production and fat burning are stimulated to take place from the gut upon ingesting Goatein. This fermentation by lactic acid bacteria is essential for well-maintained pH balance of the GI tract and other bodily tissues. In his text, *The Milk of Human Kindness Is not Pasteurized*, William Campbell Douglass, M.D., states that protein contained in cultured (lacto-fermented) dairy products is the very highest quality available for human consumption.[52]

Research among the Vilcabambans high in the Andes mountains of Ecuador and other long-lived populations on Earth indicates that they consume lacto-fermented dairy products mainly from goat's milk. It is from just such consumption that Los Viejos' (the old ones) longevity arises. An individual's regular consumption of cultured (lacto-fermented) dairy products such as Goatein tends to lower serum cholesterol and protect the skeleton against osteoporosis. Anyone healing from a bone fracture or some osteoporotic break should be consuming this powdered goat's milk product. Goatein is abundant in digestive enzymes created by the probiotics which include protease, amylase, lipase, and lactase. Such enzymes contribute to the health of the digestive tract.

Goatein IG with Goat's Milk Colostrum

At Garden of Life, we are now also producing Goatein IG caplets (the "IG" represents immunoglobulins), a protein source that also incorporates pure goat's milk colostrum in a lacto-fermented, enzymatically pre-digested form, designed to increase nutrient absorption and bioavailability two to five times. Colostrum is the fluid manufactured by the body prior to the production of mother's milk during the first 24 to 48 hours after birth. Studies have shown that colostrum has powerful, life-supporting immune and growth factors that ensure the health and vitality of the newborn. It brings the body into a natural state of equilibrium called "homeostasis," vital to health and well-being. While supporting healthy immune function, colostrum also enables us to resist the harmful effects of pollutants, contaminants and allergens. In addition, the growth factors in colostrum enhance the ability of a healthy organism to burn fat, build lean muscle mass and rejuvenate skin and cellular structure.

Colostrum is highly beneficial in the unique manner in which it provides the body with numerous immune factors. According to medical research, the presence of a wide spectrum of immunoglobulins, antibodies, and potent immune and growth factors found in colostrum offers tremendous therapeutic potential for overall health and wellness. Laboratory studies confirm that colostrum has the unique ability to support normal cell growth and tissue repair, yielding exciting, new possibilities for system-wide rejuvenation. Aging and illness occur with the gradual loss of immune and growth factors in the body after maturity. The onset of almost all infection and degenerative disease is preceded or accompanied by lowered immune system function. Colostrum contains powerful immune factors (immunoglobulin, lactoferrin, cytokines, etc.) that work to restore optimal immune functioning.

Colostrum also contains Proline-rich polypeptide (PRP), shown in clinical analysis to both enhance an underactive immune system and balance an overactive tendency. Doctors recognize that most pathogens enter the body through the mucous membranes in the bowel, then through to the intestinal tract. The majority of antibodies and immunoglobulins in colostrum are not absorbed, but remain in the intestinal tract where they attack these pathogens before they can penetrate the body's defenses. "Immunoglobulins (found in colostrum) are able to neutralize even the most harmful bacteria, viruses, and yeasts," states Dr. Per Brandtzaeg. Goatein IG contains a virtual army of immunoproteins, including PRP, which supports and regulates the thymus gland, lactoferrin, a protein that transports essential iron to the red blood cells and prevents harmful bacteria from utilizing the iron they require to grow and flourish, and lactalbumins, which research indicates may be highly effective against numerous viruses. This powerful combination of dietary peptides and growth factors makes Goatein IG an extremely important supplement for the elderly, people with compromised digestion, and those suffering from malnutrition and muscle wasting.

Goatein IG contains bioactive peptides. Dietary peptides have been shown to suppress abnormal immune cell activity and minimize the damaging side effects of radiation and chemotherapy. The amino acid L-tryptophan can be effective in cases of insomnia and depression. Glutamine, an important amino acid for building lean body mass and immune health, is not effectively absorbed when taken in combination with other amino adds due to competitive absorption. However, Goatein IG bonds glutamine with a peptide, increasing absorption many hundreds of times. The glutamine contained in Goatein IG aids in the body's ability to repair itself after intense workouts or injury. Medical studies have shown that growth factors in colostrum can help the body regenerate normal growth of muscle, bone, cartilage, skin, collagen and nerve tissue; help burn fat for fuel instead of muscle tissue during dieting; help build and retain lean muscle; synthesize DNA and RNA; balance and regulate blood sugar levels; heal burns, cuts, abrasions and mouth sores with topical application; and help regulate blood glucose levels and "brain chemicals," providing alertness and better concentration.

The manufacturing of Goatein takes place in a farming facility outside of Olympia, Washington. I had contacted many of the largest organic dairies in this country, but none were capable of producing a low-temperature processed, chemical-free protein powder. Then I found a small goat farm outside of Olympia Washington. I challenged the dairy personnel to meet my high standards of protein manufacturing; fortunately, they were already practicing or surpassing those standards. I looked at how they handle their animals—avoiding pesticides in their feed, not subjecting them to antibiotics or hormones, minimally heating our products, and routinely creating the highest quality goat's milk products available anywhere for human consumption.

Goat's milk is digested readily because its protein molecule is tiny in size and floculant. This makes the milk's molecule easily attacked by digestive juices for rapid absorption through the gut wall. The protein molecule in cow's milk, being large and dense, is much less digestible by humans.

In Washington, D.C., Susana Galle, N.D., Ph.D., directs the Body-Mind Center where she practices clinical psychology combined with her unique form of body-mind science. Dr. Galle incorporates Goatein as an integral part of her nutritional treatment program for both the body and mind.

"I utilize the goat's milk product in many ways for improving an individual's brain-behavior relationship. Most people need more absorbable protein, and I custom-make recipes for children and adult clients, especially for someone suffering from a cow's milk allergy. I appreciate the fact that Goatein is no ordinary protein powder; it possesses more friendly fat molecules which provide me with excellent therapeutic results," says Dr. Galle. "It is a main pillar in my treatment structure because of the free-form amino acids present—they are easily digested and allow for excellent absorption.

"I have created Goatein recipes in which the goat's milk protein powder becomes a part of muffins and waffles. That way an individual receives a quantity of protein in a subtle way that's absolutely delicious. Consuming the Goatein in such a recipe furnishes high levels of energy."

The medical director of South Coast Medical and Anti-aging Institute in Newport Beach, California, Leigh Erin Connealy, M.D., says, "Most patients who consult me show signs that they are not getting an adequate amount of protein in their diets. And there is controversy as to what should be the source of protein—soy, whey, cow's milk, fish, meat, eggs, etc. Because there is so much genetically altered protein, which often contains too many additives, I've solved the controversy for myself. My recommendation is that a person's main protein source should be goat's milk from organically raised goats in the convenient powder form of Goatein. I am definitely not an exponent of soy because of its carcinogenic aspects for the breast, and because it usually tastes bad. If people must eat soy, they should take it from an organic source. But my rule is to generally avoid soy and other types of designer proteins.

"As the mother of three children, it was my standard practice to feed them liquid goat's milk, but now I'm happy to recommend powdered Goatein as the liquid's handy substitute. Garden of Life, Inc. provides consumers with an excellent protein supplement," affirms Dr. Connealy. "I advise my patients to make a shake with the powder and add fruit, nuts, seeds, and other foods, especially peaches, berries, and so forth that they wish to include. Such combinations are highly nutritious and taste wonderful. I love to recommend Goatein and take it myself.

"The basic philosophy of my South Coast Medical and Anti-aging Institute is to treat illnesses affecting people without drugs but rather use nontoxic and natural remedies. Goatein fits that description beautifully," concludes Dr. Connealy.

GOOD FAT, BAD FAT

America is suffering from fear—some might say pure unadulterated hatred—of fat. Sure, we know that the wrong fats will cause you to gain weight, clog your arteries, and promote cancer. But we also know that too little fat is also a killer.

Most people have it all wrong and they hate *all* fat. Fat hatred is dogma among many still today. Mary Enig and others have written very persuasively that the studies done in the 1950s that formed the basis of the lipid hypothesis were flawed. The original researchers failed to distinguish between different kinds of fat. They concluded all fat to be bad—saturated, monounsaturated, or polyunsaturated.[53]

I believe the real culprits in heart disease are obscenely elevated intakes of human-made trans fatty acids, polyunsaturated fats high in omega-6 fatty acids and the overconsumption of carbohydrates.

Let's go to Greece for a moment and get a clearer picture of this good fat/bad fat concept. In Greece, the typical diet consists of 40 percent fat (the same percentage as in the United States), but Greek men and women have significantly lower rates of heart disease, prostate and breast cancer.

It isn't fat *per se* that is the enemy—but the type of fat. The Greek diet is loaded with omega-3 and monounsaturated (omega-9) fatty acids, conjugated linoleic acid (CLA), as well as healthy saturated fats. These are the good fats that come from salmon, walnuts, purslane, olives, lamb and goat meat, and goat's and sheep's milk and cheese, and other properly prepared dairy products—the fats that we don't get enough of from our American diet anymore. Dr. Murray has commented on more than one occasion,

"Most people have decreased their consumption of natural, unadulterated essential fatty acids and drastically increased their consumption of refined and adulterated fats and oils."[54]

Our ingestion of omega-6 fatty acids has skyrocketed with the advent of seed extraction technology during the industrial revolution. Oils such as sunflower, safflower, peanut, and corn oil are dominant in omega-6 fatty acids, while being virtually void of beneficial omega-3 fatty acids.

Saturated fats are solid at room temperature. They are stable and do not go rancid even when they are heated, which makes them ideal for cooking even at high temperatures. Saturated fats are found mostly in animal and dairy products, as well as tropical oils such as coconut, palm and palm kernel oils. These saturated fats also contain healing short-chain and medium-chain fatty acids that are very important to our health. Traditional foods contain appreciable amounts of other beneficial fats, including conjugated linoleic acid, caprylic acid, lauric acid, butyric acid and omega-3 fatty acids. These fatty acids are extremely beneficial to the health of the immune system and digestive tract. They can supply a significant portion of our energy requirements. But today our cloven-hoofed friends are fed terrible diets, rarely graze on grass, and, as a result, no longer contain appreciable amounts of beneficial omega-3 fatty acids or other healthy fats.

Dramatic scientific research shows that excess amounts of trans-fatty acids (manmade molecules created from hydrogenating vegetable oils) are killers, increasing risk for heart disease, cancer, diabetes, and other age-related maladies. You'll find these bad fats in margarines, many baked goods and other processed foods.

Until World War II, much of the added fat or oil in the diet, other than the animal, poultry, and dairy fats, came either from small presses such as those used for flaxseed oil in Eastern Europe or larger presses used for olive oil. But following World War II, the food industry capitalized on its ability to turn liquid oils, which were plentiful, but not sufficiently marketable, into solid fats for the budding fast-food industry and for the expanding baking and snack food industries.

It was the beginning of a nutritional disaster. Profits made in the ensuing years came at the expense of public health. Scientists' main concern about their health effects arise because of the structural similarity of these isomers to saturated fatty acids yet their paradoxical lack of specific metabolic functions, and competition with essential fatty acids. Today, researchers consider trans fatty acids to be a major cause of heart disease. Trans fatty acids, for example, increase circulating levels of lipoprotein(a), a non-dietary-related risk of atherogenesis.

If the ingredients list on a food includes partially hydrogenated vegetable oil, then the food contains trans fats. Trans fats are found only in foods that have been altered and conform neither to the primitive diet nor the intent of our Maker.

On the other hand, accumulating evidence from molecular and cellular biology experiments, experimental studies, and human clinical trials suggests omega-3 fatty acids, as well as short- and medium-chain fatty acids, may potentially confer important health benefits related to cardiovascular disease, cancer prevention, and reducing inflammation. These potential health benefits are consistent with epidemiological evidence that rates of heart disease, various cancers, bone fractures in people with osteoporosis, and menopausal symptoms are much less prevalent among populations that consume diets rich in omega-3, short- and medium-chain fatty acids.[55]

Omega-3 fatty acids fight heart disease by lowering dangerous LDL cholesterol and triglycerides, as well as decreasing the viscosity of thick blood, and reducing the build up of atherosclerotic plaque on artery walls. "Population studies demonstrate that people who consume a diet rich in omega-3 oils from either fish or vegetable sources have a significantly reduced risk of developing heart disease," says Dr. Murray.[56] "Over 60 double-blind studies show that either fish oil supplements or flaxseed oil [both rich in omega-3 fatty acids] are very effective in lowering blood pressure."

There may not be a single nutritional supplement or pharmacological drug today that can offer the same level of protection against cancer and other diseases as delivered with the combination of the good fats, including the omega-3 fatty acids and the saturated fats, particularly those rich in medium- and short-chain fatty acids that I describe below.

Unfortunately, modern processing has eliminated the good fats from our diet. "Most researchers describe a healthy balance of omega-6 to omega-3 oils as anywhere from 1: 1, to 3 or 4: 1," notes nutritionist Lalitha Davis, author of *10 Essential Foods*. "You probably won't be surprised to learn that the balance of these two essential fatty acids in the body of the average American is about 20:1! This basic nutrient imbalance (much more omega-6 than is healthy in balance with omega-3) is caused by a diet high in processed and refined foods, grains and grocery store vegetable oils which are highly refined with toxic chemicals, and domestic animal meats fed mostly grain."

'Good' Saturated Fats

But I want to go beyond simply telling you about omega-3 fatty acids because truthfully, many other fats are also important to your health and so many people know next to nothing about them. As I mentioned, the modern health experts tell us to avoid fat and especially saturated fat. The modern health expert tells us fat consumption is responsible for heart disease, obesity and cancer. They have been especially harsh on the use of tropical oils such as coconut, palm and palm kernel oil. "While this claim has been widely disproved in many scientific studies and journals, unfortunately this perception is still around," notes Dr. Enig. "The tropical oils were very popular in the [United States] food industry prior to World War II. With the war and the shortages of imported tropical oils, an effort was made to promote local oils, like soybean and corn oil. The [U.S.] is the largest exporter of soybeans. Studies were done to show that coconut oil, and all saturated fats, were bad for one's health because they raised serum cholesterol levels. However, these studies were done on hydrogenated coconut oil, and *all hydrogenated oils produce higher serum cholesterol levels*, whether they are saturated or not. Recent research shows that it is the presence of *trans fatty acids* that causes health problems, as they are fatty acid chains that have been altered from their original form in nature by the oil refining process."

Among saturated fats that have taken the worst beating is butter. Coconut oil has also been routinely criticized. We have been told that soy, corn, canola, safflower, sunflower and cottonseed oils were the preferred oils—or, at least, these are the ones our major food companies are using in products today. And, of course, margarine is king. Again, we have long been told that margarine is healthier. Once again, our so-called nutritional and health experts have steered us upon a bitter course. Butter, coconut oil, and animal fats have nourished human beings for several thousands of years. Yet, nowadays, these healthy foods have been relegated and replaced by new-fangled concoctions of very questionable nutritional value.

Saturated animal fat is an essential and vital part of many diets. The Masai, and related tribes in East Africa, consume a diet almost completely composed of beef, milk, and blood (which neither the Bible nor I recommend), note experts. At some parts of the year, a typical Masai warrior will consume up to 10 quarts of whole, raw cow's milk a day. The Masai are noted for their tall stature and great endurance. Heart disease, obesity, diabetes, osteoporosis, and cancer are unknown to the Masai. The Masai are also the most feared warriors, as they are healthier than virtually any of their surrounding neighbors who eat a much more vegetarian diet.

The Eskimos are another good example of a people who have historically thrived with a diet comprised largely of animal products, including huge amounts of blubber (fat) from various marine animals. Given the climate they live in, Eskimos are not frequent consumers of grains, fruits, or vegetables. Eskimos who have not abandoned their native diet have virtually no incidence of heart disease, cancer, arteriosclerosis, osteoporosis, or diabetes. Some studies have appeared in recent years attempting to show that Eskimos suffer from bone loss due to their high protein diets, but such studies have been discredited when researchers note that only those Eskimos who abandoned their native diet for "civilized" food and alcohol suffered from calcium loss.

More examples could be provided to prove that saturated fat consumption, even when very high, is not implicated in heart disease or cancer. Despite this, the prevailing dietary opinion is that saturated fat is bad and should be avoided.

Let's look at sources of some of the healthy saturated fats.

Butter

As an excellent source of fat-soluble vitamins, butter is rich in lecithin (needed for fat metabolism), trace minerals (particularly selenium), arachidonic acid (needed for prostaglandin production), and short- and medium-chain fatty acids that the body uses for energy. Two of these fatty acids, butyric and lauric acids both have anti-tumor, antifungal, and antimicrobial properties. Studies have shown that vitamins and minerals from vegetables are better absorbed when eaten with butter. Butter also provides the intestines with the fatty material needed to convert carotenes from plants into vitamin A. It is best to choose butter that is from goat's or sheep's milk or from cow's milk free from growth hormones and from grass-fed animals.

Lamb and Beef

Mostly found in lamb and beef tallow, stearic acid is the preferred fuel source for the heart. That's right, despite current dietary wisdom telling us that saturated fat is bad for the heart, the heart excels at converting fatty acids into energy for itself. Lamb tallow is also rich in oleic acid, another very beneficial fat for the cardiovascular system. Palm oil and olive oil are also rich in oleic acid.

Extra Virgin Coconut Oil

Extra virgin coconut oil is perhaps the most avoided miracle food, and I'm going to be devoting a major portion of my time to telling more and more people about its benefits. Coconut has been used as cooking oil for thousands of years. Popular cookbooks advertised it at the end of the nineteenth century. Then came the campaign against saturated fats and in favor of vegetable-sourced polyunsaturated fats such as canola, soybean, safflower, corn, and other seed and nut oils, plus their partially hydrogenated counterparts (such as margarine; some of us recall the "I can't believe it's not butter" advertising campaigns). I certainly can believe it isn't!

Although saturated fats have never been linked to heart disease in well-designed, honest epidemiological studies, nearly all commercial foods today avoid saturated fats, instead relying on polyunsaturated or partially hydrogenated vegetable fats. These may be "all vegetarian," "no-cholesterol" foods. But they're not necessarily better for your health. Indeed, for the last four decades, Americans have increased their consumption of unsaturated fats and partially hydrogenated fats and have decreased their consumption of saturated fatty acids and butter and the rate of deaths caused by heart disease has increased, as has obesity and many immune system disorders.

Here's why I recommend coconut oil:

- Foods cooked in coconut oil taste better longer. If left at room temperature unsaturated oils turn rancid fairly quickly. However, even after one year at room temperature, coconut oil shows no evidence of rancidity. Coconut oil is packed with antioxidants, and it also reduces the body's need for vitamin E.
- Coconut oil stimulates thyroid function which, in turn, stimulates conversion of production of low-density lipoprotein cholesterol into the anti-aging prohormones and hormones pregnenolone, progesterone and dehydroepiandrosterone (DHEA). These valuable agents prevent heart disease, senility, obesity, cancer and other diseases associated with premature aging, as well as chronic, degenerative diseases.
- Another benefit from coconut oil's unique ability to support thyroid function is weight loss. In the 1940s, farmers tried coconut oil to fatten their animals but discovered that it made them lean and active and increased their appetite, notes an expert. Whoops! Then they tried an anti-thyroid drug. It made the livestock fat with less food but was found to be a carcinogen (cancer-causing drug). In the late 1940s, it was found that the same anti-thyroid effect could be achieved by simply feeding animals soybeans and corn.
- Coconut oil protects against cancer. Generally speaking, animals fed unsaturated oils develop more tumors.

• Coconut oil has tremendous antiviral properties. Coconut oil contains medium-chain fatty acids such as lauric, caprylic and capric acids. Of these three, coconut oil contains 40-55 percent lauric acid, which has the greatest antiviral activity of these three fatty acids. Lauric acid is so adept at fighting viral pathogens it is present in large quantities in breast milk. The body converts lauric acid to a fatty acid derivative (monolaurin), which is the substance that protects infants and adults alike from viral, bacterial or protozoal infections.

It's important to prefer extra virgin coconut oil using fresh coconut meat or what is called non-copra (see below for a definition of copra). Chemicals and high heating are not used in further refining. The method used in the Philippines to produce extra virgin coconut oil from coconut milk is fermentation. The coconut milk expressed from the freshly harvested coconuts is fermented for 24 to 36 hours. During this time, the water separates from the oil. The oil is then slightly heated for a short time to remove moisture, and filtered. The result is a clear coconut oil that retains the distinct scent and taste of coconuts. This is a traditional method of coconut oil extraction that has been used in the Philippines for hundreds of years. Laboratory tests show that this is a very high-quality coconut oil, with the lauric acid content being 50 to 53 percent. This oil is not mass produced, but made by hand just as it has been done for hundreds of years. Since the producers of the oil live in the community where the coconuts grow, they personally guarantee that the best organic coconuts available are used in producing this extra virgin coconut oil, and that no chemicals whatsoever are used in the growing or processing of the coconuts.

Most commercial grade coconut oils are made from copra, which is the dried kernel (meat) of the coconut. Copra is made by smoke drying, sun drying, kiln drying, or a combination of these methods. If standard copra is used as a starting material, the unrefined coconut oil extracted from copra is not suitable for consumption and must be further refined. This is because the way most copra is dried is very unsanitary. Most of the copra is dried under the sun in the open air, where it is exposed to insects and molds. The standard end product made from copra is RBD coconut oil. RBD stands for refined, bleached, and deodorized. Both high heat and chemical solvents are used in this method.

The RBD oil is also often hydrogenated or partially hydrogenated. Thus, it is not a very good product.

Another difference between extra virgin coconut oil and refined coconut oils is the scent and taste. Extra virgin retains the fresh scent and taste of coconuts, whereas the copra-based refined coconut oils have no taste at all due to the refining process.

Promising studies have been done on patients suffering from immune deficiency diseases. So you can see that I'm a big fan of the healing properties of coconut oil. As you will read in the protocol section, I recommend virtually everyone consume coconut oil on a daily basis. I truly believe that coconut oil is the best widely available oil to use for cooking and baking and is even great when used externally to promote smooth and supple skin.

Dairy Products

Another important source of fats in the diet is dairy. Although not all peoples of the world consumed dairy products in abundance, primitive nomads drank the milk of their cattle, goats and sheep. Primitive people, however, fermented milk products as a means of preserving them. Archeologists have found Sumerian tablets dating to six thousand years ago that explain how to ferment milk to prepare cheese. Yogurt has been a food staple of the Middle East and Caucasian Mountains for many thousands of years. The Godly men of the Bible were shepherds and herdsmen. Abel, Job, Abraham, Isaac, Jacob, Jacob's twelve sons, David, and others all had very large numbers of livestock. In fact, in Biblical times the amount of wealth and stature one had was measured in the number of livestock kept. Jacob's entire household was in the profession of animal husbandry. That is why they settled in Goshen, for the Egyptians did not like keepers of animals. No doubt, the chosen people of God ate and enjoyed dairy products, as well as meat.

The biggest difference between our milk and the milk that primitive people drank can be seen in the destructive processes of pasteurization, homogenization and the removal of fat or the skimming process. Today, the non-organic milk that most people drink comes from cows that have been fed hormones and antibiotics. A century ago, a Holstein, a popular breed of dairy cow produced 400 to 500 pounds of milk annually. Today, the average Holstein produces 20,000 to 30,000 pounds! This high milk production is due in part to use of bovine growth hormone and other factory farm methods. Such hormone-treated cows produce milk that is high in a protein called insulin-like growth factor-1 (IGF-1). This protein stimulates cell growth and has been associated with certain kinds of cancer, especially prostate cancer. Cows are often raised in close quarters and are therefore subject to infectious diseases. Due to excessive milking, their udders are usually excoriated and infected. For those reasons, cows are fed antibiotics.

Most people cannot conceive of drinking milk or taking any milk product unless it has been pasteurized. Pasteurization is named for Louis Pasteur, the French scientist who invented the process. In pasteurization, milk is heat-treated to destroy disease-causing bacteria. Some have argued that stainless steel tanks and other sanitizing innovations in the milk production industry have made pasteurization unnecessary. Here are some of the drawbacks of pasteurized milk:

- Like antibiotics, pasteurization kills good as well as harmful bacteria. Raw milk contains lactic-acid-producing bacteria. Lactic acid can kill certain pathogens and thereby prevent disease.
- Pasteurization kills the enzymes in milk. The lack of these enzymes makes milk harder to digest.
- Pasteurization lowers the potency of some vitamins in milk, chiefly vitamin C and B12. It also makes calcium, magnesium, phosphorus, and sulfur less bioavailable.
- The U.S. Government reports that 30 percent of commercial milk samples contain measurable levels of contaminants such as pesticides and antibiotic residues. Pasteurization does not rid milk of these contaminants from industrial milk production.

Only California and a few other states currently permit raw, unpasteurized milk to be sold in markets, and raw milk is rare even in those states. However, in many areas of this country one can find people raising goats and selling fresh, raw goat's milk. Raw milk is delicious and has a consistency closer to cream than milk. Mixed with fruit, it makes a delicious dessert. For reasons explained throughout this book, I am a huge advocate of consuming goat's milk instead of cow's milk.

Raw milk, by the way, is fresh milk. The pasteurized milk in grocery stores may be three to four weeks old. It goes from the dairy to a processor to a wholesaler and then to the retail grocery story where it is sold. Some cheeses, especially the imported ones, are made with raw milk. Look for "raw milk" on the label.

Health Benefits of Fermented Dairy Products

The best dairy products are the lacto-fermented kind—yogurt, kefir, hard cheeses, cultured cream cheese, cottage cheese, and cultured cream. People who normally can't consume dairy products because they are lactose-intolerant can oftentimes tolerate fermented dairy products because the enzyme lactase is produced by the lactic acid bacteria found in those products. They can break down and digest lactose, the milk-sugar found in dairy products. What's more, properly prepared cultured dairy products should contain little or no residual lactose because the bacteria feeds on this sugar during the fermentation process. In its wake, the bacteria leave galactose, an easy-to-digest monosaccharide-type sugar.

Fermentation increases the vitamin B and C content of milk. Most importantly, fermentation is good for intestinal health. It supplies beneficial bacteria to the intestinal tract and produces lactic acid, a substance that aids the absorption of calcium, copper, iron, magnesium, and manganese. By acidifying the gut, and making it easier for proteins to be absorbed in the small intestine, the *Lactobacillus* bacteria in fermented dairy products make minerals more bioavailable. Some *Lactobacillus* strains in fermented dairy products produce natural antibiotics that are useful against infections.

The best dairy source of all is goat's milk.

FIBER

Fiber, which is also known as roughage, is the indigestible remnants of plant cells in food. Fiber is made chiefly of plant cellulose, but these substances are also fibers: hemicellulose, pectin, lignans, gums, and mucilages. Sources of fiber include vegetables, fruits, whole grains, and beans. Fiber is necessary for regular bowel movements. It prevents constipation. Fiber increases the elimination of waste matter in the large intestine and pressures the rectum muscles to loosen and expel waste. There are two kinds of fiber. Insoluble fiber cannot be broken down at all, whereas soluble fiber dissolves in water. Most fibrous foods contain both types of fiber. Insoluble fiber is believed to reduce the risk of colon cancer. Weight-loss programs recommend fiber because it gives people the feeling that they are filled up without contributing more calories to their diet.

Primitive people ate far more fiber than we do. Although Americans are constantly being reminded to eat more fiber, the average American eats approximately eight grams per day. In 1850, the average

American ate 20 to 30 grams daily, which happens to be what the National Cancer Institute recommends eating. In pioneering studies made in the 1970s, a British missionary surgeon named Dr. Dennis Burkitt observed that rural Africans who ate high-fiber diets had far less colon cancer than people in the west. They had almost no diabetes, constipation, or irritable bowel syndrome as well. Dr. Burkitt observed that Africans who ate a Western diet suffered from these diseases. He concluded that the Africans' high fiber intake accounted for their good intestinal health.

Dr. Burkitt's studies marked the beginning of "the fiber hypothesis," the idea that eating large amounts of fiber and decreasing fat intake can prevent colon cancer as well as diverticulosis, hemorrhoids, and colonic polyps. For thirty years, the fiber hypothesis was considered the gospel truth, but the hypothesis has been refined in recent years. Fiber is a carbohydrate. Many people, eager to improve their health by eating more fiber, eat high-fiber, high-carbohydrate foods such as bran, fibrous breakfast cereals, whole wheat bread, brown rice, and potatoes. However, as this book points out time and time again, the overconsumption of these carbohydrates is a primary cause of intestinal and other diseases.

The kind of fiber that promotes colon health is found as low-carbohydrate, high-fiber foods, such as broccoli, cauliflower, soaked or sprouted seeds and nuts, berries and other small fruits, celery, and lettuce. Fruits and vegetables with edible skins are especially high in fiber. Besides providing fiber, these foods are rich in vitamins, minerals and antioxidants.

Meanwhile, mucilaginous fiber decreases transit time, the amount of time that food spends in the colon before it is expelled. Lowered transit times mean that food has less time to ferment or putrefy in the colon. Toxins are quickly flushed out. Mucilaginous fiber soothes inflamed tissue in the lining of the gut. It can be found in psyllium seeds, marshmallow root, slippery elm, chia seeds, and flax seeds, many of which you will find in the products recommended in this book such as Perfect Food and Super Seed™.

Unfortunately, many people with gut disorders have a hard time with fiber, particularly insoluble fiber. Usually, cooking, juicing, pureeing, or fermenting vegetables and fruits is necessary before they can be eaten. I recommend going to the extra trouble to prepare vegetables. They are a very healthy source of fiber.

CONDIMENTS AND SALT

Go into most restaurants and you will see a selection of condiments on the table—salt, pepper, ketchup, and mustard. Most people keep a small supply in their pantry or refrigerator. Condiments have been a part of the human diet for many centuries, but their purpose has been lost in modern times. Originally, condiments were digestive aids. They were meant to be taken in small amounts with a meal to encourage proper digestion. Unlike the condiments of today, almost all the original condiments were fermented.

Next time you are dressing up your hamburger at the neighbor's barbeque, consider the pedigree of ketchup. From the Chinese *ke-tsiap*, ketchup started out as a fermented fish-brine sauce. Sailors brought it from China to England, where the locals added pickled cucumbers, kidney beans, and oysters to the mix. New Englanders made tomatoes the chief feature of ketchup in the late 1700s. Sadly, our modern commercialized ketchup is no longer fermented. Today's ketchup, however, is loaded with sugar and corn syrup.

Lacto-fermentation is difficult to achieve on an industrial scale. For that reason, the makers of modern condiments use vinegar in the brine. This makes condiments more acidic. Worse, many condiments are pasteurized. Pasteurization kills the beneficial lactic acid bacteria that naturally occur in properly prepared condiments. Condiments have ceased to be aids to digestion. They are used to dress up prepared food and give it a little more tang. Ironically, dietitians recommend cutting back on condiments, the foods that people ate originally to promote good health. For recipes to make your own lacto-fermented condiments be sure to read the world's greatest cookbook, *Nourishing Traditions* by Sally Fallon with Mary Enig.

More so than any condiment, most people put salt on their food. Salt is one of the oldest food additives. Even people who lived far from the ocean obtained salt by burning sodium-rich grasses and mixing the ash into their food. Although some have argued that salt raises blood pressure, this controversial idea is still open to debate. Salt provides chloride for the manufacturing of hydrochloric acid, the stomach acid that breaks down food. It stimulates salivation. It is an enzyme activator. It is required for proper functioning of the adrenal gland. And, of course, it makes food taste better.

Conventional table salt like the kind you buy in most stores is processed. Aluminum compounds are added to keep the salt dry. The trace minerals and iodine salts that occur naturally in sea salt are removed during processing. To make the salt a pristine white, it is exposed to bleaching agents.

I recommend a natural, unrefined salt called Celtic sea salt. This light-gray salt comes from Brittany in France, where it is gathered in clay-lined ponds as part of a two thousand-year-old tradition. Celtic sea salt is high in organic iodine from plants and the tiny skeletons of ancient marine life. It includes many trace minerals, including sodium chloride and magnesium salts. Herbamare, a combination of sea salt, spices, herbs and vegetables all steeped together for over a year, is my personal favorite seasoning. It is great on everything. I have consumed Herbamare for years, and I never tire of it. Appendix A tells where to obtain these products.

FERMENTED FOODS

The Austrians and Germans have sauerkraut. The Japanese have pickled ginger. There is kefir and a porridge called podji. We used to have real catsup, real mayonnaise, real sourdough—real fermented foods. In one sense, for all its benefits (and there are plenty), we can also say the miracle of refrigeration has ruined the health of modern men and women. Refrigeration, at least in America, has replaced our need for fermented foods. So have modern processing methods that no longer allow for the fermentation of foods. In spite of technological advancements, our bodies still cry out for such foods.

RAW FOODS

Enzymes are proteins that act as catalysts for chemical reactions in the body. They are the labor force of the body. They speed up the rate of chemical reactions. They initiate chemical reactions but are not themselves changed by those reactions. Enzymes take the food we eat and turn it into chemical structures that are able to pass through the cell membranes of the small intestine and into the bloodstream. Enzymes are found in all living organisms.

I have included a discussion of enzymes in this chapter about the Maker's Diet to introduce the subject of raw food. Raw food contains enzymes that assist with digestion. As soon as you put raw food in your mouth, the enzymes begin digesting it, and they continue to do so in the cardia (upper) portion of the stomach after the food is swallowed. These digestive enzymes—*proteases* to digest protein, *amylases* to digest carbohydrates, and *lipases* to digest fat—break down food so it can be absorbed in the small intestine.

Our primitive ancestors knew the value of raw food to digestion. Not only did primitive people eat raw fruits and vegetables, they ate raw meat. The Inuit, for example, ate raw fat from seals, whale blubber, and raw fish. These foods contain an abundance of the enzyme lipase. (The Inuit were formerly known as the Eskimo, a derogatory term from the Cree language that means "he eats it raw.") Some Pygmies devouring the decomposing carcass of a dead elephant in equatorial Africa, when asked how they tolerated such unsavory food, replied that they were eating the meat of the elephant, not its odor. Does eating raw meat seem repulsive to you? In genteel Victorian London, physicians prescribed sandwiches made from raw thyroid glands to aging patients to help rejuvenate them.

Prolonged heat over 118 degrees F. kills all enzymes. Therefore, cooking destroys the digestive enzymes in raw food. So do food processing methods and pasteurization. Seeing as most people eat cooked food, processed food, or pasteurized food, the modern diet is empty of vital enzymes. Raw food, you could say, is alive. Unless you make a point of eating more raw food, you lose the benefits of live food and its digestive enzymes.

In his classic *Enzyme Nutrition*, Dr. Edward Howell proposed the idea that everyone is born with a finite store of enzymes. Enzymes, he noted, fall into three classes: metabolic enzymes that direct body functions; digestive enzymes secreted by the pancreas for digesting food; and enzymes found in raw food that assist with digestion. Dr. Howell believed that eating too much cooked food depleted the body's store of finite enzymes. To digest cooked food, the body must draw upon its own enzymes, and that leaves fewer enzymes for other functions—for operating the brain, muscles, organs and tissues. Dr. Howell believed in eating more raw food in order to keep the body's store of enzymes from being depleted. He wrote:

> A certain amount of raw, uncooked food in the diet is indispensable to the highest degree of health. Assuming that the proteins, fats, carbohydrates, minerals, and vitamins are equally available for nutrition in raw and cooked food, any demonstrable nutritional superiority of raw food must then be ascribed to the "live" quality of raw food, and when this live quality is subjected to analysis, it is shown to consist of... no other property than that possessed by enzymes.

The enzymes in fruits and vegetables fully develop when the fruits and vegetables are ripe. A ripe banana, for example, has far more digestive enzymes than a green banana. For this reason, you should try to eat naturally ripened fruits and vegetables that have not been truck- or gas-ripened. What's more, some seeds and nuts contain enzyme inhibitors. These substances prevent seeds and nuts from sprouting until they are nestled deeply enough in the soil. Enzyme inhibitors serve an important role in Nature, but they also make the enzymes in fruits and nuts unavailable. You can, however, free the enzymes in seeds and nuts by soaking them before eating.

Besides raw food, you can obtain digestive enzyme supplements (see Chapter 6). In my experience, digestive enzyme supplements have helped patients with gastrointestinal disorders immensely. The supplements aid digestion and also reduce inflammation in the colon.

STOCKS, BROTHS, AND GELATIN

Unfortunately for our health, stocks, bone soups and broths, which require several hours of careful simmering, are no longer an important part of the modern diet. People believe they are too busy to make these foods; yet they are some of the most nutritious foods you can eat. "Good broth resurrects the dead," according to a South American proverb. Stocks, broths, and non-pork gelatins are a folk remedy for colds and the flu in almost every culture. There's a reason for this.

Stocks and broths are especially beneficial to people who have intestinal diseases because they are very high in nutrients the gastrointestinal tract can absorb without having to do a lot of work. Gelatin, the odorless, tasteless substance extracted by boiling bones, animal tissues, and hoofs is especially easy to digest. Broth from meat and animal bones is an excellent source of many important minerals, including iodine, chloride, sodium, magnesium, and potassium. Iodine is especially plentiful in stock made from fish bones and heads.

Dr. Francis Pottenger believed that stocks, broths, and gelatin are easy to digest because they contain hydrophilic colloids. Colloids are large molecules. Hydrophilic means "water-loving." Normally, the colloids in cooked food are the opposite of hydrophilic—they are hydrophobic. They don't attract liquids. But stocks, broths, and gelatins, although they have been cooked, attract digestive liquids. This explains why they are easier to digest than other cooked food.

BEVERAGES

The modern diet is insufficient in water, and the beverages that are in the diet are often more harmful than healthy. In most cases, our primitive ancestors were able to obtain drinking water straight from the source—from a river, creek, or spring. Natural water is extremely healthy. This water is mineral-rich and "structured." That is, the water has a strong electrical charge and low surface tension. It is not as dense as conventional tap water. No one knows precisely why people in some cultures live, on average, longer than others, but many attribute longevity to drinking copious amounts of healthy water.

Whenever possible, it is important to consume such structured waters. Structured water is known to exist in regions of the living organism where there are transitions between more lipophilic and more hydrophilic areas, such as at the surface of the cell membrane and around enzymes, notes a report in the Spring 2001 issue of *The AAO Journal*, a publication of the American Academy of Osteopathy. "Structured water facilitates the activity of enzymes and receptivity of cell membranes to activators of cellular function," says the journal. Since structured water has a high solubility for the body's minerals and vitamins, which are potentiated with structured water, they tend to go from the digestive tract and bloodstream into the tissues much more efficiently. It also is located around the membranes of the nucleus and the endoplasmic reticulum, a network of cellular tubules, vesicles and sacs that are interconnected and serve specialized functions within cells, including protein and lipid synthesis, sequestration of calcium, production of steroids, storage and production of glycogen, and insertion of membrane proteins. It is known that structured water carries information of the "images" of molecules. This type of information plays a critical role in all metabolic activities of the body.

There are some great water supplements available that simply make drinking water an even healthier experience. This is a new area of health for many consumers. But it is a very interesting one indeed.

Our Springs of Life™ is not water as we might think of water but rather a concentrated liquid supplement to add to water—an energizing, life-supporting liquid concentrate that rapidly and effectively penetrates through to the cells walls, dispersing its nutrients directly into the cell's interior.

Understanding that the mission of Garden of Life is to aid our return to the primitive diet of our ancestors, Springs of Life is a combination of biologically active enzymes, minerals and trace elements that naturally energizes and transforms water, returning it to the pristine quality that indigenous people drank hundreds of years ago.

Consumed on an empty stomach, it is thought to provide fast-acting absorption while preserving and potentiating the delicate, biological components of any supplement you take with it.

Springs of Life utilizes structured water principles that serve as a catalyst that helps to accelerate the healing process, assimilate nutrients more efficiently, increase enzyme activity, and strengthen the immune system. In essence, the naturally occurring compounds in Springs of Life replicate the activity of a young healthy cell, sounding a wake-up call throughout the entire body, resulting in vitalizing, youthful energy.

What about other beverages? Soda pop is marketed aggressively to the young. Soda pop has been rightfully called a "sweet poison." The ubiquitous vending machine that sells soda pop can even be found in schools. I just read an interesting article that reported the Los Angeles Unified School District, one of the largest in the nation, is finally prohibiting soft drink vending machines on campuses. I think it is outrageous that soft drinks ever found their way into schools.

Girls in their early teens who often drink soda pop have an increased risk of getting fractures and osteoporosis. The culprit is probably the phosphoric acid in soda pop, which impedes the absorption of magnesium and calcium. Soda pop represents yet another inroad made by sugar into the American diet. It is often blamed for the increase in obesity among children. Americans drink twice the amount of soft drinks as they did only 25 years ago.

In order to avoid the calories imparted by sugar, many soda drinkers are turning to sugar-free beverages. However, aspartame, the artificial sweetener found in most sugar-free soda pop brands, may be worse than sugar. Aspartame has been implicated in seizures, depression, and neurological disorders such as dizziness and muscle aches. In an American Cancer Society study of 78,000 women, those who consumed artificially sweetened foods gained more weight over a one-year period than those who consumed sugar-sweetened products. The researchers speculated that the sugar substitutes may have stimulated the women's appetites.

The other beverage that has gained in popularity in recent years is coffee. This substance injures the stomach and esophagus. It relaxes the sphincter muscle that controls the passage of food from the esophagus to the stomach and may permit hydrochloric acid from the stomach to splash into the esophagus and cause heartburn. On account of its caffeine content, coffee can tax the adrenal glands and can lead to adrenal gland exhaustion, a condition in which the adrenal glands fail to release adrenaline. Some believe that adrenal gland exhaustion weakens the immune system and makes the body more susceptible to disease and infection. Coffee also raises blood pressure and impairs one's ability to cope with stress (probably via its effects on the adrenal glands).

Concentrated fruit juices and sports drinks are also better avoided. They contain copious amounts of sugar. These drinks present all the problems that a diet high in sugar presents. They cause a sudden surge of blood sugar that disrupts hormonal functions and can contribute to diabetes and other health problems.

By the way, almost as important as what to drink is when to drink. I think you should avoid drinking liquids with meals because the fluid may dilute digestive enzymes. Drink between meals instead. Avoid ice-cold beverages as well. Traditional societies simply did not drink ice-cold beverages. The body must use enzymes to raise the temperature of ice-cold beverages before it can absorb them. Ice-cold drinks may shock the system and temporarily shut down digestion. In Asian cultures, cold drinks are almost never consumed.

Think teas and vegetables juices. Teas such as maitake, ginseng, green tea and teas made from other herbs have a wonderful tonifying and relaxing effect on the body and are much healthier than coffee, soda pop or even fruit juices. Vegetable juices made from low-sugar vegetables such as greens, celery, or spinach mixed with super green foods such as chlorella, spirulina, and wheat grass are also good choices.

━━━◇◇◇━━━

The Maker's Diet
in Your Daily Life

Lists of "Super," "Healthy," "Neutral," and "Dangerous" foods follow. Obviously, listing every type of food is impossible, but you can follow this rule of thumb to determine which category a food belongs in: If a food is overly processed, non-organic, or altered in any major way from the way it was created, you can be pretty sure that it belongs in the "Neutral" or "Dangerous" category.

Do your very best to choose foods exclusively from the "Super" and the "Healthy" category in a 75 percent to 25 percent ratio. Only after you are free of symptoms for at least three months can you more than occasionally eat foods in the "Neutral" food category.

Try to avoid foods in the "Dangerous" category altogether. These foods do not impart any beneficial qualities and actually cause harm to the body. They should be avoided by everyone whether healthy or ill.

"SUPER" FOODS

Foods that fall in the "Super" category are optimal foods for optimal wellness. They supply the body with the building blocks it needs to heal itself and maintain vibrant health. These foods are highly nutritious and life-giving. They have kept people healthy and disease-free for thousands of years. They have a moderate amount of calories per serving. Generally speaking, foods in the "Super" category are well tolerated even by people with gastrointestinal diseases, food allergies and food sensitivities. These foods contain the same naturally occurring nutrients that they contained hundreds of years ago. In their organic form, they contain little or no residues from pesticides, herbicides, hormones, or antibiotics. The utmost care is taken in their growth and they are grown in accordance with self-sustaining agricultural practices. I selected each food on the "Super" list according to its level of vitamins, minerals, healthy fats, enzymes, and probiotics. These foods truly exemplify the principles of the Maker's Diet.

Sources of many foods in the "Super" category can be found in Appendix A.

Protein	Meats and fowl raised organically beef, lamb, chicken, turkey, duck… (no antibiotics or hormones). Grass-fed meat and fowl is preferable.
	Game (venison, buffalo, elk).
	Eggs (at the very least free-range, fertile or organic, but preferably eggs that are high in omega-3 fats).
	Fish with fins and scales. Deep water ocean fish, not farm-raised. The best ocean fish are salmon, halibut, tuna, cod, sea bass, and sardines (canned sardines packed in water or olive oil but not soy bean oil; look for a fat content of 16-22 grams per serving).
	Organ meats (liver and heart) only from organic sources.
	Goat's Milk protein powder (Goatein; see Appendix B)
Fats	Raw, organic/chemical-free butter from goat's milk (milk from grass-fed animals is preferable). Do not heat.
	Pasteurized goat's milk butter from organically raised animals.
	Organic extra virgin coconut oil (the best oil for cooking), coconut milk and cream, extra virgin olive oil, unrefined, expeller-pressed; flax seed oil, hemp seed oil, pumpkin seed oil, hazel nut oil. Except for the occasional use of extra virgin olive oil, other liquid oils should not be used for cooking. Olives in water, coconut, and avocado. (To be in this category, all foods should be certified organic, or locally grown, and/or herbicide- and pesticide-free.)
Dairy	Organic, cultured dairy products (yogurt, *crème Bulgare*, kefir) from whole goat's milk (cultured for 30 hours or more). See Appendix A
Beverages	Filtered, non-carbonated, high mineral or catalyst altered, structured water (Springs of Life), meat stocks and vegetable broths, raw vegetable juices, and lacto-fermented beverages.
Condiments	Celtic sea salt, Herbamare (see Appendix A), lacto-fermented sauces and condiments, raw homemade salsa, guacamole, homemade salad dressing, apple cider vinegar (look for the words "with the mother" on the label) and organic herbs and spices with no added starches, sugars or stabilizers.
CARBOHYDRATES	
Grains and Starches	Certified organic, sprouted or yeast-free sourdough whole grain breads (Ezekial bread, sprouted bread, manna bread, etc.).
	Soaked non-gluten whole grains and soaked whole grain meals and flours (quinoa, amaranth, millet, buckwheat, and brown rice).

continued on next page

Vegetables	*Vegetables (raw, frozen or cooked), organic or unsprayed and non-genetically modified are best, including squash (winter and summer), broccoli, artichoke (French not Jerusalem), asparagus, beets, cauliflower, Brussels sprouts, cabbage, carrots, celery, cucumber, eggplant, pumpkin, garlic, onion, kale, collard greens, okra, lettuce and greens of all kinds, mushrooms, peas, peppers, string beans, tomatoes, turnips, watercress, sprouts (broccoli, sunflower, pea shoots, etc.). *Avoid* bean and alfalfa sprouts, corn, potatoes, yams, and sweet potatoes.
	*Unheated lacto-fermented vegetables including sauerkraut (See resource section).
	*Raw vegetable juices made from recommended vegetables, including wheat grass juice (field grown is preferred). If using commercially grown vegetables, wash the vegetables thoroughly to remove pesticide residues and chemicals.
Fruits	Organic, unsprayed (fresh, frozen or cooked), fully ripened fruits (fruits should be limited to 2 to 3 pieces per day).
Sweeteners	Raw unheated, unpasteurized honey (in moderation), filtered or unfiltered.
Legumes/Beans	Small amounts of the fermented soy product miso (used in soup).
Nuts and Seeds	Organic soaked or sprouted nuts and seeds (no cashews or peanuts).
	Certified organic raw nut and seed butters; organic raw nut and seed flours (no cashews or peanuts).

"HEALTHY" FOODS

Foods in the "Healthy" category should make up about 25 percent of your diet, especially during your first year on the program.

Protein	Conventional meat and poultry.
	Fish (farm-raised, fresh-water); canned tuna and salmon in spring water.
	Eggs (common supermarket eggs not raised organically).
	Fresh deli turkey, chicken, and roast beef from free-range sources with no preservatives, and smoked fish without preservatives.

continued on next page

Fats	Expeller-pressed, unrefined organic or chemical-free sesame oil, peanut oil, grapeseed oil, walnut oil, conventional virgin olive oil, unrefined palm oil, palm kernel oil, avocado oil.
	Non-organic coconut, olives in water, and avocado.
	Chicken, goose, duck, lamb, and beef fat (not cover fat) from free-range animals.
Dairy	Raw goat's milk, pasteurized cultured dairy (yogurt or kefir) from whole goat's milk, organic hard goat milk cheeses (cheddar, Swiss, Havarti, Colby), made from raw or pasteurized goat's milk, dry curd cottage cheese from goat's milk.
Beverages	Fresh raw fruit juices.
	Organic, unpasteurized dry red wine.
	Purified reverse osmosis water.
	Organic herbal teas (sweetened with honey) including green tea.
	Naturally carbonated mineral waters.
Condiments	Organic wheat-free soy sauce (tamari), organic mustard, organic mayonnaise, mayonnaise mixed with flax, fish sauce, ketchup, organic tomato sauce, wasabi, organic salsa, organic salad dressings, organic carob or cocoa powder (raw, if possible), non-organic spices with no added starches, sugars or stabilizers (see Appendix A for sources for these condiments).
CARBOHYDRATES	
Grains and Starches	Soaked whole grains, meals and flours (Spelt, Kamut, Barley, Oat, Rye, etc.).
Vegetables	Heated, fermented vegetables (sauerkraut, pickles with no vinegar).
	Organic canned vegetables, including tomato products. Fresh vegetables including sweet potatoes, yams, sea vegetables, parsnips, and jicama.
Fruits	Conventional fruits raw or cooked and fully ripened, organic dried fruits with no added sugar or sulfites, organic canned fruits in their own juices without added sugars.
Sweeteners	Filtered or heated honey.
Legumes/Beans	White beans, lentils, split peas, lima beans soaked for more than eight hours or fermented.

continued on next page

Nuts and Seeds	Conventional nuts and seeds raw, soaked or sprouted.
	Organic roasted nut and seed butters (including cashew).
	Organic peanut butter (*no letters please—I know it's really a legume!*).

"NEUTRAL" FOODS

Foods in the "Neutral" category should be avoided or consumed in strict moderation during the first six to twelve months of the program. And when the first twelve months have passed, make these foods a small part of your diet. When consuming "Neutral" foods, it is important to consume good quantities of Omega-Zyme with your meal or snack.

Protein	Supermarket deli meat (conventional turkey breast, chicken, and roast beef cold cuts).
	Free-range, health food store-bought chicken, turkey or beef products such as bologna, sausage, hot dogs, bacon (due to the added fat) No Pork Products.
	Natural preservative-free, sugar-free jerky.
	Egg-whites only.
	Whey protein and milk protein powders (from hormone-free sources).
	Tofu.
Fats	Cow's milk butter and cream.
	Chicken, goose, duck, lamb, and beef fat (not cover fat) from conventional farms.
	Expeller-pressed sunflower and safflower oils, and olive oil.
Dairy	Cow's milk: cultured, full fat. Cow's milk hard and soft cheeses.
	Sour cream, cream cheese, non-organic dry curd cottage cheese.
	Pesticide-free dairy products (kefir and yogurt) without added sweeteners.
Beverages	Distilled water, organic coffee freshly ground, organic black tea, non-organic herbal teas sweetened with honey, pasteurized 100-percent juice not from concentrate, unpasteurized beer, white wine, and carbonated beverages with carbonation added.
Condiments	Condiments with organic sugar, canola mayonnaise, unflavored gelatin, non-organic spices containing added sugar, starch and stabilizers.

continued on next page

CARBOHYDRATES	
Grains and Starches	Organic whole grains (not soaked or sprouted), whole grain flours, and whole grain pastas.
Vegetables	Canned non-organic vegetables and tomato products. Organic white potatoes. Heated, fermented vegetables with vinegar. Organic corn.
Fruits	Canned non-organic fruits in their own juices with no added sugar, non-organic dried fruits with no added sugar or sulfites.
Sweeteners	Organic cane sugar (sucanat, rhapadura), organic maple syrup, and stevia.
Legumes/Beans	Garbanzo beans, black eyed peas, azuki, kidney, and soy soaked for more than eight hours or fermented.
Nuts and Seeds	Unsoaked nuts and seeds, roasted nuts and seeds, and non-organic nut and seed butters.

"DANGEROUS" FOODS

Foods in the "Dangerous" category should be strictly avoided by all individuals who want to attain and maintain health. Eating any of these foods will significantly increase your risk of illness or, if you've been ill, relapse. Each food in this category should read ***Caution: consumption of this food may cause damage to your health.*** In fact, many of these foods when mentioned in the Bible were described by a word meaning "not food." If you do consume these foods, it is prudent to consume extra digestive enzymes with the food and increase your consumption of probiotics for three days after the food is eaten.

Protein	Shellfish (crab, lobster, shrimp, oysters, scallops, muscles and clams cooked and from clean waters). Pork and pork products including ham, bacon, commercial hot dogs and sausage, cured meats. Imitation shellfish, organ meats from non-organically raised animals, farm-raised smoked fish, smoked meats, and nitrite-preserved jerky. Imitation eggs. Soy protein and other vegetable proteins. Any and all soy imitation protein foods (soy bacon, soy deli meats, soy burgers, meatloaf, turkey, and so on). Deep-fried and breaded chicken and fish. Frozen prepared meals.

continued on next page

Fats	All refined vegetable and seed oils from supermarkets (corn, safflower, canola, sunflower oil). Lard. Any hydrogenated or partially hydrogenated oil, margarine, shortening, any refined oil, and non-dairy creamer
Dairy	All reduced fat or nonfat dairy products. All fluid dairy products pasteurized or UHT (ultra heat-treated), whether organic or commercial, as well as non-organic, homogenized dairy products. Powdered milk, acidophilus milk, buttermilk, imitation milk (rice, soy, oat, and almond milks). Sour cream and processed cheese products, including American cheese, processed cheese food, conventional cream cheese, cottage cheese, ricotta, and mozzarella. Ice cream and frozen yogurt.
Beverages	Concentrated fruit juices and frozen concentrates, sodas, tap water, diet drinks, non-organic coffee, wine with sulfites, pasteurized beer, and hard liquor.
Condiments	Condiments with sugar, preservatives, MSG, textured vegetable protein, soy protein isolate, artificial sweeteners. Pickled ginger with sugar, bouillon cubes, instant soups, agar, carrageen, commercial mayonnaise with processed soybean or other oils, bean dips and other dips.
Miscellaneous Items	Liquid medications and elixirs that contain sugars or artificial sweeteners (ask your pharmacist).
CARBOHYDRATES	
Grains and Starches	Unbleached, bleached, and fortified white flours and subsequent products—dried cereals, packaged grain products, grain flours, tapioca, arrowroot, and corn starch. Most commercially made crackers, cookies, pastries, and cakes fall into this category.
Vegetables	Deep-fried or processed vegetables.
Sweeteners	Malt, barley malt, corn syrup, sugar, artificial sweeteners (aspartame, acesulfame K, sucrulose, saccharin), rice syrup, fruit juice concentrate, fructose, glucose, dextrose, fructooligosaccharide, inulin, and dahulin.

continued on next page

Fruits	Canned fruits with heavy or light syrup or added sugar, dried fruits with added sugar and sulfites.
Legumes/Beans	Unsoaked legumes and beans.
Nuts and Seeds	Non-organic peanut products, nuts and seeds roasted in vegetable oil, honey-roasted nuts and seeds, and soy nut butter.

SAMPLE THREE-DAY PLAN

Here is a sample three-day meal and supplement plan for the Maker's Diet.

On Day 1:

- **Upon rising:** 1) Cleansing Drink: Dissolve one to two tablespoons of Super Seed whole food fiber blend in 12 ounces of water and add 12 drops of structured water concentrate such as Springs of Life. Drink immediately.
  - *Morning Supplements (approximately 20 minutes after cleansing drink):* Drink 8 to 16 ounces of vegetable juice or purified water with two tablespoons of an organic green food such as Perfect Food and add 12 drops of Springs of Life. Take $1/2$ of the daily serving of the recommended supplements (Primal Defense, RM-10, FYI; see individual protocols in Chapter 12).
- **Breakfast:** Synergy Smoothie (see Chapter 11).
  - *Supplements:* one to three Omega-Zyme digestive enzyme caplets.
- **Lunch:** Grilled salmon with organic stir-fried vegetables (broccoli, onion, yellow squash, and garlic stir fried in extra virgin coconut oil).
  - Supplements: one to three Omega-Zyme digestive enzyme caplets.
- **Dinner:** Green salad with high omega-3 salad dressing (see the recipe in Chapter 11) and meatloaf made from grass-fed beef with roasted or steamed vegetables.
  - *Supplements:* one to three Omega-Zyme digestive enzyme caplets.
- **Snack:** Balanced veggie juice (see recipe in Chapter 11).
  - *Evening supplements (at least one hour after dinner):* $1/2$ of the daily serving of the recommended supplements (Primal Defense, RM-10, FYI).
  - *Bedtime supplements:* Cleansing Drink: mix one to two tablespoons of Super Seed whole food fiber and a green superfood such as Perfect Food in 12 ounces of water and add 12 drops of structured water concentrate such as Springs of Life. Drink immediately.
- **Beverages:** Drink purified water with 12 drops of structured water concentrate per glass, a lacto-fermented beverage, or balanced veggie juice (see the recipes in Chapter 11). Drink beverages between meals.

On Day 2:

- **Upon rising:** Cleansing Drink: Dissolve one to two tablespoons of Super Seed whole food fiber blend in 12 ounces of water and add 12 drops of structured water concentrate such as Springs of Life. Drink immediately.
  - *Morning Supplements (approximately 20 minutes after cleansing drink):* Drink 8 to 16 ounces of vegetable juice or purified water with two tablespoons of an organic green food such as Perfect Food and add 12 drops of Springs of Life. Take $1/2$ of the daily serving of the recommended supplements (Primal Defense, RM-10, FYI; see individual protocols in Chapter 12).
- **Breakfast:** Three poached high omega-3 eggs and two ounces of raw sauerkraut. For the remainder, either steamed organic vegetables topped with olive oil, extra virgin coconut oil, or goat's milk butter and Celtic sea salt or Herbamare; or one piece of sprouted or natural sourdough bread with Better Butter (see Chapter 11 for the Better Butter recipe).
  - *Supplements:* one to three Omega-Zyme digestive enzyme caplets.
- **Lunch:** Green salad with chicken, tuna or salmon; or free-range chicken served with steamed or stir-fried vegetables.
  - *Supplements:* one to three Omega-Zyme digestive enzyme caplets.
- **Dinner:** Organic green salad with high omega-3 dressing (see the recipes in Chapter 11) and chicken soup with chicken and vegetables.
  - *Supplements:* one to three Omega-Zyme digestive enzyme caplets.
- **Snack:** Creamy high enzyme dessert (see the recipes in Chapter 11).
  - *Evening supplements (at least one hour after dinner):* $1/2$ of the daily serving of the recommended supplements (Primal Defense, RM-10, FYI).
  - *Bedtime supplements:* Cleansing Drink: Mix one to two tablespoons of Super Seed whole food fiber and a green drink such as Perfect Food in 12 ounces of water and add 12 drops of structured water concentrate such as Springs of Life. Drink immediately.
- *Beverages:* Drink purified water with 12 drops of structured water concentrate per glass, a lacto-fermented beverage, or balanced veggie juice (see the recipes in Chapter 11). Drink beverages between meals.

On Day 3:

- **Upon rising:** 1) Cleansing Drink: Dissolve one to two tablespoons of Super Seed whole food fiber blend in 12 ounces of water and add 12 drops of structured water concentrate such as Springs of Life. Drink immediately.
  - *Morning Supplements (approximately 20 minutes after cleansing drink):* Drink 8 to 16 ounces of vegetable juice or purified water with two tablespoons of an organic green food such as Perfect Food and add 12 drops of Springs of Life. Take $1/2$ of the daily serving of the recommended supplements (Primal Defense, RM-10, FYI; see individual protocols in Chapter 12).

- **Breakfast:** Three soft-boiled or fried eggs (in extra virgin coconut oil) with sliced oranges, apples or grapefruit, and one tablespoon of raw nut or seed butter.
  - *Supplements:* one to three Omega-Zyme digestive enzyme caplets.
- **Lunch:** Roasted chicken with broccoli, squash and onions.
  - *Supplements:* one to three Omega-Zyme digestive enzyme caplets.
- **Dinner:** Green salad with high omega-3 dressing or fruit and soft goat's milk chevre. Grilled fish (salmon, tuna, snapper, or cod) with steamed or stir-fried vegetables.
  - *Supplements:* one to three Omega-Zyme digestive enzyme caplets.
- **Snack:** Raw organic celery and carrots dipped in raw organic almond or sesame butter or organic apple slices spread with organic almond or sesame butter.
  - *Evening supplements (at least one hour after dinner):* $1/2$ of the daily serving of the recommended supplements (Primal Defense, RM-10, FYI).
  - *Bedtime supplements: Cleansing Drink:* Mix one to two tablespoons of Super Seed whole food fiber and a green drink such as Perfect Food in 12 ounces of water and add 12 drops of structured water concentrate such as Springs of Life. Drink immediately.
- **Beverages:** Drink purified water with 12 drops of structured water concentrate per glass, a lacto-fermented beverage, or balanced veggie juice (see the recipes in Chapter 11). Drink beverages between meals.

If you are on a restricted budget, I recommend consuming canned tuna, sardines, and salmon instead of fresh fish. You can also eat conventionally grown fruits and vegetables that have been treated with a special wash (see Appendix C).

NOTES

Mercury is an issue in the case of deep-water fish. However, wild Pacific salmon, red snapper, cod, and halibut are four types of fish known to be relatively low in mercury. Fish is generally rich in vitamins A and D. Fish also provide zinc and iodine, two minerals that are found in abundance in the ocean but have been depleted from the soil.

All cooking oils should be certified organic or chemical free. Processed oils are produced under high heat. They are subject to rancidity. Most include deodorizing chemicals that disguise their rancidity. When you heat process oil as you fry food, you release the chemicals. It has been said that the chemicals that are released are the equivalent of smoking cigarettes. Prefer extra virgin coconut oil for frying.

Organic fruit and vegetables are excellent, but they are also expensive. Do your best to obtain organic vegetables and fruit as long as you stay within your budget. If you have to make compromises, I would reluctantly recommend compromising on organic fruits and vegetables before grass-fed meat and free-range poultry. In other words, it is better to spend the money on high-quality meat than organic fruit and vegetables. When you buy commercial, non-organic produce, it is important to treat it with a vegetable wash (available at most health food stores and some grocery stores) to remove pesticide residues.

It is important to carry digestive enzyme supplements with you at all times. This way, when you eat at someone else's house or in a restaurant that offers only "Neutral" or "Dangerous" foods, you can take the enzymes and hope to digest the food properly.

A GUIDE TO EATING OUT AND TRAVELING

Besides the usual challenge of keeping your self-discipline, you will encounter a new set of difficulties when you are traveling. You don't know where the stores that sell healthy food are. You find yourself in restaurants where "Neutral " and "Dangerous " foods are served.

When you go to restaurants on the road, stick with the proteins—fish, chicken and beef. Ocean fish is usually the best chance to get protein from the "super" category. Ask the waiter if the food is cooked in butter or margarine and choose food items prepared in butter. Always order vegetables instead of potatoes. If your budget allows, higher-end restaurants offer more "Super" and "Healthy" choices (such as ocean fish) than, for example, fast-food restaurants would. Typically, they offer the healthiest food. Most importantly, avoid the bread and the dessert. These foods are loaded with carbohydrates and calories. Usually, the simpler the meal, the better it is for your health.

Here are some meal suggestions for tourists and business travelers:

- **Breakfast:** Eggs, fruit, and lean meats such as breakfast steak are the best choices. Ask the waiter if the eggs are prepared in margarine or shortening, and if they are, avoid them. Skip the traditional toast and hash browns that are served in so many roadside diners.
- **Lunch:** Salads, lean meats, fish, and fresh fruit are available on most luncheon menus. Stay with olive oil-based dressings. That means no ranch or thousand island or similar sweet-tasting dressings. These dressings usually contain added sugar, or worse.
- **Dinner:** Ask for seafood or a lean meat as the main course, and remember to keep it simple. Avoid rich sauces. As a side dish, get the steamed vegetables or have the salad.
- Be sure to pack digestive enzyme supplements when you are on the road. No matter where your travels take you and what food you eat, digestive enzymes can help you digest the food. They make it less likely that you will suffer heartburn, diarrhea, or worse.

FOODS ESSENTIAL TO HEALING

The last part of this chapter concerns foods that are essential to healing and good health. You are encouraged to fall in love with these foods. They can be your best friends. These foods are nutritious and soothing to the gastrointestinal tract which, after all, is the center of your health universe. They have been eaten since primitive times for their nutritional qualities, not to mention their good flavor. Sources for these foods can be found in Appendix A.

30-Hour Cultured Goat's Milk Products

Goat's milk yogurt that has been fermented for 30 hours is a rich source of probiotics, enzymes, and short-chain fatty acids. It is virtually free of lactose, which means that people who are lactose intolerant can consume it. It is a rich source of selenium. It does not contain *Streptococcus thermophilus*, the bacterial strain that has been known to exacerbate certain autoimmune disorders, or *Mycobacterium avium paratuberculosis* (MAP), the micro-organism that some believe may be involved in the development of Crohn's disease.

Not only does goat's milk yogurt have no negative effects, it is very beneficial for a healthy immune system. Everybody who can obtain this excellent healing food should take full advantage of it. I have consumed cultured goat's milk products for the last seven years and believe it to be one of the secrets that helped me overcome my own illness.

The Potential Dangers of Streptococcus Thermophilus

I recommend choosing cultured dairy products that do not contain the bacterial strain Streptococcus thermophilus. Studies have shown that people who suffer from autoimmune diseases such as rheumatoid arthritis run the risk of aggravating the symptoms of their disease if they consume more than two cups of yogurt that contains *Streptococcus thermophilus*. What's more, *Streptococcus thermophilus* can cause a shift in immune function known as a Th2 dominated immune system. People with Th2 mediated immune systems have higher incidences of allergies and other illnesses (see Chapter 3).

People suffering from digestive problems usually have imbalanced or weak immune systems. For this reason, avoiding products that may contribute to immune system dysfunction is wise if you have an intestinal disease.

Most commercial yogurts and probiotic supplements, even those found in health food stores, contain *Streptococcus thermophilus*. I have found a goat's milk yogurt cultured for 30 hours that does not contain *Streptococcus thermophilus* but is cultured using *Lactobacillus bulgaricus*, *Lactobacillus acidophilus*, and other friendly strains. Information is available about these yogurts in Appendix A.

High Omega-3 Eggs

Eggs from chickens, turkeys and ducks who are truly free to roam and eat a diet high in insects and worms, as well as eggs from chickens fed certain strains of algae, contain large amounts of important omega-3 fatty acids. Eggs from these birds usually contain a ratio of omega-3 to omega-6 fatty acids between 1:1–1:4, whereas eggs from battery-raised hens have a ratio of omega-3 to omega-6 fatty acids of 1:20. Studies show that omega-3 fatty acids are helpful against high blood pressure, heart disease, blood clotting, diabetes, colitis, and inflammatory diseases. So-called battery-raised hens are kept in coops where a light is always burning. This confuses the hens into thinking it is daytime, which makes them lay more eggs.

In addition to containing docosahexaenoic acid (DHA), omega-3 eggs contain significant amounts of vitamin E and B_{12}, as well as the antioxidants lutein and beta carotene. By eating two high omega-3 eggs, you can get as much as 150 mg of DHA. Eggs are healthiest when they are poached, soft boiled, or consumed raw in smoothies. Frying and scrambling eggs can damage some of the nutrients contained in the yolk. Omega-3 eggs make a wonderful addition to any diet.

Extra Virgin Coconut Oil

Extra virgin coconut oil is an extremely healthy fat. It contains large amounts of lauric acid, one of the chief fatty acids in breast milk. According to scientific and clinical research, consuming extra virgin coconut oil can reduce the risk of deadly degenerative diseases such as cancer, heart disease, and diabetes. Extra virgin coconut oil supports the immune system and helps prevent bacterial, viral, and fungal infections. Reportedly, it reduces the symptoms of Crohn's disease, ulcerative colitis, diverticulosis, irritable bowel syndrome, and constipation. Extra virgin coconut oil is one of the best oils to cook with because it can withstand heat without oxidation. People who suffer from digestive disorders often notice an improvement in symptoms after they substitute extra virgin coconut oil for whatever cooking oil they use.

Grass-Fed Red Meat

Grass-fed red meat, including beef, venison, buffalo and lamb, is an excellent source of high-quality protein, vitamin B_{12}, and iron. Grass-fed red meat provides protective nutrients such as CLA (conjugated linoleic acid), carnitine, and creatine. Grass-fed meat also has a much higher omega-3 fatty acid content than grain-fed meat.

Unheated Honey

Raw, unheated honey is Nature's only predigested food. Unheated honey supplies a rich array of nutrients, including amino acids and enzymes. The body uses pure honey for quick energy. Consumed in small amounts, honey does not contribute to blood sugar imbalances. Raw, unheated honey is the only sweetener we recommend. Nevertheless, you should consume it in moderation.

Fatty Fish

High-fat ocean fish such as salmon, sardines, mackerel, herring and tuna are Nature's richest source of the omega-3 fatty acids eicosapentaenoic acid (EPA) and DHA. Dr. Weston Price found that cultures that relied on fish as their main source of protein were the healthiest among all the indigenous groups he studied. Fish provides easily absorbable protein and minerals and is great for the heart. Eating fresh fish is best, but canned sardines and herring (with skin and bones) may be the exception to the rule. Canned sardines contain healthy levels of omega-3 fatty acids, are high in calcium, and are one of Nature's richest sources of nucleic acids.

Grass-Fed/Organic Organ Meat

Almost all of the ancient cultures that Dr. Weston Price studied prized organ meats for their ability to build strength and vitality. Organ meats are a rich source of fat-soluble vitamin A and D. They contain a great balance of B vitamins and are one of the best sources of minerals, including zinc. It is important to note that organ meats must come from organic or free-range animals. Toxins tend to concentrate in the organs of animals that are given growth hormones and pesticides. For that reason, eating organ meats from animals that were not properly raised is very harmful.

Cod Liver Oil

For those who can't stomach organ meats, and even those who can, cod liver oil is the next best thing. Cod liver oil contains large amounts of fat-soluble vitamin A and D, as well as the essential fatty acids EPA and DHA. You will be glad to know that you can obtain an extremely high quality flavored cod liver oil that actually tastes pretty good. It is called Olde World Icelandic Cod Liver Oil. See Appendix A.

Organic Berries

Berries are some of Nature's richest sources of antioxidants. Organic blueberries, strawberries, raspberries and blackberries contain powerful disease-fighting phytochemicals such as ellagic acid, quercetin, vitamin C, and anthocyanins. Berries are also high in fiber. A great way to enjoy the antioxidant power of berries is to incorporate them into smoothies, or top them with yogurt. That's why I designed Fruits of Life™.

This delicious-tasting antioxidant fruit blend contains certified organic, low temperature-dried concentrates of blueberry, raspberry, strawberry, blackberry, prunes and raisins—as well as a "live food" blend of biologically active alkalizing minerals, enzymes and probiotics from goat's milk. Fruits of Life is a whole food concentrate—and it's power-packed. It isn't me saying so. These results come from the U.S. Department of Agriculture. Here's the story.

There is a test conducted at Tufts University called **ORAC**—short for Oxygen Radical Absorbance Capacity—that measures the ability of foods, blood plasma, and just about any substance to subdue oxygen free radicals in the test tube. Studies at the Jean Mayer USDA Human Nutrition Research Center on Aging at Tufts University in Boston suggest that consuming fruits and vegetables with a high-ORAC value may help slow the aging process in both body and brain. Early evidence indicates that this antioxidant activity translates to animals, protecting cells and their components from oxidative damage. Getting plenty of the foods with a high-ORAC activity, such as spinach, strawberries, and blueberries, has so far raised the antioxidant power of human blood, prevented some loss of long-term memory and learning ability in middle-aged rats, maintained the ability of brain cells in middle-aged rats to respond to a chemical stimulus, and protected rats' tiny blood vessels—capillaries—against oxygen damage.

The ORAC values of fruits and vegetables cover such a broad range, you can pick seven with low values and get only about 1,300 ORAC units. Or, you can eat seven with high values and reach 6,000 ORAC units or more. One cup of blueberries alone supplies 3,200 ORAC units. Based on the evidence so far, experts at the USDA and Tufts University suggest that daily intake be increased to between 3,000 and 5,000 ORAC units to have a significant impact on plasma and tissue antioxidant capacity.

It is notable that Fruits of Life is the first and only product to contain the six top fruit antioxidant foods on the planet in one whole food concentrate. Dried Plums may be an important defense against aging and its associated diseases, according to researchers at the Center on Aging at Tufts. Their antioxidant ORAC score was 5,770, more than double the next highest fruit antioxidant.

Fruit Antioxidant Scores (as ranked by USDA scientists at Tufts University)

Fruit	ORAC Score	Fruit	ORAC Score	Fruit	ORAC Score
Dried Plums*	5770	Strawberries*	1546	Pink Grapefruit	483
Raisins*	2830	Raspberries*	1220	Cantaloupe	252
Blueberries*	2400	Plums	949	Apples	218
Blackberries*	2036	Oranges	750	Pears	134

*Contained in Fruits of Life an antioxidant product from Garden of Life

Cultured Vegetables

Raw, cultured vegetables are a great source of naturally occurring probiotics and enzymes. Cultured vegetables can aid in the digestion of meals that contain cooked animal protein. The daily consumption of raw, cultured vegetables, including sauerkraut, kim chi, or fermented beets, carrots and ginger can help keep the digestive tract healthy and even eliminate harmful microorganisms such as Candida albicans.

Vegetable Juice

Vegetable juice, especially green juices, is a potent source of enzymes, vitamins, and trace minerals. Vegetable juices are easy to assimilate. They supply many of the nutrients that are needed to rebuild health.

Cereal Grass Juice

Cereal grass juices from the young leaves of wheat, oat and barley are nutrient powerhouses. Wheatgrass juice has been consumed around the world and taken as a primary therapy for digestive disorders such as irritable bowel syndrome, ulcers, and inflammatory bowel disease (Crohn's and ulcerative colitis). The minerals in wheatgrass are easy to assimilate. Wheatgrass contains minerals, lightweight vegetable proteins, and chlorophyll. It is Nature's richest source of trace minerals. Many people with digestive sensitivities cannot handle fresh wheatgrass juice, but many do well with powder juice extracts as contained in Perfect Food.

Stocks

Properly prepared soup stocks from meat, fish, and poultry contain many life-giving nutrients, including minerals, gelatin, and electrolytes from vegetables. Many people are unaware of the research that has been done on the naturally occurring gelatin found in stocks. Gelatin acts as a digestive aid. It has been used successfully in the treatment of many intestinal disorders, including non-ulcerative dyspepsia (sour stomach), irritable bowel syndrome, ulcers, and Crohn's disease. Stocks also contain cartilage and collagen, both of which have been used to aid in the health of those suffering from arthritis and other inflammatory conditions. Consumption of stocks such as chicken soup can help heal the digestive lining and reduce the inflammation that occurs in many severe digestive disorders.

Fiber

The consumption of dietary fiber from sources such as properly prepared seeds, legumes and grains is extremely important. Dr. Dennis Burkitt was the first individual to bring the importance of consuming adequate dietary fiber to the forefront. In his travels around the world, Dr. Burkitt found that natives who consumed high amounts of fiber between 35 to 75 grams per day were free from many of today's common ailments including constipation, hemorrhoids, IBS, heart disease, inflammation, and more. We recommend adding a whole food fiber supplement such as Super Seed to everyone's daily regime.

Cultured Beverages

Cultured beverages such as kvass are great sources of probiotics, enzymes, and electrolytes. Consuming cultured beverages between meals strengthens the digestive tract and can aid in the restoration of the proper acidic balance of the colon. Cultured beverages provide electrolytes that help to rapidly hydrate the body.

CHAPTER ELEVEN

The Maker's Diet Recipes

Please don't take shortcuts with these recipes. The ingredients in these recipes contain healing compounds. Do your best to obtain the ingredients as they are listed. Appendix A lists sources for these foods. The Chicken Soup recipe, for example, is not just chicken soup out of a can. This soup recipe was specifically designed to deliver micronutrients and minerals that will assist the healing process. Especially in the case of the broth, following the recipe to a tee is necessary. For more great recipes, read *Nourishing Traditions* by Sally Fallon and Mary Enig, Ph.D.

Chicken Soup (adapted from *Nourishing Traditions* by Fallon and Enig)

1 medium whole chicken, organic, free-range or kosher
  (if you want, you may substitute turkey, or any poultry for chicken)
3-4 quarts filtered water
4-6 tablespoons extra virgin coconut oil
2-4 chicken feet (See Appendix A)
8 organic carrots
6 stalks of organic celery
2-4 organic zucchinis
4 medium-size organic white or yellow onions
1 tablespoon apple cider vinegar
4 inches of grated ginger
5 cloves of garlic
1 large bunch of parsley (added 30 minutes before the soup is finished)
3-5 tablespoons of moist high-mineral Celtic sea salt

Fill the largest stainless steel pot you can find with 3 quarts of purified water. Add 1 tablespoon of apple cider vinegar. Let stand for 10 minutes. Fill the pot with chicken, vegetables, sea salt and other ingredients, and bring to a boil. Let boil for 60 seconds and lower heat. Simmer soup for 12 to 24 hours. Add parsley 30 minutes before the soup is finished.

Remove chicken from the bones and place the chicken meat back in the soup. Remove and discard chicken feet.

For acute situations with high inflammation, allow the soup to cool, and blend or puree all ingredients in a high-powered blender or food processor.

A word for the budgetary challenged: Each ingredient in the soup is very important to your health. Most of the ingredients in the broth are available in supermarkets. However, if you are on a restricted budget, using non-organic vegetables and kosher or conventional chicken instead of free-range chicken is acceptable. You may also substitute sea salt for the moist Celtic sea salt.

Synergy Smoothie

Combine the following ingredients in a high-speed blender (see Appendix C):

10 ounces 30-hour raw, cultured goat's milk dairy product (Probiogurt™; see Appendix A),
    or 10 ounces of full fat coconut milk (see Appendix A)

1 tablespoon extra virgin coconut oil

1-2 raw high omega-3 whole eggs

1 tablespoon cold-pressed flax seed oil

1-2 tablespoons of unheated honey

1 tablespoon goat's milk protein powder (optional if using a raw dairy product)

1/2-1 cup fresh or frozen fruit (berries, bananas, pineapple, etc.), preferably organic

Vanilla extract (optional)

Properly prepared, this smoothie is an extraordinary source of easy-to-absorb nutrition. It contains large amounts of "live" enzymes, probiotics, vitally important "live" proteins, and a full spectrum of essential fatty acids. It can be consumed one to two times per day. It should be consumed within 24 hours after it is blended.

For those who are underweight and wasting, it is best to use *Crème Bulgare* or a combination of 5 ounces of 30-hour yogurt and 5 ounces of coconut milk and cream as the first ingredient in the smoothie. We have seen people who were severely undernourished consume this smoothie on a daily basis and gain phenomenal amounts of weight.

During my healing process, I consumed this smoothie one to two times per day with raw eggs (contrary to popular belief, eggs from healthy free-range chickens are almost always free of Salmonella). For added protection it is best to wash the eggs in the shell with a mild alcohol or hydrogen peroxide solution or a fruit and vegetable wash (available in health food stores). For those who can't stand the thought of consuming raw eggs in their smoothies (did you know that egg yolks are one of the secrets of Haagen Dazs ice cream's great taste?), the smoothie can still be beneficial without the eggs. However, it may take longer to see positive results. If you choose to leave out the eggs you should add 1 additional tablespoon of extra virgin coconut oil.

Creamy High Enzyme Dessert

4 ounces of Probiogurt, quark or cultured goat's milk cream (see Appendix A)

1 tablespoon unheated honey

1 teaspoon of flax seed oil

$1/2$ cup organic fresh or frozen berries

Mix quark, honey and flax seed oil and top with berries.

Salad Dressing

Cold-pressed flax seed oil or hemp seed oil (garlic-chili flax from Omega is my favorite)

Extra virgin olive oil

Apple cider vinegar

Lemon juice

Sea salt or spice blend (see Appendix A)

Mix equal parts of 8 ounces flax seed oil and 8 ounces olive oil and add 2 tablespoons of apple cider vine-gar and 1 teaspoon lemon juice with sea salt or seasoning. Blend to taste. Combine all ingredients and blend slowly. Keep refrigerated and use as a salad dressing or marinade.

Lactic Acid Wine

2 quarts fresh, pressed grape juice from organic dark grapes

4-6 ounces goat's milk yogurt or continental liquid acidophilus (plain)

Mix fresh, pressed grape juice with fermented whey or liquid acidophilus (see resource section) in a glass mason jar. Cover and let stand at room temperature for 4-6 days, and transfer to refrigerator. The taste should be slightly sweet and sour and slightly carbonated. Alcoholic content should be kept to a minimum. If juice is fermented too long alcohol content will increase.

This lactic acid wine is believed to be similar to the "new wine" consumed during Biblical times. It is very refreshing and extremely healthy.

Fermented Veggie Drink

3 red beets

1 carrot

1 ounce grated ginger

2-4 tablespoons fermented whey or continental liquid acidophilus (plain)

1 teaspoon sea salt

purified water

32 drops or 1 teaspoon structured water concentrate (see Appendix B)

Peel and chop beets and carrot and combine with peeled and grated ginger. Place in a 1-2 quart glass con-tainer with a seal. Cover with water and add whey, salt, and structured water concentrate. Stir well and cover.

Keep at room temperature for 2-3 days before transferring to the refrigerator. Taste should be sour but pleasant. If product smells offensive, discard and start over.

This drink is a great source of probiotics and enzymes and can be consumed several times per day.

Balanced Veggie Juice

As long as you are not suffering from diarrhea, vegetable juices are a great source of essential nutrients. Here is a great staple vegetable juice blend.

50% carrot juice

10% beet juice

30% celery juice

10% parsley or other green juice

Optional: 1-2 tablespoons of Perfect Food

Optional: 1 teaspoon of goat's milk yogurt, quark, *crème Bulgare*, or coconut milk and cream
   (see Appendix A)

Note the following about this recipe:

- It is better to consume a higher amount of green juice in relation to carrot and beet juice to ensure stable blood sugar levels.
- The addition of a quality fat like quark or coconut helps ensure balanced blood sugar levels and adds a creamy taste to the drink.
- When time does not permit, simply mixing one to two tablespoons of an enzyme-enhanced, whole-food mineral blend such as Perfect Food makes a great substitute for fresh vegetable juice.

Better Butter

Combine equal parts of the following ingredients: the highest quality goat's milk butter you can find (see Appendix A), extra virgin coconut oil, and cold-pressed flax seed oil. Let the butter and coconut oil soften at room temperature and combine it with cold-pressed flax seed oil. Refrigerate it to harden and use as a spread.

Never use Better Butter for cooking. The enzymes and essential fats will be damaged by heat.

Part IV–
Health & Healing

CHAPTER TWELVE

Healing Protocols

This chapter presents protocols, or plans of treatment, for many of the common diseases, disorders and health conditions that we face today. Using these protocols, the vast majority of patients have improved their health, whether suffering from allergies, eczema, irritable bowel syndrome, or far more serious conditions. Once again, taking care of your gastrointestinal health is key to your overall health—whether your battle is with heart disease, cancer, diabetes or any of the other myriad conditions detailed in this chapter.

Patients who have followed these healing protocols have dramatically improved their absorption and assimilation of foods and nutrients. They improved their elimination of toxins, clarity of mind, vitality and immune function. In short, they have dramatically improved their overall health.

Many patients have been able to overcome long-standing symptoms and remain free of disease by following these healing protocols. They have been able to reduce or discontinue medications (in consultation with their physician).

Under each disease description are specific instructions and practical techniques to help resolve the condition and alleviate the symptoms that are associated with it. All protocols refer to the foods and supplements mentioned throughout this book.

As part of each protocol, you will find recommendations in these categories:
- *Diet:* Which foods will promote optimal health and initiate your body's healing response.
- *Therapeutic Foods:* These are specific foods that should be consumed as often as possible and can positively contribute to the health of the immune system and digestive tract.
- *Supplements:* The health supplements I recommend should help to alleviate symptoms and improve your overall health, as well as address specific health issues.

The focus of this book is to help you to enjoy super health and even regain your health if you have lost it, and I believe that the health of the gastrointestinal tract and immune system, both interlinked themselves, are fundamental to your overall well-being. If you follow these protocols diligently, you should see improvement in the first month of the program—perhaps even in the first few hours; your body is a wonderfully sensitive machine and it will respond to beneficial changes in your dietary and lifestyle habits almost immediately. What's more, you might experience many other benefits. You will have more energy, attain and maintain proper weight for your body type, experience increased lean muscle mass and improved skin tone. Your memory and ability to concentrate will improve. However, if you are suffering from a severe illness, you may not notice any significant improvement for as long as 90 days. If after that period you see little or no results and you can honestly say that you followed the program diligently, this program may not be right for you. I would advise that you seek help elsewhere.

LIFESTYLE THERAPIES

Throughout this chapter, I explain therapeutic foods you can eat to improve your health. I will also list supplements you can take to supercharge your body's healing response. However, changing your lifestyle is an important part of an optimal health program. Following are some lifestyle therapies that I recommend. Where a therapy requires obtaining a product of some kind, you will find sources for the product in Appendix C.

Squatting for elimination: Squatting aligns the colon properly for elimination and empties the colon more completely. Using an elimination bench to raise the legs during elimination can help to fully detoxify the colon. This is essential for those suffering from digestive problems including IBS, constipation and hemmorhoids.

Exercise: As well as toning and strengthening muscles, exercising encourages peristalsis, the wavelike expanding and contracting of the digestive system that eliminates waste. Exercise also enhances the health of the lymphatic system, which is important for proper detoxification and immune system function. If your condition allows it, I recommend taking some form of moderate daily exercise (something as simple as walking can be very healthy). In fact, for some conditions, as with weight problems, exercise has been shown to markedly synergize the benefits of your nutritional supplements.

Avoiding hormonal contraceptives (females): Evidence shows that hormonal contraceptives, whether taken orally, implanted or administered by injection, can lead to imbalanced intestinal flora and contribute to yeast overgrowth (candidiasis), as well as increase the risk for developing ulcerative colitis, breast and liver cancer.

Sunlight: Spend approximately 20 minutes each day in the sun. Most of the vitamin D you obtain comes from sunlight. Many people with chronic diseases including digestive disorders have less than optimal levels of vitamin D. Getting proper levels of vitamin D is crucial for proper calcium absorption and utilization.

Breathing properly: Performing 5 to 15 minutes of deep breathing exercises can be very beneficial. Inhale through your nose for three to seven seconds and exhale quickly through your mouth. Deep breathing can enhance oxygen utilization and improve the functioning of the immune system.

Sauna/steam detoxification: Spend at least 20 to 30 minutes daily in a sauna or steam bath, especially during periods of detoxification. Use adequate hydration and mineral replenishment (e.g., Springs of Life and/or Perfect Food mixed in purified water). Be sure to use low-heat saunas (temperatures ranging from

120 to 140 degrees F.). Raising the temperature of your body helps it to detoxify and expel foreign substances such as bacteria and viruses, as well as heavy metals, pesticides, and industrial chemicals.

Detoxification baths: Take baths with essential oils, clays, and other healing compounds. Doing so aids the body's ability to detoxify harmful chemicals. To make a clay bath, fill the tub with hot water (as hot as you can tolerate) and add one-half to one cup of powdered clay (available in the cosmetic section of most health food stores). Stay in the bath for 5 to 30 minutes. These baths may cause a temporary feeling of weakness and other detoxification symptoms, so you may have to stay in the bath for short periods of time at first. After the bath, consume 16 ounces of structured water, vegetable juice, or water mixed with one to two tablespoons of Perfect Food.

Skin brushing: Skin brushing removes dead skin, improves circulation, and aids in the detoxification of harmful chemicals.

Sleep: Getting enough sleep is essential, especially if you have a digestive disorder. Nighttime is when the body detoxifies and regenerates. When you sleep matters as much as how much sleep you get. Try to get at least one to three hours of sleep before midnight. Groundbreaking research on health and regeneration has shown that sleep before midnight is up to four times more beneficial than sleep after midnight. It is important to note that in Biblical times and throughout ancient history people would rise and retire with the rising and setting of the sun. I believe this to be the healthiest way for us to function today, resulting in improved digestion, immune system health and mood. It is my experience that the amount and quality of your sleep, as well as the times you retire and rise, are as important to your health as diet, supplements, and exercise.

Chewing properly: Chew each bite of food 30 to 50 times to ensure proper digestion and absorption. Eating slowly and chewing properly greatly decreases indigestion.

Eating smaller meals: Eat small meals instead of overstuffing yourself. Many foods recommended in this program greatly enhance metabolism. When large portions are consumed, however, metabolism slows down, digestion is stressed, and feelings of weakness and lethargy ensue.

Avoiding ice-cold foods and beverages: Ice-cold foods and beverages may shock the digestive tract and shut down digestive function. The body must work very hard to raise the temperature of the food or beverage to body temperature. People in eastern cultures never consume ice cold foods because they "weaken digestive fire." Even foods from the refrigerator can be left at room temperature for ten minutes or so to help dispel the cold. Our ancestors rarely consumed cold food due in part to the fact that refrigeration has only existed for the past hundred years or so.

A-Z GUIDE TO THE CONDITIONS

ACNE...see *Skin Health*
ADDICTION...see *Mental Disorders*
ALZHEIMER'S DISEASE...see *Brain Health*
AGORAPHOBIA...see *Mental Disorders*

ANGINA…see *Cardiovascular Health*
ANKYLOSING SPONDYLITIS…see *Joint Disorders*
ANXIETY…see *Mental Disorders*
ASTHMA…see *Upper Respiratory Health*
ATHEROSCLEROSIS/ARTERIOSCLEROSIS…see *Cardiovascular Health*
ATOPIC DERMATITIS (ECZEMA)…see *Skin Health*
ATTENTION DEFICIT/HYPERACTIVITY DISORDER…see *Children's Health*
AUTISM…see *Children's Health*

AUTOIMMUNE DISEASE

- Diabetes Type I
- Grave's Disease
- Lupus
- Multiple Sclerosis
- Myasthenia Gravis
- Rheumatoid Arthritis
- Scleroderma

Overview

The word *auto* is the Greek word for self. The immune system is a complicated network of cells and cell components (called *molecules*) that normally work to defend the body and eliminate infections caused by bacteria, viruses, and other invading microbes. When a person has an autoimmune disease, the immune system mistakenly attacks self, targeting the cells, tissues, and organs of a person's own body. A collection of immune system cells and molecules at a target site is broadly referred to as inflammation.

There are many different autoimmune diseases, and they can each affect the body in different ways. For example in multiple sclerosis, the autoimmune reaction is directed against the myelin sheath of the nervous system; the joints are targeted in rheumatoid arthritis; and, the skin and internal organs in scleroderma. In other autoimmune diseases such as systemic lupus erythematosus (lupus), affected tissues and organs may vary among individuals with the same disease. One person with lupus may have affected skin and joints whereas another may have affected skin, kidneys, and lungs. Ultimately, damage to certain tissues by the immune system may be permanent, as with destruction of insulin-producing cells of the pancreas in Type 1 diabetes mellitus.

Many of the autoimmune diseases, such as Myasthenia gravis (a chronic autoimmune neuromuscular disease characterized by varying degrees of weakness of the voluntary muscles of the body) are rare. As a group, however, autoimmune diseases afflict millions of Americans. Most autoimmune diseases strike women more often than men; in particular, they affect women of working age and during their childbearing years. Some autoimmune diseases occur more frequently in certain minority populations. For example, lupus is more common in African-American and Hispanic women than in Caucasian women of European ancestry. Rheumatoid arthritis and scleroderma affect a higher percentage of residents in some Native American communities than in the general U.S. population. Multiple sclerosis seems to be more prevalent in the northern latitudes.

Diet

Follow the diet prescribed in Chapters 9 through 11 diligently for 6 to 12 months. After symptoms are completely gone for at least three months, you may gradually add foods from the "Neutral" or "Dangerous" categories, if you desire. Because people with autoimmune diseases appear to have a predisposed weakness in their immune systems, I strongly recommend that they adhere to a diet of foods in the "Super" and "Healthy" categories for the rest of their lives.

Therapeutic Foods

These therapeutic foods will help you get well. Appendix A lists sources where you can obtain these foods.

- *Cultured goat's milk dairy products:* Consume 8 to 32 ounces of the highest quality cultured dairy products from goat's milk. I recommend a 30 hour fermented yogurt called Probiogurt (see resource section). Try to find yogurt that does not contain the organism *Streptococcus thermophilus*, a bacterial microbe that has been known to make immune-system disorders worse.
- *Grass-fed red meat:* Red meat from grass-fed cattle, buffalo, and lamb is very healthy and can be eaten a few times per week. This meat is a great source of protein, minerals, vitamin B_{12}, vitamins A and D, omega-3 fats, and CLA.
- *Omega-3 eggs:* Consume as many as one to three eggs high in omega-3 fatty acids each day. These eggs contain DHA, vitamins E and B_{12}, and antioxidants including lutein.
- *Extra virgin coconut oil:* This oil is perhaps the healthiest of the widely available oils. I recommend cooking almost exclusively with extra virgin coconut oil. Consume as much as two to four tablespoons per day of the oil in cooking, smoothies, or right off the spoon. It contains large amounts of lauric acid, a potent antimicrobial and one of the chief fatty acids found in breast milk.
- *Ocean-caught fish:* This type of fish is perhaps the healthiest of all protein sources. Salmon, sardines, mackerel, herring and albacore tuna are high in the omega-3 fatty acids eicosapentaenoic acid (EPA) and docosahexaenoic acid (DHA). Ocean-caught fish can be consumed every day to enhance digestive and immune system health.
- *Cod liver oil:* Take one to three teaspoons of flavored Olde World Icelandic Cod Liver Oil each day. The amount consumed should be based upon the amount of sunlight you receive. People in colder climates generally need to consume larger amounts. Cod liver oil is a fantastic source of the omega-3 fats DHA and EPA, as well as fat-soluble vitamins A and D.
- *Vegetable juice:* Consume vegetable juices that are low in carbohydrates, such as celery and green juices mixed with a small amount of higher carbohydrate veggies such as carrot or beet. Mix in some form of healthy fat with each glass of the juice. One to three teaspoons of cultured goat's milk, extra virgin coconut oil, canned or fresh coconut milk and cream, or flaxseed oil enhances absorption of minerals and prevents spikes in blood sugar.

- **Fermented vegetables:** Consume a few tablespoons of fermented vegetables such as sauerkraut with each meal to aid in digestion. Fermented vegetables are an excellent source of naturally occurring probiotics and enzymes.
- **Stocks:** It is a great idea to consume stocks on a regular basis, especially when you have a cold or flu. Stocks made from the bones of chicken, fish, lamb and beef contain minerals, gelatin, cartilage, collagen, and electrolytes from the vegetables. Stocks are an excellent source of proteins, especially collagen. They help to heal the gut lining and reduce inflammation.

Supplements

Take these health supplements to alleviate symptoms and get well. Appendix B explains where to obtain these supplements.

- **Primal Defense:** Start with one caplet per day on an empty stomach, 30 minutes before or one hour after meals. Increase usage by adding one additional caplet per day (i.e., one caplet the first day, two the second day, three the third day and so on). Once your dosage is up to 12 caplets per day, stay on that amount for a minimum of three months or until health has greatly improved and there are no visible signs of autoimmune disease, and then begin to gradually decrease to a maintenance dosage of between three to six caplets per day. Primal Defense is best taken first thing in the morning and right before bedtime with eight ounces pure water. Primal Defense may be taken with other nutritional supplements, but should be taken one hour apart from medications. If you experience symptoms of detoxification (i.e., increased elimination, loose stools, constipation, excess gas, flu-like symptoms or fever), reduce the dosage and work up slowly to 12 per day.
- **RM-10:** Take five caplets twice per day, morning and evening, until diagnostic markers have improved. Once improvement is noted the dosage can be reduced to two to five caplets daily. This formula may be taken with Primal Defense, FYI, or Perfect Food.
- **Omega-Zyme:** Take one to three caplets with each meal or snack.
- **FYI:** Take six FYI first thing in the morning and six before bed (with Primal Defense) for three to six months or until health has greatly improved, and then reduce to a maintenance level of three to six caplets per day.
- **Perfect Food:** Take one to two tablespoons twice daily with eight ounces water or fresh vegetable juice. You may take Perfect Food together with Primal Defense, FYI or RM-10. Best taken on an empty stomach away from food.
- **Springs of Life:** Consume at least eight, eight-ounce glasses per day of purified water mixed with 12 drops of Springs of Life living water concentrate.
- **Goatein:** The only protein powder on the market made from organically produced goat's milk. This protein powder is partially pre-digested, low temperature dried and is usually well tolerated by those with food allergies and digestive problems. Take one to four tablespoons per day mixed in water, juice, smoothies, yogurt or can be used in baking.

Additional Therapies

For people who have or may have imbalanced immune systems, avoiding contact with chlorinated water is of the utmost importance. That includes bathing water and drinking water. Chlorine kills bacteria, friendly and unfriendly, in the intestines. It can be absorbed through the skin. I recommend installing a shower filter to remove chlorine (see Appendix C). Avoid swimming in chlorinated water as well.

BENIGN PROSTATIC HYPERTROPHY…see *Male Health*
BLOOD PRESSURE (ELEVATED)…see *Cardiovascular Health*

BLOOD SUGAR IMBALANCES

- Diabetes Type II
- Hypoglycemia
- Syndrome X

Overview

There are two tragedies associated with adult onset diabetes today. The first is that by the time a person has been diagnosed with this condition, they've most likely already had it several years or longer. Extensive damage to the nervous and circulatory systems and even their vision may have already occurred.

The second tragedy is that diabetes is striking baby boomers with a vengeance. About six percent of our population presently has diabetes. Many experts believe that percentage will increase significantly as the boomers enter their fifties and sixties. And they say that diet and nutrition will be crucial to helping persons with diabetes maintain their health and reduce their risk of complications. The prevalence of diabetes is increasing four to five percent annually with an estimated 40 to 45 percent of people over 65 years of age at most risk.[57] These estimates were recently further confirmed by a study in the November 2001 issue of *Diabetes Care*. The number of Americans with diagnosed diabetes is expected to increase 165 percent over the next 50 years, says the U.S. Centers for Disease Control and Prevention in a report in *USA Today*.[58]

And even if frank diabetes isn't a concern, many other individuals—perhaps a quarter of the adult population—will experience a related condition called Syndrome X. This is a sinister-sounding term for a cluster of conditions that, when occurring together, indicate a predisposition to diabetes, hypertension, heart disease and other common deadly diseases. The term was first coined by a group of researchers at Stanford University to describe a cluster of disease-causing symptoms, including high blood pressure, high triglycerides, decreased high-density lipoprotein (HDL, the "good" cholesterol), insulin resistance, and obesity, which tend to appear together in some individuals and increase their risk for diabetes and heart disease and, possibly, cancer as well as many other disease processes.

In fact, Type II diabetes and Syndrome X have much in common. Both are very complex conditions where insulin deficiency is not the problem. Rather, the problem is the body's *resistance* to insulin. The body 〔ma〕y be producing plenty of insulin, but the hormone isn't being metabolized for optimal use. This condi〔tion i〕s known as peripheral insulin resistance. It is difficult to treat, even with our best medical drugs.[59]

Clearly, the underlying theme of effective diabetes treatment is that for most adult cases of diabetes, front line therapy should consist of improved diet with a reduction in carbohydrates and an increase in healthy fats, exercise, and, for additional help, the inclusion of whole food nutritional products.

Diet

Follow the diet prescribed in Chapters 9 to 11 diligently for 6 to 12 months. People with blood sugar imbalances (either diabetes or hypoglycemia) should do very well following the Maker's Diet. One should choose more high protein and low carbohydrate foods until blood sugar levels are under control. The consumption of healthy fats and proteins along with low glycemic carbohydrates should lead to tremendous improvements in health and far better insulin sensitivity. After symptoms are completely gone for at least three months, you may gradually add foods from the "Neutral" or "Dangerous" categories, if you desire. I recommend that people with a propensity to blood sugar imbalances choose most of their foods from the "Super" and "Healthy" categories.

Therapeutic Foods

These therapeutic foods will help you get well. Appendix A lists sources where you can obtain these foods.

- *Cultured goat's milk dairy products:* Consume 8 to 16 ounces of the highest quality cultured dairy products from goat's milk. I recommend a 30 hour fermented yogurt called Probiogurt (see resource section). Try to find yogurt that does not contain the organism *Streptococcus thermophilus*, a bacterial microbe that has been known to make immune-system disorders worse.
- *Grass-fed red meat:* Red meat from grass-fed cattle, buffalo, and lamb is very healthy and can be eaten a three to five times per week. This meat is a great source of protein, minerals, vitamin B_{12}, vitamins A and D, omega-3 fats, and CLA.
- *Omega-3 eggs:* Consume as many as two eggs high in omega-3 fatty acids each day. These eggs contain DHA, vitamins E and B_{12}, and antioxidants including lutein.
- *Extra virgin coconut oil:* This oil is perhaps the healthiest of the widely available oils. I recommend cooking almost exclusively with extra virgin coconut oil. Consume as much as two to four tablespoons per day of the oil in cooking, smoothies, or right off the spoon. It contains large amounts of lauric acid, a potent antimicrobial and one of the chief fatty acids found in breast milk.
- *Ocean-caught fish:* This type of fish is perhaps the healthiest of all protein sources. Salmon, sardines, mackerel, herring and albacore tuna are high in the omega-3 fatty acids EPA and DHA. Ocean-caught fish can be consumed every day to enhance digestive and immune system health.
- *Cod liver oil:* Take one to three teaspoons of Olde World Icelandic Cod Liver Oil each day. The amount consumed should be based upon the amount of sunlight you receive. People in colder climates generally need to consume larger amounts. Cod liver oil is a fantastic source of the omega-3 fats DHA and EPA, as well as vitamins A and D.

- **Vegetable juice:** Consume vegetable juices that are low in carbohydrates, such as celery and green juices mixed with a small amount of higher carbohydrate veggies such as carrot or beet. Mix in some form of healthy fat with each glass of the juice. One to three teaspoons of cultured goat's milk, extra virgin coconut oil, canned or fresh coconut milk and cream, or flaxseed oil enhances absorption of minerals and prevents spikes in blood sugar.
- **Fermented vegetables:** Consume a few tablespoons of fermented vegetables such as sauerkraut with each meal to aid in digestion. Fermented vegetables are an excellent source of naturally occurring probiotics and enzymes.
- **Stocks:** It is a great idea to consume stocks on a regular basis, especially when you have a cold or flu. Stocks made from the bones of chicken, fish, lamb and beef contain minerals, gelatin, cartilage, collagen, and electrolytes from the vegetables. Stocks are an excellent source of proteins, especially collagen. They help to heal the gut lining and reduce inflammation.

Supplements

Take these health supplements to alleviate symptoms and get well. Appendix B explains where to obtain these supplements.

- **Primal Defense:** Start with one caplet per day on an empty stomach, 30 minutes before or one hour after meals. Increase usage by adding one additional caplet per day (i.e., one caplet the first day, two the second day, three the third day and so on). Once your dosage is up to 12 caplets per day, stay on that amount for a minimum of three months and then begin to gradually decrease to a maintenance dosage of between three to six caplets per day. Primal Defense is best taken first thing in the morning and right before bedtime with eight ounces pure water. Primal Defense may be taken with other nutritional supplements, but should be taken one hour apart from medications. If you experience symptoms of detoxification (i.e., increased elimination, loose stools, constipation, excess gas, flu-like symptoms or fever), reduce the dosage and work up slowly to 12 per day.
- **FYI:** Take six FYI first thing in the morning and six before bed (with Primal Defense) for three to six months or until health has greatly improved, and then reduce to a maintenance level of three to six caplets per day.
- **RM-10:** Take five caplets twice per day, morning and evening, until diagnostic markers have improved. Once improvement is noted the dosage can be reduced to two to five caplets daily. This formula may be taken with Primal Defense, FYI, or Perfect Food.
- **Omega-Zyme:** Take one to three caplets with each meal or snack.
- **Perfect Food:** Take one to two tablespoons twice daily with eight ounces water or fresh vegetable juice.
- **Springs of Life:** Consume at least eight, eight-ounce glasses per day of purified water mixed with 12 drops of Springs of Life living water concentrate.
  - **Seed:** Consume one two-tablespoon serving twice per day, morning and evening, with eight re ounces of purified water.

- *Goatein:* The only protein powder on the market made from organically produced goat's milk. This protein powder is partially pre-digested, low temperature dried and is usually well tolerated by those with food allergies and digestive problems. Take one to four tablespoons per day mixed in water, juice, smoothies, yogurt or can be used in baking.

Additional Therapies

For people who have or may have imbalanced intestinal flora or a weakened immune system, avoiding contact with chlorinated water is of the utmost importance. That includes bathing water and drinking water. Chlorine kills bacteria, friendly and unfriendly, in the intestines. It can be absorbed through the skin. I recommend installing a shower filter to remove chlorine (see Appendix C). Avoid swimming in chlorinated water as well.

BRAIN HEALTH

- Alzheimer's Disease
- Dementia
- Memory Loss
- Parkinson's

Overview

The ability to think creatively, react quickly to new intellectual challenges and circumstances, remember phone numbers, addresses, even where we parked our car are just some of the valuable functions of a brain operating at peak efficiency. In a very real sense, our intelligence is perhaps our greatest gift.

Yet, the cells of the brain are under siege daily from both the inexorable and natural processes of aging, including exposure to cell-damaging free radicals, age-related decrease in activity of important neurotransmitters, as well as from exposure to toxic chemicals found in a wide range of consumer products, especially petroleum-based household cleaners, paints, and home and garden pesticides.

It is not surprising that experts have found the brain measurably loses function starting as early as age 45. Many otherwise healthy adults will lose a full 50 percent of their brain function related to memory, learning and concentration over the course of their lives. A recent survey of 1,000 French adults found that two-thirds complained of memory problems.[60] These problems are becoming more and more common in the 35 to 50 age group.

A decline in mental function can have a significant impact on both our physical and emotional health. Psychologist John Barefoot, of Duke University Medical Center, reports that in a study, which began in 1964 and followed people for several decades, those persons with the highest scores for despair, poor self-esteem, difficulty concentrating and low motivation had a seventy percent higher risk of heart attack and sixty percent higher risk of overall death compared to men and women with the lowest scores.[61]

"We are living in a graying world," notes Ursula Lehr, Ph.D., of the University of Heidelberg and former Secretary of Health of the Federal Republic of Germany. "Never before in the world could so many people reach such an advanced age. Many studies have found that people who are mentally more active, have higher IQs, a wider range of interests, a farther-reaching perspective and a greater number of social contacts, reach old age with greater feelings of psycho-physical well-being. It has been established that cognitive activity is essential for healthy aging."

Diet

Follow the diet prescribed in Chapters 9 to 11 diligently for 6 to 12 months. After symptoms are completely gone for at least three months, you may gradually add foods from the "Neutral" or "Dangerous" categories, if you desire. Because people with brain disorders (Parkinson's, Alzheimer's, dementia) appear to have a predisposed weakness which presents itself as a brain disorder, I strongly recommend that they adhere to a diet of foods in the "Super" and "Healthy" categories for the rest of their lives.

Therapeutic Foods

These therapeutic foods will help you get well. Appendix A lists sources where you can obtain these foods.

- *Cultured goat's milk dairy products:* Consume 8 to 32 ounces of the highest quality cultured dairy products from goat's milk. I recommend a 30 hour fermented yogurt called Probiogurt (see resource section). Try to find yogurt that does not contain the organism *Streptococcus thermophilus*, a bacterial microbe that has been known to make immune-system disorders worse.
- *Grass-fed red meat:* Red meat from grass-fed cattle, buffalo, and lamb is very healthy and can be eaten a few times per week. This meat is a great source of protein, minerals, vitamin B_{12}, vitamins A and D, omega-3 fats, and CLA.
- *Omega-3 eggs:* Consume as many as two eggs high in omega-3 fatty acids each day. These eggs contain DHA, vitamins E and B_{12}, and antioxidants.
- *Extra virgin coconut oil:* This oil is perhaps the healthiest of the widely available oils. I recommend cooking almost exclusively with extra virgin coconut oil. Consume as much as two to four tablespoons per day of the oil in cooking, smoothies, or right off the spoon. It contains large amounts of lauric acid, a potent antimicrobial and one of the chief fatty acids in breast milk.
- *Ocean-caught fish:* This type of fish is perhaps the healthiest of all protein sources. Salmon, sardines, mackerel, herring and albacore tuna are high in the omega-3 fatty acids EPA and DHA. Ocean-caught fish can be consumed every day to enhance digestive and immune system health.
- *Cod liver oil:* Take one to three teaspoons of Olde World Icelandic Cod Liver Oil each day. The amount consumed should be based upon the amount of sunlight you receive. People in colder climates generally need to consume larger amounts. Cod liver oil is a fantastic source of the omega-3 fats DHA and EPA, as well as vitamins A and D.
- *Vegetable juice:* Consume vegetable juices that are low in carbohydrates, such as celery and green ... mixed with a small amount of higher carbohydrate veggies such as carrot or beet. Mix in some ... f healthy fat with each glass of the juice. One to three teaspoons of cultured goat's milk, extra

virgin coconut oil, canned or fresh coconut milk and cream, or flaxseed oil enhances absorption of minerals and prevents spikes in blood sugar.

- *Berries:* Berries such as blueberries, raspberries, blackberries and strawberries are perhaps the greatest sources of dietary antioxidants available. Scientists at Tufts University have shown that blueberries serve as the premiere dietary source of antioxidants and may reduce the damaging effects of age-related memory loss.
- *Fermented vegetables:* Consume a few tablespoons of fermented vegetables such as sauerkraut with each meal to aid in digestion. Fermented vegetables are an excellent source of naturally occurring probiotics and enzymes.
- *Stocks:* It is a great idea to consume stocks on a regular basis, especially when you have a cold or flu. Stocks made from the bones of chicken, fish, lamb and beef contain minerals, gelatin, cartilage, collagen, and electrolytes from the vegetables. Stocks are an excellent source of proteins, especially collagen. They help to heal the gut lining and reduce inflammation.

Supplements

Take these health supplements to alleviate symptoms and get well. Appendix B explains where to obtain these supplements.

- *Primal Defense:* Start with one caplet per day on an empty stomach, 30 minutes before or one hour after meals. Increase usage by adding one additional caplet per day (i.e., one caplet the first day, two the second day, three the third day and so on). Once your dosage is up to 12 caplets per day, stay on that amount for a minimum of three months and then begin to gradually decrease to a maintenance dosage of between three to six caplets per day. Primal Defense is best taken first thing in the morning and right before bedtime with eight ounces pure water. Primal Defense may be taken with other nutritional supplements, but should be taken one hour apart from medications. If you experience symptoms of detoxification (i.e., increased elimination, loose stools, constipation, excess gas, flu-like symptoms or fever), reduce the dosage and work up slowly to 12 per day.
- *FYI:* Take six FYI first thing in the morning and six before bed (with Primal Defense) for three to six months or until health has greatly improved, and then reduce to a maintenance level of three to six caplets per day.
- *RM-10:* Take five caplets twice per day, morning and evening, until diagnostic markers have improved. Once improvement is noted the dosage can be reduced to two to five caplets daily. This formula may be taken with Primal Defense, FYI, or Perfect Food.
- *Omega-Zyme:* Take one to three caplets with each meal or snack.
- *Fruits of Life:* Take one to two servings of Fruits of Life powder or caplets per day. Fruits of Life contains foods such as blueberries which are rich in antioxidants and may play a role in relieving symptoms of premature aging. Follow directions on the label.
- *Perfect Food:* Take one to two tablespoons twice daily with eight ounces water or fresh vegetable juice.
- *Springs of Life:* Consume at least eight, eight-ounce glasses per day of purified water mixed with 12 drops of Springs of Life living water concentrate.

- **Super Seed:** Consume one serving twice per day, morning and evening, with eight or more ounces of purified water.
- **Goatein:** The only protein powder on the market made from organically produced goat's milk. This protein powder is partially pre-digested, low temperature dried and is usually well tolerated by those with food allergies and digestive problems. Take one to four tablespoons per day mixed in water, juice, smoothies, yogurt or can be used in baking.

Additional Therapies

For people who have or may have imbalanced intestinal flora, avoiding contact with chlorinated water is of the utmost importance. That includes bathing water and drinking water. Chlorine kills bacteria, friendly and unfriendly, in the intestines. It can be absorbed through the skin. I recommend installing a shower filter to remove chlorine (see Appendix C). Avoid swimming in chlorinated water as well.

Also consider limiting exposure to the following consumer products:

Food additives. Some food additives, such as artificial colors, contain lead which impairs mental function, reports *The Safe Shopper's Bible* (Hungry Minds 1995). Other types of food additives, known as excitotoxins, can actually kill brain cells; examples of excitotoxins are monosodium glutamate (often found in hydrolyzed vegetable protein) and aspartame (Nutrasweet).

Excess alcohol. While a single serving of alcohol daily appears to be protective against heart disease, excess alcohol intake can result in destruction of brain cells and cause long-term irreversible brain damage.

Hazardous chemicals. Household cleaning products, paints, auto products, and home and garden pesticides often contain toxic solvents and other chemicals that damage the nervous system. Consult *The Safe Shopper's Bible* for safe brands.

BURSITIS…*see Inflammatory Conditions*

CANCER

- Bladder
- Brain
- Breast
- Colorectal
- Endometrial
- Leukemia
- Lung
- Lymphoma
- Melanoma
- Ovarian
- Prostate

Cancer is one of the leading killers in the world today. Greater than one in three Americans will be stricken with cancer in their lifetime. Cancer is actually many diseases characterized by uncontrolled cell division, starting with a single cell that has begun to uncontrollably multiply.

The body is made up of many types of cells. Normally, cells grow and divide to produce more cells only when the body needs them. This orderly process helps keep the body healthy. Sometimes, however, cells keep dividing when new cells are not needed. These extra cells form a mass of tissue, called a growth or tumor. Tumors can be benign or malignant.

Benign tumors are not cancer. They can often be removed and, in most cases, they do not come back. Cells from benign tumors do not spread to other parts of the body. Most important, benign tumors are rarely a threat to life.

Malignant tumors are cancerous. Cells in these tumors are abnormal and divide without control or order. They can invade and damage nearby tissues and organs. Also, cancer cells can break away from a malignant tumor and enter the bloodstream or the lymphatic system. That is how cancer spreads from the original cancer site to form new tumors in other organs. The spread of cancer is called metastasis.

Most cancers are named for the organ or type of cell in which they begin. For example, cancer that begins in the lung is lung cancer, and cancer that begins in cells in the skin known as melanocytes is called melanoma. Leukemia and lymphoma are cancers that arise in blood-forming cells. The abnormal cells circulate in the bloodstream and lymphatic system. They may also invade (infiltrate) body organs and form tumors.

When cancer spreads (metastasizes), cancer cells are often found in nearby or regional lymph nodes (sometimes called lymph glands). If the cancer has reached these nodes, it means that cancer cells may have spread to other organs, such as the liver, bones, or brain. When cancer spreads from its original location to another part of the body, the new tumor has the same kind of abnormal cells and the same name as the primary tumor. For example, if lung cancer spreads to the brain, the cancer cells in the brain are actually lung cancer cells. The disease is called metastatic lung cancer (it is not brain cancer).

Because cancer is a generic term for many individual diseases, it is beyond the scope of this work to tailor an individual program for every single person. However, the constituents of RM-10, Primal Defense and FYI have been shown to be effective at controlling the over-proliferation (growth) of many common cancers and should be part of your complementary cancer program.

Diet

Follow the diet prescribed in Chapters 9 to 11 diligently for 6 to 12 months. Once there is no trace of cancer, you may begin to consume certain foods from the "Neutral" and "Dangerous" categories occasionally, but it is best to make the "Super" and "Healthy" foods the largest part of your diet.

Therapeutic Foods

These therapeutic foods will help you get well. Appendix A lists sources where you can obtain these foods.

- *Cultured goat's milk dairy products:* Consume 8 to 32 ounces of the highest quality cultured dairy products from goat's milk. I recommend a 30 hour fermented yogurt called Probiogurt (see resource

section). Try to find yogurt that does not contain the organism *Streptococcus thermophilus*, a bacterial microbe that has been known to make immune-system disorders worse.

- **Grass-fed red meat:** Red meat from grass-fed cattle, buffalo, and lamb is very healthy and can be eaten a few times per week. This meat is a great source of protein, minerals, vitamin B_{12}, vitamins A and D, omega-3 fats, and CLA.
- **Omega-3 eggs:** Consume as many as two eggs high in omega-3 fatty acids each day. These eggs contain DHA, vitamins E and B_{12}, and antioxidants including lutein.
- **Extra virgin coconut oil:** This oil is perhaps the healthiest of the widely available oils. I recommend cooking almost exclusively with extra virgin coconut oil. Consume as much as two to four tablespoons per day of the oil in cooking, smoothies, or right off the spoon. It contains large amounts of lauric acid, a potent antimicrobial and one of the chief fatty acids in breast milk.
- **Ocean-caught fish:** This type of fish is perhaps the healthiest of all protein sources. Salmon, sardines, mackerel, herring and to a lesser extent tuna are high in the omega-3 fatty acids EPA and DHA. Ocean-caught fish can be consumed every day to enhance digestive and immune system health.
- **Cod liver oil:** Take one to three teaspoons of Olde World Icelandic Cod Liver Oil each day. The amount consumed should be based upon the amount of sunlight you receive. People in colder climates generally need to consume larger amounts. Cod liver oil is a fantastic source of the omega-3 fats DHA and EPA, as well as vitamins A and D.
- **Vegetable juice:** Consume vegetable juices that are low in carbohydrates, such as celery and green juices mixed with a small amount of higher carbohydrate veggies such as carrot or beet. Mix in some form of healthy fat with each glass of the juice. One to three teaspoons of cultured goat's milk, extra virgin coconut oil, canned or fresh coconut milk and cream, or flaxseed oil enhances absorption of minerals and prevents spikes in blood sugar.
- **Fermented vegetables:** Consume a few tablespoons of fermented vegetables such as sauerkraut with each meal to aid in digestion. Fermented vegetables are an excellent source of naturally occurring probiotics and enzymes.
- **Stocks:** It is a great idea to consume stocks on a regular basis, especially when you have a cold or flu. Stocks made from the bones of chicken, fish, lamb and beef contain minerals, gelatin, cartilage, collagen, and electrolytes from the vegetables. Stocks are an excellent source of proteins, especially collagen. They help to heal the gut lining and reduce inflammation.

Supplements

Take these health supplements to alleviate symptoms and get well. Appendix B explains where to obtain these supplements.

- **Primal Defense:** Start with one caplet per day on an empty stomach, 30 minutes before or one hour after meals. Increase usage by adding one additional caplet per day (i.e., one caplet the first day, two the second day, three the third day and so on). Once your dosage is up to 12 to 18 caplets per day, stay on that amount for a minimum of three months or until health has greatly improved and there are no visible signs of cancer and then begin to gradually decrease to a maintenance dosage of between three to six caplets per day. Primal Defense is best taken first thing in the morning and right before bedtime with eight ounces pure water. Primal Defense may be taken with other nutritional supplements, but should be taken one hour apart from medications. If you experience symptoms of detoxification (i.e., increased elimination, loose stools, constipation, excess gas, flu-like symptoms or fever), reduce the dosage and work up slowly to 12 per day.

- *RM-10:* Take five caplets twice per day, morning and evening, until cancer markers have improved. Once improvements are noted, you may decrease dosage to two to five caplets per day. May be taken with Primal Defense, FYI and Perfect Food.
- *FYI:* Take six FYI first thing in the morning and six before bed (with Primal Defense) for three to six months or until health has greatly improved, and then reduce to a maintenance level of three to six caplets per day.
- *Omega-Zyme:* Take one to three caplets with each meal or snack.
- *Perfect Food:* Take two tablespoons twice daily with eight ounces water or fresh vegetable juice. You may take Perfect Food together with Primal Defense, FYI or RM-10. Best taken on an empty stomach away from food.
- *Super Seed:* Consume one serving twice per day, morning and evening, with eight or more ounces of purified water.
- *Springs of Life:* Consume at least eight, eight-ounce glasses per day of purified water mixed with 12 drops of Springs of Life living water concentrate.
- *Goatein:* The only protein powder on the market made from organically produced goat's milk. This protein powder is partially pre-digested, low temperature dried and is usually well tolerated by those with food allergies and digestive problems. Take one to four tablespoons per day mixed in water, juice, smoothies, yogurt or can be used in baking.

Additional Therapies

For people who have or may have a weakened immune system, avoiding contact with chlorinated water is of the utmost importance. That includes bathing water and drinking water. Chlorine kills bacteria, friendly and unfriendly, in the intestinal tract. It can be absorbed through the skin. I recommend installing a shower filter to remove chlorine (see Appendix C). Avoid swimming in chlorinated water as well.

CANDIDIASIS

Candida albicans, a common yeast, is part of the regular flora (bacteria) in the digestive tract. In a healthy state, they live in a ratio of about one candida cell to one million other microorganisms . However, due to our modern lifestyles, women who take birth control pills and men or women who consume large amounts of carbohydrates, especially refined carbohydrates (e.g., refined sugars and fruit juices), or have used antibiotics or corticosteroids might experience candida overgrowth. Women might also experience yeast overgrowth premenstrually or during pregnancy since progesterone levels seem to enhance yeast growth. Stress is also a cause of yeast overgrowth.

When this happens, yeast overgrowth-related disorders may then develop, such as yeast infections, rectal itch, constipation, bloating and weight gain, skin problems, brain "fog," and many others.

With long-term infestation, candida shifts into a fungal form that develops roots called rhizoids. These can grow right into the intestinal wall and cause the intestine to become porous, allowing toxins and undigested proteins and carbohydrates to flow through the bowel wall, to be absorbed into the body and the blood stream. This condition is called Leaky Gut Syndrome. So many seemingly untreatable health problems start with candida overgrowth, which can evolve into Leaky Gut Syndrome.

The next step in this vicious cycle is that the immune system of the individual makes antibodies (proteins) that attempt to neutralize the candida overgrowth. These antibodies can cause the body to become hypersensitive to certain foods and molds, and can create a wide variety of food allergies. They can also interfere with hormonal activity and cause nutritional deficiencies.

The yeast syndrome is characterized by patients saying they "feel sick all over." Major symptoms include: fatigue or lethargy; feeling "drained"; poor memory; feeling "spacey" or "unreal"; depression; numbness; burning or tingling; muscle aches and weakness; pain and/or swelling in the joints; abdominal pain and bloating; constipation and/or diarrhea; persistent vaginal itch or burning; endometriosis; cramps and other menstrual irregularities including premenstrual tension; erratic vision including spots in front of eyes; allergies; immune system malfunction; chemical sensitivities; and digestive disturbances.

The best method for diagnosing chronic candidiasis is clinical evaluation by a physician knowledgeable about yeast-related illness. The manner in which the doctor will diagnose the yeast syndrome will probably be based on clinical judgment from a detailed medical history and patient questionnaire. The doctor may also employ laboratory techniques, such as stool cultures for candida, and measurement of antibody levels to candida or candida antigens in the blood.

Once diagnosed, most physicians prescribe drugs such as nystatin, ketoconazol and diflucan as well as various natural anticandida agents, but these rarely produce significant long-term results because they fail to address the underlying factors that promote candida overgrowth.

Therefore, a holistic and integrative approach, involving diet, lifestyle and whole food nutritional supplements, is essential for long-term improvement and prevention.

Diet

Follow the diet prescribed in Chapters 9 to 11 diligently for 6 to 12 months. For the first 30 days it is best to limit or even restrict fruit and honey consumption. Make sure that if you do consume fruit it is the less sweet, high-nutrient, high-fiber fruits such as berries, apples or grapefruit.

After symptoms are completely gone for at least six months, you may gradually add foods from the "Neutral" or "Dangerous" categories, if you desire. Many people suffering from systemic yeast overgrowth will need to eliminate almost all grains and fruit for the first three months of the program. Because people with fungal and parasitic overgrowth appear to have a predisposed weakness in their intestinal tracts, I strongly recommend that they adhere to a diet of foods in the "Super" and "Healthy" categories for the rest of their lives.

Therapeutic Foods

These therapeutic foods will help you get well. Appendix A lists sources where you can obtain these foods.

- *Cultured goat's milk dairy products:* Consume 8 to 32 ounces of the highest quality cultured dairy products from goat's milk. I recommend a 30 hour fermented yogurt called Probiogurt (see resource section). Try to find yogurt that does not contain the organism *Streptococcus thermophilus*, a bacterial microbe that has been known to make immune-system disorders worse.

- *Grass-fed red meat:* Red meat from grass-fed cattle, buffalo, and lamb is very healthy and can be eaten a few times per week. This meat is a great source of protein, minerals, vitamin B_{12}, vitamins A and D, omega-3 fats, and CLA.

- *Omega-3 eggs:* Consume as many as two eggs high in omega-3 fatty acids each day. These eggs contain DHA, vitamins E and B_{12}, and antioxidants including lutein.

- *Extra virgin coconut oil:* This oil is perhaps the healthiest of the widely available oils. I recommend cooking almost exclusively with extra virgin coconut oil. Consume as much as four to six tablespoons of the oil in cooking, in smoothies, or right off the spoon. Extra virgin coconut oil contains large amounts of lauric, capric and caprylic acids, which are potent antifungal compounds.

- *Ocean-caught fish:* This type of fish is perhaps the healthiest of all protein sources. Salmon, sardines, mackerel, herring and albacore tuna are high in the omega-3 fatty acids EPA and DHA. Ocean-caught fish can be consumed every day to enhance digestive and immune system health.

- *Cod liver oil:* Take one to three teaspoons of Olde World Icelandic Cod Liver Oil each day. The amount consumed should be based upon the amount of sunlight you receive. People in colder climates generally need to consume larger amounts. Cod liver oil is a fantastic source of the omega-3 fats DHA and EPA, as well as vitamins A and D.

- *Vegetable juice:* Consume vegetable juices that are low in carbohydrates, such as celery and green juices mixed with a small amount of higher carbohydrate veggies such as carrot or beet. Mix in some form of healthy fat with each glass of the juice. One to three teaspoons of cultured goat's milk, extra virgin coconut oil, canned or fresh coconut milk and cream, or flaxseed oil enhances absorption of minerals and prevents spikes in blood sugar.

- *Fermented vegetables:* Consume a few tablespoons of fermented vegetables such as sauerkraut with each meal to aid in digestion. Fermented vegetables are an excellent source of naturally occurring probiotics and enzymes.

- *Stocks:* It is a great idea to consume stocks on a regular basis, especially when you have a cold or flu. Stocks made from the bones of chicken, fish, lamb and beef contain minerals, gelatin, cartilage, collagen, and electrolytes from the vegetables. Stocks are an excellent source of proteins, especially collagen. They help to heal the gut lining and reduce inflammation.

Supplements

Take these health supplements to alleviate symptoms and get well. Appendix B explains where to obtain these supplements.

- *Fungal Defense:* Follow the 14-day protocol as directed on label.
- *Primal Defense:* Following the 14-day Fungal Defense protocol, take 12 caplets of Primal Defense per day; stay on that amount for three to six months or when tests for candida overgrowth are negative. Then begin to gradually decrease to a maintenance dosage of between three to six caplets per day. Primal Defense is best taken first thing in the morning and right before bedtime with eight ounces pure water. Primal Defense may be taken with other nutritional supplements, but should be taken one hour apart from medications. If you experience symptoms of detoxification (i.e., increased elimination, loose stools, constipation, excess gas, flu-like symptoms or fever), reduce the dosage and work up slowly to 12 per day.
- *Perfect Food:* Take two tablespoons twice daily with eight ounces water or fresh vegetable juice. You may take Perfect Food together with Primal Defense. Best taken on an empty stomach away from food.
- *Omega-Zyme:* Take one to three caplets with each meal or snack.
- *Springs of Life:* Consume at least eight, eight-ounce glasses per day of purified water mixed with 12 drops of Springs of Life living water concentrate.
- *Super Seed:* Consume one serving twice per day, morning and evening, with eight or more ounces of purified water. (Consuming a fiber supplement is essential during the first two weeks of the program. Thereafter, consume fiber as needed.)
- *Goatein:* The only protein powder on the market made from organically produced goat's milk. This protein powder is partially pre-digested, low temperature dried and is usually well tolerated by those with food allergies and digestive problems. Take one to four tablespoons per day mixed in water, juice, smoothies, yogurt or can be used in baking.

Additional Therapies

For people who have or may have imbalanced intestinal flora, avoiding contact with chlorinated water is of the utmost importance. That includes bathing water and drinking water. Chlorine kills bacteria, friendly and unfriendly, in the intestines. It can be absorbed through the skin. I recommend installing a shower filter to remove chlorine (see Appendix C). Avoid swimming in chlorinated water as well.

In treating chronic candidiasis, a comprehensive approach is more effective than simply trying to kill the candida with a drug or a natural anticandida agent. For example, most physicians fail to recognize that a number of dietary factors appear to promote the overgrowth of candida. It is also important to increase digestive secretions; enhance immunity; promote detoxification and elimination; and use a comprehensive nutritional supplement program, including the use of the natural anti-yeast herbal extracts contained in Fungal Defense. Follow these guidelines:

Limit sugar. Sugar is the chief nutrient for *Candida albicans*. Restriction of sugar intake is an absolute necessity in the treatment of chronic candidiasis. Most people do well by simply avoiding grains, flours, pasta, refined sugar and large amounts of honey, maple syrup and fruit juice and limiting overall consumption of carbohydrates to less than 100 grams per day.

Limit milk and dairy products. There are several reasons to restrict or eliminate the intake of milk in chronic candidiasis. Milk's high lactose content promotes the overgrowth of candida. Milk is also one of the most common food allergens and may even contain trace levels of antibiotics, which can further disrupt the gastrointestinal bacterial flora and promote candida overgrowth. The consumption of a 30-hour cultured goat's milk yogurt is very beneficial to those suffering from candidiasis.

Avoid mold- and yeast-containing foods. It is generally recommended by many experts that individuals with chronic candidiasis avoid foods with a high content of yeast or mold, including alcoholic beverages, grains, cheeses, dried fruits, and peanuts.

Increase digestive secretions. In many cases, an important step in treating chronic *candidiasis* is improving digestive secretions. Gastric hydrochloric acid, pancreatic enzymes, and bile all inhibit the overgrowth of candida and prevent its penetration into the absorptive surfaces of the small intestine. Decreased production of any of these important digestive components can lead to overgrowth of Candida albicans in the gastrointestinal tract. Therefore, restoration of normal digestive secretions through the use of supplemental digestive enzymes (e.g., Omega-Zyme) is critical in the treatment of chronic candidiasis.

Restoring immune function. Restoring proper immune function is one of the key goals in the treatment of chronic candidiasis. Consuming immune enhancing products such as Primal Defense and RM-10 can greatly aid in the body's fight against candida overgrowth.

Promoting detoxification. Candida patients usually exhibit multiple chemical sensitivities and allergies, an indication that detoxification reactions are stressed. Therefore, the liver function of the candida patient needs to be supported. In fact, improving the health of the liver and promoting detoxification may be one of the most critical factors in the successful treatment of candidiasis.

Damage to the liver is often an underlying factor in chronic candidiasis as well as chronic fatigue. When the liver is even slightly damaged by a toxic chemical, immune function is severely compromised. Liver injury is also linked to candida overgrowth, as evident in studies of mice demonstrating that when the liver is even slightly damaged, candida runs rampant through the body. Consuming a high quality green food supplement such as Perfect Food can greatly enhance the liver's ability to properly detoxify the body.

Promoting elimination. In addition to directly supporting liver function, proper detoxification involves proper elimination. A diet that focuses on high-fiber plant foods should be sufficient to promote proper elimination by supplying an ample amount of dietary fiber. If additional support is needed, fiber formulas can be taken. These formulas are composed of natural plant fibers derived from seeds, vegetables and grains. I have designed a high-fiber, low-carbohydrate formula called Super Seed, which is ideal for those suffering from yeast overgrowth.

Natural antiyeast compounds. There are a number of natural agents with proven activity against Candida albicans. Among natural agents recommended to treat Candida albicans are garlic and wild oregano, both contained in Fungal Defense.

Garlic has demonstrated significant antifungal activity. In fact, its inhibition of *Candida albicans* in both animal and test tube studies has shown it to be more potent than nystatin, gentian violet, and six other reputed antifungal agents.

The most recent "new wave" natural anti-candida formulas are wild spices such as oregano. A recent study compared the anti-candida effect of oregano oil to that of caprylic acid. The results indicated that oregano oil is over 100 times more potent than caprylic acid against candida. Since the volatile oils contained in wild oregano are quickly absorbed and associated with heartburn, we include the whole herb not just the isolated oil fraction. The use of the whole wild oregano allows for the inclusion of the beneficial water-soluble fractions of the herb.

There is no doubt that candida overgrowth is a major health problem today among men and especially women. It is also equally clear that conventional treatments fail to address the underlying condition that allowed the overgrowth to occur. By following the steps in this natural program, you can overcome candida and start feeling great all over.

CARDIOVASCULAR HEALTH

- Angina
- Arteriosclerosis/Atherosclerosis
- Blood Pressure (Elevated)
- Cholesterol (Elevated)
- Homocysteine Levels (Elevated)
- Triglycerides (Elevated)

Overview

Cardiovascular disease (CVD), principally heart disease and stroke, is the nation's leading killer for both men and women among all racial and ethnic groups. More than 960,000 Americans die of CVD each year, accounting for more than 40 percent of all deaths. About 58 million Americans (almost one-fourth of the nation's population) live with some form of cardiovascular disease. Heart disease is the leading cause of premature, permanent disability among working adults. Stroke alone accounts for disability among more than one million people nationwide. Almost six million hospitalizations each year are due to cardiovascular disease. Congestive heart failure, one form of cardiovascular disease, is the single most frequent cause of hospitalization for people aged 65 years or older.

Angina

Angina pectoris (angina) is a recurring pain or discomfort in the chest that happens when some part of the heart does not receive enough blood. It is a common symptom of coronary heart disease (CHD), which occurs when vessels that carry blood to the heart become narrowed and blocked due to athero-sclerosis (see below). Angina is usually precipitated by exertion.

Arteriosclerosis/Atherosclerosis

Arteriosclerosis is a group of diseases characterized by the thickening of the artery wall—the hardening and calicifciation of the arteries—and in the narrowing of its lumen. Hardening of the arterial wall is due to various depositions within the plaque including lipids, cholesterol crystals, and calcium salts. These depositions make the arteries bone-like rigid tubes. They are most prominently found in the disease, atherosclerosis.

Atherosclerosis is a specific type of arteriosclerosis involving fatty deposits that affect large arteries, and the underlying pathologic condition in most cases of coronary heart disease, aortic aneurysm, peripheral vascular disease and stroke.

Blood Pressure (Elevated)

Blood pressure is the force of blood against the walls of arteries. Blood pressure rises and falls during the day. When blood pressure stays elevated over time, it is called high blood pressure or hypertension.

Blood pressure is typically recorded as two numbers—the systolic pressure (as the heart beats) over the diastolic pressure (as the heart relaxes between beats). A consistent blood pressure reading of 140/90 mm Hg or higher is considered high blood pressure.

Systolic pressure is the force of blood in the arteries as the heart beats. It is shown as the top number in a blood pressure reading. High blood pressure is 140 mm Hg and higher for systolic pressure. Diastolic pressure does not need to be nearly as high (usually over 80 mm Hg) for you to have high blood pressure.

If left uncontrolled, high blood pressure can lead to stroke, heart attack, congestive heart failure, kidney damage, blindness, or other conditions. Yet, most Americans do not have their systolic pressure under control.

Cholesterol (Elevated)

We can all agree on the American Heart Association's description of cholesterol as a soft, waxy substance found among the lipids (fats) in the bloodstream and in all your body's cells. We can even all agree that it's normal to have cholesterol. After all, cholesterol is an important part of a healthy body because it's used to form cell membranes, some hormones and serve other needed bodily functions.

With this in mind, it is disturbing that cholesterol has been given such a terrible beating by the medical establishment. It doesn't deserve its evil reputation. Keep in mind the following points so eloquently summarized by Danish physician Uffe Ravnskov, M.D., Ph.D.:

• A high cholesterol is not dangerous by itself, but may reflect an unhealthy condition, or it may be totally innocent.

- High blood cholesterol is said to promote atherosclerosis and thus also coronary heart disease. But many studies have shown that people whose blood cholesterol is low become just as atherosclerotic as people whose cholesterol is high.
- The body produces three to four times more cholesterol than you eat. The production of cholesterol increases when you eat little cholesterol and decreases when you eat much. This explains why the "prudent" diet or "low saturated fat" diet cannot lower cholesterol more than on average a few percent.
- There is no evidence that too much animal fat and cholesterol in the diet promotes atherosclerosis or heart attacks. For instance, more than twenty studies have shown that people who have had a heart attack haven't eaten more fat of any kind than other people, and degree of atherosclerosis at autopsy is unrelated with the diet.
- The new cholesterol-lowering drugs, the statins, do prevent cardiovascular disease, but this is due to other mechanisms than cholesterol-lowering. Unfortunately, they also stimulate cancer in rodents.
- Many of these facts have been presented in scientific journals and books for decades but are rarely told to the public by the proponents of the use of cholesterol-lowering drugs since these drugs represent major profits to corporate interests.
- The reason why laymen, doctors and most scientists have been misled is because opposing and disagreeing results are systematically ignored or misquoted in the scientific press.

Homocysteine (Elevated)

A more likely culprit in heart disease is elevated homocysteine. In the optimally functioning body, homocysteine is only an intermediate point in a metabolic pathway that starts with consumption of foods rich in the essential amino acid methionine. At the end of this pathway, methionine generally is metabolized to cysteine. For this conversion to be completed, however, requires the help of an enzyme called cystathionine synthetase, and the coenzyme pyridoxal phosphate. If this metabolic pathway is stymied, homocysteine accumulates in the blood and exerts a toxic effect on the inner linings of the body's vessels, causing low-density lipoprotein cholesterol to accumulate. J.C. Tsai and co-investigators report in a 1994 study, published in the *Proceedings of the National Academy of Sciences*, that homocysteine stimulates the proliferation of smooth-muscle cells, a key factor in narrowing of the arteries. Another potential mechanism of toxicity is impaired production of endothelium-derived relaxing factor.

There are several causes of elevated homocysteine levels. The most dramatic elevation, which leads to life-threatening vascular abnormalities at a young age, is due to rare genetic enzymatic defects at various points in the metabolic pathway. A far more common cause is diet. In particular, three members of the vitamin B complex family—folate (also known as folic acid), vitamin B_6, and vitamin B_{12}—enable this full conversion to take place. Foods rich in folate include deep green leafy vegetables, carrots, liver, egg yolk, cantaloupe, apricots, pumpkins, avocados, beans, and whole dark rye flour. Vitamin B6-rich foods are brewer's yeast, wheat germ, liver, fermented soy foods, cantaloupe, cabbage, blackstrap molasses, brown rice, eggs, oats, peanuts, and walnuts; those rich in vitamin B_{12} include animal foods such as liver, beef, eggs, milk, and cheese. A 1998 study published in the *Netherland Journal of Medicine* reports that vegetarians and vegans have higher levels of homocysteine compared to people who have high fat and meat intakes.

It is also quite clear that the homocysteine theory of heart disease might someday displace the fat/cholesterol theory. What makes the homocysteine theory even more appealing is that Kilmer McCully, M.D., the doctor/scientist who must be credited with its founding, is also a pathologist. He found the smoking gun—signs of homocysteine toxicity—even in arteries of people with normal to low cholesterol levels who have been felled by heart disease.[62]

Triglycerides (Elevated)

Triglycerides are the form in which fat exists in meats, cheese, fish, nuts, vegetable oils, and the greasy layer on the surface of soup stocks or in a pan in which bacon has been fried. In a healthy person, triglycerides and other fatty substances are normally moved into the liver and into adipose cells to provide energy for later use. Triglycerides are the chemical form in which most fat exists in the body.

The current conventional wisdom is high levels of triglycerides create a high risk for a heart attack or stroke. No less a publication than *Circulation* from the American Heart Association has been in the forefront of exposing the triglyceride-heart disease link. There is merit to this work. But I see high triglycerides as symptomatic of a diet that is too high in carbohydrates and refined foods and low in protein and the good fats. I think this truly is the key issue.

The latest epidemiological studies from Harvard University make it clear that the good fats are not only benign when it comes to heart disease but actually reduce risk. Therefore, the Maker's Diet, with adequate protein and fats from the proper foods, is beneficial in healing heart disease. The real culprit in heart disease is our overly processed, carbohydrate-rich food supply. The promoters of low-protein, low-fat diets remain oblivious to many factors, but most important is that no amount of supplementation can substitute for the proper balance of fat and protein that is obtained from eating healthy foods, the way our Maker intended.

Diet

Follow the diet prescribed in Chapters 9 to 11 diligently for 6 to 12 months.

After symptoms are completely gone for at least three months, you may gradually add foods from the "Neutral" or "Dangerous" categories, if you desire. Because people with cardiovascular disorders appear to have a predisposed weakness which manifests as a cardiovascular condition, I strongly recommend that they adhere to a diet of foods in the "Super" and "Healthy" categories for the rest of their lives.

Therapeutic Foods

These therapeutic foods will help you get well. Appendix A lists sources where you can obtain these foods.

- *Cultured goat's milk dairy products:* Consume 8 to 32 ounces of the highest quality cultured dairy products from goat's milk. I recommend a 30 hour fermented yogurt called Probiogurt (see resource section). Try to find yogurt that does not contain the organism *Streptococcus thermophilus*, a bacterial microbe that has been known to make immune-system disorders worse.
- *Grass-fed red meat:* Red meat from grass-fed cattle, buffalo, and lamb is very healthy and can be eaten a few times per week. This meat is a great source of protein, minerals, vitamin B_{12}, vitamins A and D, omega-3 fats, and CLA.
- *Omega-3 eggs:* Consume as many as two eggs high in omega-3 fatty acids each day. These eggs contain DHA, vitamins E and B_{12}, and antioxidants including lutein.
- *Extra Virgin Coconut Oil:* This oil is perhaps the healthiest of the widely available oils. I recommend cooking almost exclusively with extra virgin coconut oil. Consume as much as two to four tablespoons per day of the oil in cooking, smoothies, or right off the spoon. It contains large amounts of lauric acid, a potent antimicrobial and one of the chief fatty acids in breast milk.
- *Ocean-caught fish:* This type of fish is perhaps the healthiest of all protein sources. Salmon, sardines, mackerel, herring and albacore tuna are high in the omega-3 fatty acids EPA and DHA (which are critically important to prevention of heart attack and stroke). Ocean-caught fish can be consumed every day to enhance digestive and immune system health.
- *Cod liver oil:* Take one to three teaspoons of Olde World Icelandic Cod Liver Oil each day. The amount consumed should be based upon the amount of sunlight you receive. People in colder climates generally need to consume larger amounts. Cod liver oil is a fantastic source of the omega-3 fats DHA and EPA, as well as vitamins A and D.
- *Vegetable juice:* Consume vegetable juices that are low in carbohydrates, such as celery and green juices mixed with a small amount of higher carbohydrate veggies such as carrot or beet. Mix in some form of healthy fat with each glass of the juice. One to three teaspoons of cultured goat's milk, extra virgin coconut oil, canned or fresh coconut milk and cream, or flaxseed oil enhances absorption of minerals and prevents spikes in blood sugar.
- *Fermented vegetables:* Consume a few tablespoons of fermented vegetables such as sauerkraut with each meal to aid in digestion. Fermented vegetables are an excellent source of naturally occurring probiotics and enzymes.
- *Stocks:* It is a great idea to consume stocks on a regular basis, especially when you have a cold or flu. Stocks made from the bones of chicken, fish, lamb and beef contain minerals, gelatin, cartilage, collagen, and electrolytes from the vegetables. Stocks are an excellent source of proteins, especially collagen. They help to heal the gut lining and reduce inflammation.

Supplements

Take these health supplements to alleviate symptoms and get well. Appendix B explains where to obtain these supplements.

- *Primal Defense:* Take three to six caplets per day on an empty stomach.
- *Omega-Zyme:* Take one to three caplets with each meal or snack.
- *RM-10:* Take nine caplets per day of RM-10 for 120 days on an empty stomach. Thereafter consume a maintenance dosage of two to five caplets per day.
- *FYI:* Take two to three caplets twice per day first thing in the morning (with Primal Defense).
- *Perfect Food:* Take one to two tablespoons twice daily with eight ounces of water or fresh vegetable juice.
- *Springs of Life:* Consume at least eight, eight-ounce glasses per day of purified water mixed with 12 drops of Springs of Life living water concentrate.
- *Super Seed:* Consume one serving twice per day, morning and evening, with 8 ounces of purified water.
- *Goatein:* The only protein powder on the market made from organically produced goat's milk. This protein powder is partially pre-digested, low temperature dried and is usually well tolerated by those with food allergies and digestive problems. Take one to four tablespoons per day mixed in water, juice, smoothies, yogurt or can be used in baking.

Additional Therapies

In order to maintain a healthy balance of intestinal flora, avoiding contact with chlorinated water is of the utmost importance. That includes bathing water and drinking water. Chlorine kills bacteria, friendly and unfriendly, in the intestines. It can be absorbed through the skin. I recommend installing a shower filter to remove chlorine (see Appendix C). Avoid swimming in chlorinated water as well.

Many researchers now believe that heart disease can be caused by infections that originate in the oral cavity. While the diet outlined in this book is sure to improve dental health, I recommend that you find and use a toothbrush, mouthwash and dental floss that contains anti-microbial essential oils. It may be helpful to use a tongue cleaner. Natural toothpaste, mouthwash, dental floss and tongue cleaners are available at your local health food store.

CELIAC DISEASE…see *Chronic Digestive Disease*

CHILDREN'S HEALTH

- Attention Deficit Disorder (ADD)
- Attention Deficit/Hyperactivity Disorder (ADHD)
- Autism
- Pervasive Developmental Disorders (PDD)

Overview

Attention Deficit Disorder/Attention Deficit/Hyperactivity Disorder

Attention deficit hyperactivity disorder (ADHD) and attention deficit disorder (ADD) are characterized by developmentally inappropriate inattention and impulsivity, with or without hyperactivity. ADHD is implicated in learning disorders and is diagnosed four times more frequently in boys than girls. Despite the frequent references to ADHD as a neurobiological disorder, the cause of ADHD remains unknown.

The primary signs of ADD with or without hyperactivity are the display of inattention and impulsivity. ADHD with hyperactivity is diagnosed when signs of overactivity are obvious. Inattention is described as a failure to finish tasks started, easy distractibility, seeming lack of attention, and difficulty concentrating on tasks requiring sustained attention. Impulsivity is described as acting before thinking, difficulty taking turns, problems organizing work, and constant shifting from one activity to another. Hyperactivity is described as difficulty staying seated and sitting still, and running or climbing excessively.

Autism

Autism symptoms usually manifest within the first two to four years of life. Once considered a rare disorder with an incidence of only one to three cases per 10,000 births, autism is now reaching epidemic proportions with an incidence of 20 to 40 cases per 10,000 births and clusters of one case per 150 children reported in New Jersey and California. Autism now ranks third among childhood developmental disorders, making it more common than Down's syndrome, multiple sclerosis, and cystic fibrosis.

Almost all of us have been told about the benefits of childhood vaccinations. Many recall receiving their first polio vaccine at school. The revolution in disease prevention touched most of our lives.

But less well known is the fact that some childhood vaccines expose children to potentially toxic levels of heavy metals, including mercury. One of the most notorious culprits is thimerosol, a preservative that contains 49.6 percent methyl mercury, one of the most dangerous nervous system toxins known today.

Thimerosol is used in many common childhood vaccines. In June 1999, Food and Drug Administration officials noted, "Infants who receive thimerosol containing vaccines at several visits may be exposed to more mercury than recommended by Federal guidelines for total mercury exposure."

A growing number of doctors and researchers are concerned that increased rates of autism, a neurological disorder characterized by impairments in language, cognitive and social development, may be linked with such vaccinations.

Pervasive Developmental Disorder

Autism and pervasive developmental disorder (PDD) are developmental disabilities that share many of the same characteristics. Usually evident by age three, autism and PDD are neurological disorders that affect a child's ability to communicate, understand language, play, and relate to others.

Diet

Follow the diet prescribed in Chapters 9 to 11 as diligently as possible. Many children have poor health or even illness due to poor nutrition and improper detoxification. The improvement in diet and the addition of key nutrients can keep children healthy and may even aid in the reversal of many childhood health problems, especially as we find that these disorders are exacerbated or, in some cases, caused by gastrointestinal imbalances. By following the Maker's Diet, we believe each child will have excellent health, improved learning ability and the potential to grow into a healthy adult.

Therapeutic Foods

These therapeutic foods will help you get well. Appendix A lists sources where you can obtain these foods.

- *Cultured goat's milk dairy products:* Consume 8 to 32 ounces of the highest quality cultured dairy products from goat's milk. I recommend a 30 hour fermented yogurt called Probiogurt (see resource section). Try to find yogurt that does not contain the organism *Streptococcus thermophilus*, a bacterial microbe that has been known to make immune-system disorders worse.
- *Grass-fed red meat:* Red meat from grass-fed cattle, buffalo, and lamb is very healthy and can be eaten a few times per week. This meat is a great source of protein, minerals, vitamin B_{12}, vitamins A and D, omega-3 fats, and CLA.
- *Omega-3 eggs:* Consume as many as one or two eggs high in omega-3 fatty acids each day. These eggs contain DHA, vitamins E and B_{12}, and antioxidants including lutein.
- *Extra virgin coconut oil:* This oil is perhaps the healthiest of the widely available oils. I recommend cooking almost exclusively with extra virgin coconut oil. Consume as much as two tablespoons per day of the oil in cooking, smoothies, or right off the spoon. It contains large amounts of lauric acid, a potent antimicrobial and one of the chief fatty acids in breast milk.
- *Ocean-caught fish:* This type of fish is perhaps the healthiest of all protein sources. Salmon, sardines, mackerel, herring and albacore tuna are high in the omega-3 fatty acids EPA and DHA. Ocean-caught fish can be consumed every day to enhance digestive and immune system health.
- *Cod liver oil:* Take $1/2$ to one teaspoon of Olde World Icelandic Cod Liver Oil each day. The amount consumed should be based upon the amount of sunlight you receive. People in colder climates generally need to consume larger amounts. Cod liver oil is a fantastic source of the omega-3 fats DHA and EPA, as well as vitamins A and D.
- *Vegetable juice:* Consume vegetable juices that are low in carbohydrates, such as celery and green juices mixed with a small amount of higher carbohydrate veggies such as carrot or beet. Mix in some form of healthy fat with each glass of the juice. One to three teaspoons of cultured goat's milk, extra virgin coconut oil, canned or fresh coconut milk and cream, or flaxseed oil enhances absorption of minerals and prevents spikes in blood sugar.
- *Fermented vegetables:* Consume a few tablespoons of fermented vegetables such as sauerkraut with each meal to aid in digestion. Fermented vegetables are an excellent source of naturally occurring probiotics and enzymes.
- *Stocks:* It is a great idea to consume stocks on a regular basis, especially when you have a cold or flu. Stocks made from the bones of chicken, fish, lamb and beef contain minerals, gelatin, cartilage, collagen, and electrolytes from the vegetables. Stocks are an excellent source of proteins, especially collagen. They help to heal the gut lining and reduce inflammation.

Supplements

Take these health supplements to alleviate symptoms and get well. Appendix B explains where to obtain these supplements.

- *Primal Defense:* Start with one caplet or one scoop of powder per day mixed with juice or applesauce. Increase usage by adding one additional caplet or scoop per week (i.e., one caplet/scoop the first day, two the second day, three the third day and so on). Once your dosage is up to three to six caplets or scoops per day (depending on severity), stay on that amount for a minimum of three months and then begin to gradually decrease to a maintenance dosage of between one to three caplets or scoops per day. Primal Defense is best taken first thing in the morning and right before bedtime. Primal Defense may be taken with other nutritional supplements, but should be taken one hour apart from medications. If you experience symptoms of detoxification (i.e., increased elimination, loose stools, constipation, excess gas, flu-like symptoms or fever), reduce the dosage and work up slowly to 12 per day.
- *Fruits of Life:* Use one to two tablespoons as part of a healthy diet. Fruits of Life is an excellent source of antioxidants and minerals and may be taken with water, juice, yogurt, mixed in cereal or smoothies, or even eaten right off the spoon.
- *Perfect Food:* Take one to three teaspoons once daily with eight ounces water or fruit or vegetable juice.
- *Super Seed:* Consume one to three teaspoons twice per day, morning and evening, mixed in water or juice to ensure proper fiber intake.

Additional Therapies

For children who are rapidly developing a strong immune system, avoiding contact with chlorinated water is of the utmost importance. That includes bathing water and drinking water. Chlorine kills bacteria, friendly and unfriendly, in the intestines. It can be absorbed through the skin. I recommend installing a shower filter to remove chlorine (see Appendix C). Avoid swimming in chlorinated water as well.

CHOLESTEROL (ELEVATED)... see *Cardiovascular Health*
CHRONIC CONSTIPATION...see *Functional Bowel Disorders*
CHRONIC DIARRHEA...see *Functional Bowel Disorders*

CHRONIC DIGESTIVE DISEASE
- Celiac Disease
- Crohn's Disease
- Diverticulitis
- Ulcerative Colitis
- Ulcers

Overview
Chronic digestive diseases usually involve an intestinal condition characterized by a combination of abdominal pain; constipation; diarrhea; increased secretion of colon-related mucus; and dyspeptic symp-

toms such as flatulence, nausea, anorexia and varying degrees of anxiety or depression. Each condition has specific causes and symptoms as well. Celiac disease is characterized by gluten intolerance and severe wasting. Crohn's disease is a condition in which the intestinal wall thickens and causes narrowing of the bowel channel, blocking the intestinal tract. Diverticulitis is inflammation of an abnormal pouch or sac opening from a hollow organ (as the intestine or bladder). Ulcerative colitis is a nonspecific inflammatory disease of the colon of unknown cause characterized by diarrhea with discharge of mucus and blood, cramping abdominal pain, and inflammation and edema of the mucous membrane with patches of ulceration. An ulcer involves a break in the gastrointestinal mucous membrane with loss of surface tissue, disintegration and necrosis of epithelial tissue.

The onset for chronic digestive diseases peak during young adulthood, although gastrointestinal ulcers afflict persons of all ages. Restoration of the balance of friendly bacteria to the gastrointestinal tract is essential to recovery. The complete avoidance of disaccharide-containing foods such as grains, most beans, sugar, maple syrup, noncultured fluid dairy products (milk and ice cream), potatoes and corn is a must in order to heal the digestive tract and improve the microbial balance.

Diet

Follow the diet prescribed in Chapters 9 to 11 diligently for 6 to 12 months. It is imperative to avoid all grains even those in the "Super" and "Healthy" categories which include soaked sprouted or sour leavened grains for the first six months. While the aforementioned properly prepared grains are healthy for most people, those suffering from chronic digestive disease often have problems digesting grains in any form. After symptoms are completely gone for at least three months, you may gradually add foods from the "Neutral" or "Dangerous" categories, if you desire. Because people with chronic digestive diseases (Crohn's, irritable bowel syndrome, celiac disease and ulcerative colitis) appear to have a predisposed weakness in their intestinal tracts, we strongly recommend that they adhere to a diet of foods in the "Super" and "Healthy" categories for the rest of their lives.

Therapeutic Foods

These therapeutic foods will help you get well. Appendix A lists sources where you can obtain these foods.

- *Cultured goat's milk dairy products:* Consume 8 to 32 ounces of Probiogurt, the highest quality cultured yogurt from goat's milk. Try to find yogurt that does not contain the organism *Streptococcus thermophilus*, a bacterial microbe that has been known to make immune-system disorders worse.
- *Grass-fed red meat:* Red meat from grass-fed cattle, buffalo, and lamb is very healthy and can be eaten a few times per week. This meat is a great source of protein, minerals, vitamin B_{12}, vitamins A and D, omega-3 fats, and CLA.
- *Omega-3 eggs:* Consume as many as two eggs high in omega-3 fatty acids each day. These eggs contain DHA, vitamins E and B_{12}, and antioxidants including lutein.

- *Extra virgin coconut oil:* This oil is perhaps the healthiest of the widely available oils. I recommend cooking almost exclusively with extra virgin coconut oil. Consume as much as two to four table-spoons per day of the oil in cooking, smoothies, or right off the spoon. It contains large amounts of lauric acid, a potent antimicrobial and one of the chief fatty acids in breast milk.
- *Ocean-caught fish:* This type of fish is perhaps the healthiest of all protein sources. Salmon, sardines, mackerel, herring and albacore tuna are high in the omega-3 fatty acids EPA and DHA. Ocean-caught fish can be consumed every day to enhance digestive and immune system health.
- *Cod liver oil:* Take one to three teaspoons of Olde World Icelandic Cod Liver Oil each day. The amount consumed should be based upon the amount of sunlight you receive. People in colder cli-mates generally need to consume larger amounts. Cod liver oil is a fantastic source of the omega-3 fats DHA and EPA, as well as vitamins A and D.
- *Vegetable juice:* As long as diarrhea is not active, consume vegetable juices that are low in carbohy-drates, such as celery and green juices mixed with a small amount of higher carbohydrate veggies such as carrot or beet. Mix in some form of healthy fat with each glass of the juice. One to three tea-spoons of cultured goat's milk, extra virgin coconut oil, canned or fresh coconut milk and cream, or flaxseed oil enhances absorption of minerals and prevents spikes in blood sugar.
- *Fermented vegetables:* Consume a few tablespoons of fermented vegetables such as sauerkraut with each meal to aid in digestion. Fermented vegetables are an excellent source of naturally occurring probiotics and enzymes.
- *Berries:* Berries, particularly blueberries and raspberries can be very beneficial for those suffering from chronic digestive diseases. These berries are high in antioxidant nutrients and are great sources of fiber.
- *Stocks:* It is a great idea to consume stocks on a regular basis, especially when you have a cold or flu. Stocks made from the bones of chicken, fish, lamb and beef contain minerals, gelatin, cartilage, col-lagen, and electrolytes from the vegetables. Stocks are an excellent source of proteins, especially col-lagen. They help to heal the gut lining and reduce inflammation.

Supplements

Take these health supplements to alleviate symptoms and get well. Appendix B explains where to obtain these supplements.

- *Primal Defense:* Start with one caplet per day on an empty stomach, 30 minutes before or one hour after meals. Increase usage by adding one additional caplet per day (i.e., one caplet the first day, two the second day, three the third day and so on). Once your dosage is up to 12 caplets per day, stay on that amount for a minimum of three months and then begin to gradually decrease to a maintenance dosage of between three to six caplets per day. Primal Defense is best taken first thing in the morning and right before bedtime with eight ounces pure water. Primal Defense may be taken with other nutritional supplements, but should be taken one hour apart from medications. If you experience symptoms of detoxification (i.e., increased elimination, loose stools, constipation, excess gas, flu-like symptoms or fever), reduce the dosage and work up slowly to 12 per day.

- *Omega-Zyme:* Take one to three caplets with each meal or snack.
- *FYI:* Take six caplets two times per day on an empty stomach for one to four weeks, followed by 12 caplets per day for three to six months, and then reduce to a maintenance level of three caplets per day. If a relapse or "flare-up" occurs, take 12 caplets per day for at least one week or until symptoms are under control.
- *Perfect Food:* Take two tablespoons twice daily with eight ounces water or fresh vegetable juice.
- *Springs of Life:* Consume at least eight, eight-ounce glasses per day of purified water mixed with 12 drops of Springs of Life living water concentrate.
- *Goatein:* The only protein powder on the market made from organically produced goat's milk. This protein powder is partially pre-digested, low temperature dried and is usually well tolerated by those with food allergies and digestive problems. Take one to four tablespoons per day mixed in water, juice, smoothies, yogurt or can be used in baking. (For those with known milk allergies and/or lactose intolerance it is best to add Goatein once symptoms have begun to improve.)

Additional Therapies

For people who have or may have imbalanced intestinal flora, avoiding contact with chlorinated water is of the utmost importance. That includes bathing water and drinking water. Chlorine kills bacteria, friendly and unfriendly, in the intestines. It can be absorbed through the skin. I recommend installing a shower filter to remove chlorine (see Appendix C). Avoid swimming in chlorinated water as well.

CHRONIC FATIGUE/FIBROMYALGIA
Overview

Chronic fatigue immune deficiency syndrome (CFIDS, also known as chronic fatigue syndrome, CFS, myalgic encephalomyelitis, ME and by many other names) is a complex and debilitating chronic illness that affects the brain and multiple body systems. This devastating illness affects more Americans than multiple sclerosis, AIDS or lung cancer. Although its name trivializes the illness as little more than mere tiredness, chronic fatigue immune deficiency syndrome brings with it a constellation of debilitating symptoms.

Chronic fatigue is characterized by incapacitating fatigue (experienced as profound exhaustion and extremely poor stamina) and problems with concentration and short-term memory. It is also accompanied by flu-like symptoms such as pain in the joints and muscles, unrefreshing sleep, tender lymph nodes, sore throat, and headache.

Persons with chronic fatigue have symptoms that vary from person to person and fluctuate in severity. Specific symptoms may come and go, complicating treatment and the person's ability to cope with the illness. Many symptoms are invisible to the doctor's eye, which makes it difficult for others to understand the vast array of debilitating symptoms with which such people contend.

Diet

Follow the diet prescribed in Chapters 9 to 11 diligently for 6 to 12 months. After symptoms are completely gone for at least three months, you may gradually add foods from the "Neutral" or "Dangerous" categories, if you desire. Because people suffering from chronic fatigue or fibromyalgia appear to have a predisposed weakness in their immune systems and intestinal tracts, I strongly recommend that they adhere to a diet of foods in the "Super" and "Healthy" categories for the rest of their lives.

Therapeutic Foods

These therapeutic foods will help you get well. Appendix A lists sources where you can obtain these foods.

- *Cultured goat's milk dairy products:* Consume 8 to 32 ounces of the highest quality cultured dairy products from goat's milk. I recommend a 30 hour fermented yogurt called Probiogurt (see resource section). Try to find yogurt that does not contain the organism *Streptococcus thermophilus*, a bacterial microbe that has been known to make immune-system disorders worse.
- *Grass-fed red meat:* Red meat from grass-fed cattle, buffalo, and lamb is very healthy and can be eaten a few times per week. This meat is a great source of protein, minerals, vitamin B_{12}, vitamins A and D, omega-3 fats, and CLA.
- *Omega-3 eggs:* Consume as many as two eggs high in omega-3 fatty acids each day. These eggs contain DHA, vitamins E and B_{12}, and antioxidants including lutein.
- *Extra virgin coconut oil:* This oil is perhaps the healthiest of the widely available oils. I recommend cooking almost exclusively with extra virgin coconut oil. Consume as much as two to four tablespoons per day of the oil in cooking, smoothies, or right off the spoon. It contains large amounts of lauric acid, a potent antimicrobial and one of the chief fatty acids in breast milk.
- *Ocean-caught fish:* This type of fish is perhaps the healthiest of all protein sources. Salmon, sardines, mackerel, herring and albacore tuna are high in the omega-3 fatty acids EPA and DHA. Ocean-caught fish can be consumed every day to enhance digestive and immune system health.
- *Cod liver oil:* Take one to three teaspoons of Olde World Icelandic Cod Liver Oil each day. The amount consumed should be based upon the amount of sunlight you receive. People in colder climates generally need to consume larger amounts. Cod liver oil is a fantastic source of the omega-3 fats DHA and EPA, as well as vitamins A and D.
- *Vegetable juice:* Consume vegetable juices that are low in carbohydrates, such as celery and green juices mixed with a small amount of higher carbohydrate veggies such as carrot or beet. Mix in some form of healthy fat with each glass of the juice. One to three teaspoons of cultured goat's milk, extra virgin coconut oil, canned or fresh coconut milk and cream, or flaxseed oil enhances absorption of minerals and prevents spikes in blood sugar.
- *Fermented vegetables:* Consume a few tablespoons of fermented vegetables such as sauerkraut with each meal to aid in digestion. Fermented vegetables are an excellent source of naturally occurring probiotics and enzymes.

- *Stocks:* It is a great idea to consume stocks on a regular basis, especially when you have a cold or flu. Stocks made from the bones of chicken, fish, lamb and beef contain minerals, gelatin, cartilage, collagen, and electrolytes from the vegetables. Stocks are an excellent source of proteins, especially collagen. They help to heal the gut lining and reduce inflammation.

Supplements

Take these health supplements to alleviate symptoms and get well. Appendix B explains where to obtain these supplements.

- *Primal Defense:* Start with one caplet per day on an empty stomach, 30 minutes before or one hour after meals. Increase usage by adding one additional caplet per day (i.e., one caplet the first day, two the second day, three the third day and so on). Once your dosage is up to 12 caplets per day, stay on that amount for a minimum of three months and then begin to gradually decrease to a maintenance dosage of between three to six caplets per day. Primal Defense is best taken first thing in the morning and right before bedtime with eight ounces pure water. Primal Defense may be taken with other nutritional supplements, but should be taken one hour apart from medications. If you experience symptoms of detoxification (i.e., increased elimination, loose stools, constipation, excess gas, flu-like symptoms or fever), reduce the dosage and work up slowly to 12 per day.
- *Omega-Zyme:* Take one to three caplets with each meal or snack.
- *RM-10:* Take nine caplets of RM-10 per day for 120 days on an empty stomach in divided doses. After symptoms have greatly improved slowly reduce intake to between two to five caplets per day.
- *FYI:* Take six caplets two times per day on an empty stomach for 90 days followed by a maintenance dose of three to six caplets per day.
- *Perfect Food:* Take two tablespoons twice daily with eight ounces water or fresh vegetable juice.
- *Springs of Life:* Consume at least eight, eight-ounce glasses per day of purified water mixed with 12 drops of Springs of Life living water concentrate.
- *Super Seed:* Consume one serving twice per day, morning and evening, with eight or more ounces of purified water.
- *Goatein:* The only protein powder on the market made from organically produced goat's milk. This protein powder is partially pre-digested, low temperature dried and is usually well tolerated by those with food allergies and digestive problems. Take one to four tablespoons per day mixed in water, juice, smoothies, yogurt or can be used in baking.

Additional Therapies

For people who have or may have an imbalanced immune system, avoiding contact with chlorinated water is of the utmost importance. That includes bathing water and drinking water. Chlorine kills bacteria, friendly and unfriendly, in the intestines. It can be absorbed through the skin. I recommend installing a shower filter to remove chlorine (see Appendix C). Avoid swimming in chlorinated water as well.

Just a reminder, be sure to use Primal Defense, RM-10 and FYI. Human herpesvirus-6 (HHV-6) is one of numerous causes of chronic fatigue syndrome. And it may be a big deal.

HHV-6 is a nasty virus that infects a wide range of the body's cells, including brain, immune and endothelial cells. It comes in two variants (A and B) with the A variant attracting most of the attention. Not surprisingly, HHV-6 is closely related to herpes simplex virus-1—that herpes virus most of us have heard about, which causes genital and oral herpes—but it's potentially far more devastating and might cause many different kinds of autoimmune disorders as well.

The HSOs contained in Primal Defense produce bio-surfactants that destroy lipid enveloped viruses such as HHV-6. The addition of RM-10 ensures that the immune system is brought back into balance by normalizing overproduction of compounds such as interleukins and tumor necrosis factor-alpha. FYI with its blend of foods, herbs and enzymes can reduce inflammation and may help reduce the thickened blood often caused by HHV-6.

COLD AND FLU (ALSO SEE VIRAL DISEASES)
Overview

Seasonal colds and flus can be very inconvenient to one's lifestyle. The best course of action is to use natural means and allow the body to run its course. I believe that every time one is able to overcome a cold or flu without medication they will be healthier for it.

Occasionally, we need a good cold or flu to stimulate the body's cleansing processes. Maybe there is a good reason for us to get a cold or flu every once in a while. While we admit it is no fun to be laid up in bed, aching, feverish and nauseous, your body might actually be doing something that is terrific for your long-term health. One line of thought posits that when we become feverish our body is actually doing much more than simply vanquishing a single pathogen but actually cleansing the tissues of many pathogens and even cancer cells. Thus, an occasional cold or flu is your body's natural cleansing and detoxifying response. When we take antibiotics or prevent this process altogether, we may actually be weakening our health by not allowing the body to go through this cleansing.

Diet

During a cold or flu it is important to only eat when hungry. This can give the body ample opportunity to heal itself. Consuming the foods mentioned below can insure a healthy and speedy recovery.

Therapeutic Foods

These therapeutic foods will help you get well. Appendix A lists sources where you can obtain these foods.

• *Extra virgin coconut oil:* This oil is perhaps the healthiest of the widely available oils. I recommend cooking almost exclusively with extra virgin coconut oil. Consume as much as four to six tablespoons of the oil per day during a cold or flu. Extra virgin coconut oil can be used in cooking, in smoothies, or consumed right off the spoon. Extra virgin coconut oil contains large amounts of lauric, capric and caprylic acids, which are potent antiviral and antifungal compounds.

- *Ocean-caught fish:* This type of fish is perhaps the healthiest of all protein sources. It is important to consume a high quality source of protein during a cold/flu and fish is a great source. Salmon, sardines, mackerel, herring and albacore tuna are high in the omega-3 fatty acids EPA and DHA. Ocean-caught fish can be consumed every day to enhance digestive and immune system health.
- *Cod liver oil:* Take three teaspoons of Olde World Icelandic Cod Liver Oil each day for the duration of the cold/flu. The amount consumed should be based upon the amount of sunlight you receive. People in colder climates generally need to consume larger amounts. Cod liver oil is a fantastic source of the omega-3 fats DHA and EPA, as well as vitamins A and D.
- *Vegetable juice:* Consume vegetable juices that are low in carbohydrates, such as celery and green juices mixed with a small amount of higher carbohydrate veggies such as carrot or beet. Mix in some form of healthy fat with each glass of the juice. One to three teaspoons of cultured goat's milk, extra virgin coconut oil, canned or fresh coconut milk and cream, or flaxseed oil enhances absorption of minerals and prevents spikes in blood sugar.
- *Chicken Soup/Stock:* It is a great idea to consume chicken soup on a regular basis, especially when you have a cold or flu. Going on a one to three day chicken soup fast can be extremely helpful to eliminate even the toughest cold or flu. Even if you don't go on an exclusively chicken soup diet, consuming some chicken soup daily will be very helpful.

Supplements

Take these health supplements to alleviate symptoms and get well. Appendix B explains where to obtain these supplements.

- *Cold and Flu Defense:* Follow the seven-day protocol as directed on the label. If the seven-day protocol is completed and symptoms are still lingering you may take three days off and then begin an additional seven-day protocol.
- *Primal Defense:* Take 12 caplets per day until symptoms subside. Then begin to gradually decrease to a maintenance dosage of between three to six caplets per day. Primal Defense is best taken first thing in the morning and right before bedtime with eight ounces pure water. Primal Defense may be taken with other nutritional supplements, but should be taken one hour apart from medications. If you experience symptoms of detoxification (i.e., increased elimination, loose stools, constipation, excess gas, flu-like symptoms or fever), reduce the dosage and work up slowly to 12 per day.
- *Omega-Zyme:* Take one to three caplets with each meal or snack.
- *Springs of Life:* Consume at least eight, eight-ounce glasses per day of purified water mixed with 12 drops of Springs of Life living water concentrate.
- *Super Seed:* Consume one serving twice per day, morning and evening, with eight or more ounces of purified water. (Consuming a fiber supplement is essential during a cold or flu in order to eliminate toxins from the body. Thereafter, consume fiber as needed.)

- *Goatein:* The only protein powder on the market made from organically produced goat's milk. This protein powder is partially pre-digested, low temperature dried and is usually well tolerated by those with food allergies and digestive problems. Take one to four tablespoons per day mixed in water, juice, smoothies, yogurt or can be used in baking.

Additional Therapies

For people who have or may have imbalanced intestinal flora, avoiding contact with chlorinated water is of the utmost importance. That includes bathing water and drinking water. Chlorine kills bacteria, friendly and unfriendly, in the intestines. It can be absorbed through the skin. I recommend installing a shower filter to remove chlorine (see Appendix C). Avoid swimming in chlorinated water as well.

COLON CLEANSING

I have discussed the relationship of intestinal toxemia to poor health in Chapter 3. So it should be clear that colon cleansing is not only important but essential in order to regain your health and maintain it. With daily colon cleansing, you will avoid buildup of harmful bacteria and mucus. Our colon should be cleansed daily through the consumption of foods rich in probiotics and enzymes.

Diet

Follow the diet prescribed in Chapters 9 through 11 diligently for 6 to 12 months. For those who want to thoroughly cleanse the colon, it is good to consume large amounts of vegetables as well as cleansing fruits such as figs, grapes, watermelon, stone fruits (plums, apricots, peaches) and small berries such as blueberries and raspberries. Be sure to consume cleansing beverages such as cultured goat's milk yogurt, fermented vegetables, vegetable juices and lacto-fermented beverages daily.

Therapeutic Foods

These therapeutic foods will help you get well. Appendix A lists sources where you can obtain these foods.

- *Cultured goat's milk dairy products:* Consume 8 to 32 ounces of Probiogurt, the highest quality cultured dairy product made from goat's milk.
- *Grass-fed red meat:* Red meat from grass-fed cattle, buffalo, and lamb is very healthy and can be eaten a few times per week. This meat is a great source of protein, minerals, vitamin B_{12}, vitamins A and D, omega-3 fats, and CLA.
- *Omega-3 eggs:* Consume as many as two eggs high in omega-3 fatty acids each day. These eggs contain DHA, vitamins E and B_{12}, and antioxidants including lutein.
- *Extra virgin coconut oil:* This oil is perhaps the healthiest of the widely available oils. I recommend cooking almost exclusively with extra virgin coconut oil. Consume as much as two to four table-

spoons per day of the oil in cooking, smoothies, or right off the spoon. It contains large amounts of lauric acid, a potent antimicrobial and one of the chief fatty acids in breast milk.

- *Ocean-caught fish:* This type of fish is perhaps the healthiest of all protein sources. Salmon, sardines, mackerel, herring and albacore tuna are high in the omega-3 fatty acids EPA and DHA. Ocean-caught fish can be consumed every day to enhance digestive and immune system health.
- *Cod liver oil:* Take one to three teaspoons of Olde World Icelandic Cod Liver Oil each day. The amount consumed should be based upon the amount of sunlight you receive. People in colder climates generally need to consume larger amounts. Cod liver oil is a fantastic source of the omega-3 fats DHA and EPA, as well as vitamins A and D.
- *Vegetable juice:* Consume vegetable juices that are low in carbohydrates, such as celery and green juices mixed with a small amount of higher carbohydrate veggies such as carrot or beet. Mix in some form of healthy fat with each glass of the juice. One to three teaspoons of cultured goat's milk, extra virgin coconut oil, canned or fresh coconut milk and cream, or flaxseed oil enhances absorption of minerals and prevents spikes in blood sugar.
- *Fermented vegetables:* Consume a few tablespoons of fermented vegetables such as sauerkraut with each meal to aid in digestion. Fermented vegetables are an excellent source of naturally occurring probiotics and enzymes.
- *Berries:* Consuming high-fiber berries such as blueberries and raspberries can lead to effective daily colon cleansing as well as provide the body with antioxidants.
- *Stocks:* It is a great idea to consume stocks on a regular basis, especially when you have a cold or flu. Stocks made from the bones of chicken, fish, lamb and beef contain minerals, gelatin, cartilage, collagen, and electrolytes from the vegetables. Stocks are an excellent source of proteins, especially collagen. They help to heal the gut lining and reduce inflammation.

Supplements

Take these health supplements to alleviate symptoms and get well. Appendix B explains where to obtain these supplements.

- *Primal Defense:* Start with one caplet per day on an empty stomach, 30 minutes before or one hour after meals. Increase usage by adding one additional caplet per day (i.e., one caplet the first day, two the second day, three the third day and so on). Once your dosage is up to 12 caplets per day, stay on that amount for a minimum of three months and then begin to gradually decrease to a maintenance dosage of between three to six caplets per day. Primal Defense is best taken first thing in the morning and right before bedtime with eight ounces pure water. Primal Defense may be taken with other nutritional supplements, but should be taken one hour apart from medications. If you experience symptoms of detoxification (i.e., increased elimination, loose stools, constipation, excess gas, flu-like symptoms or fever), reduce the dosage and work up slowly to 12 per day.
- *Omega-Zyme:* Take one to three caplets with each meal or snack.

- *Perfect Food:* Take two tablespoons twice daily with eight ounces water or fresh vegetable juice.
- *Springs of Life:* Consume at least eight, eight-ounce glasses per day of purified water mixed with 12 drops of Springs of Life living water concentrate.
- *Super Seed:* Consume one serving twice per day, morning and evening, with eight or more ounces of purified water.
- *Goatein:* The only protein powder on the market made from organically produced goat's milk. This protein powder is partially pre-digested, low temperature dried and is usually well tolerated by those with food allergies and digestive problems. Take one to four tablespoons per day mixed in water, juice, smoothies, yogurt or can be used in baking.

Additional Therapies

For people who have or may have imbalanced intestinal flora, avoiding contact with chlorinated water is of the utmost importance. That includes bathing water and drinking water. Chlorine kills bacteria, friendly and unfriendly, in the intestines. It can be absorbed through the skin. I recommend installing a shower filter to remove chlorine (see Appendix C). Avoid swimming in chlorinated water as well.

Be sure to read the Lifestyle Therapies section at the start of this chapter.

Crohn's Disease...see *Chronic Digestive Disease*

Dementia...see *Brain Health*

Depression...see *Mental Disorders*

Dermatitis...see *Skin Health*

DETOXIFICATION

Detoxification in our modern vernacular is usually thought of as the unburdening of the human body of chemical toxins such as pesticides, heavy metals, industrial chemicals, radiation and other toxins. It is an essential process to go through in order to relieve each individual's growing burden of toxicity, which can lead to cancer, heart disease, premature aging, and many other maladies.

Diet

Follow the diet prescribed in Chapters 9 to 11 diligently for 6 to 12 months. After the body has been properly detoxified, I strongly recommend that people adhere to a diet of foods in the "Super" and "Healthy" categories for the rest of their lives.

Therapeutic Foods

These therapeutic foods will help you get well. Appendix A lists sources where you can obtain these foods.

- *Cultured goat's milk dairy products*: Consume 8 to 32 ounces of the highest quality cultured dairy products from goat's milk. I recommend a 30 hour fermented yogurt called Probiogurt (see resource

section). Try to find yogurt that does not contain the organism *Streptococcus thermophilus*, a bacterial microbe that has been known to make immune-system disorders worse.

- *Grass-fed red meat:* Red meat from grass-fed cattle, buffalo, and lamb is very healthy and can be eaten a few times per week. This meat is a great source of protein, minerals, vitamin B_{12}, vitamins A and D, omega-3 fats, and CLA.

- *Omega-3 eggs:* Consume as many as two eggs high in omega-3 fatty acids each day. These eggs contain DHA, vitamins E and B_{12}, and antioxidants including lutein.

- *Extra virgin coconut oil:* This oil is perhaps the healthiest of the widely available oils. I recommend cooking almost exclusively with extra virgin coconut oil. Consume as much as two to four tablespoons per day of the oil in cooking, smoothies, or right off the spoon. It contains large amounts of lauric acid, a potent antimicrobial and one of the chief fatty acids in breast milk.

- *Ocean-caught fish:* This type of fish is perhaps the healthiest of all protein sources. Salmon, sardines, mackerel, herring and albacore tuna are high in the omega-3 fatty acids EPA and DHA. Ocean-caught fish can be consumed every day to enhance digestive and immune system health.

- *Cod liver oil:* Take one to three teaspoons of Olde World Icelandic Cod Liver Oil each day. The amount consumed should be based upon the amount of sunlight you receive. People in colder climates generally need to consume larger amounts. Cod liver oil is a fantastic source of the omega-3 fats DHA and EPA, as well as vitamins A and D.

- *Berries:* The daily consumption of berries including blueberries, strawberries, blackberries and raspberries can provide the body with antioxidants which can neutralize harmful toxins that can damage the body. Berries supply rich sources of dietary fiber.

- *Vegetable juice:* Consume vegetable juices that are low in carbohydrates, such as celery and green juices mixed with a small amount of higher carbohydrate veggies such as carrot or beet. Mix in some form of healthy fat with each glass of the juice. One to three teaspoons of cultured goat's milk, extra virgin coconut oil, canned or fresh coconut milk and cream, or flaxseed oil enhances absorption of minerals and prevents spikes in blood sugar.

- *Fermented vegetables:* Consume a few tablespoons of fermented vegetables such as sauerkraut with each meal to aid in digestion. Fermented vegetables are an excellent source of naturally occurring probiotics and enzymes.

- *Stocks:* It is a great idea to consume stocks on a regular basis, especially when you have a cold or flu. Stocks made from the bones of chicken, fish, lamb and beef contain minerals, gelatin, cartilage, collagen, and electrolytes from the vegetables. Stocks are an excellent source of proteins, especially collagen. They help to heal the gut lining and reduce inflammation.

Supplements

Take these health supplements to alleviate symptoms and get well. Appendix B explains where to obtain these supplements.

- *Primal Defense:* Start with one caplet per day on an empty stomach, 30 minutes before or one hour after meals. Increase usage by adding one additional caplet per day (i.e., one caplet the first day, two the second day, three the third day and so on). Once your dosage is up to 12 caplets per day, stay on that amount for a minimum of three months and then begin to gradually decrease to a maintenance dosage of between three to six caplets per day. Primal Defense is best taken first thing in the morning and right before bedtime with eight ounces pure water. Primal Defense may be taken with other nutritional supplements, but should be taken one hour apart from medications. If you experience symptoms of detoxification (i.e., increased elimination, loose stools, constipation, excess gas, flu-like symptoms or fever), reduce the dosage and work up slowly to 12 per day.
- *Omega-Zyme:* Take one to three caplets with each meal or snack.
- *Perfect Food:* Take two tablespoons twice daily with eight ounces water or fresh vegetable juice.
- *Springs of Life:* Consume at least eight, eight-ounce glasses per day of purified water mixed with 12 drops of Springs of Life living water concentrate.
- *Super Seed:* Consume one serving twice per day, morning and evening, with eight or more ounces of purified water.
- *Goatein:* The only protein powder on the market made from organically produced goat's milk. This protein powder is partially pre-digested, low temperature dried and is usually well tolerated by those with food allergies and digestive problems. Take one to four tablespoons per day mixed in water, juice, smoothies, yogurt or can be used in baking.

Additional Therapies

In order to properly detoxify the body, avoiding contact with chlorinated water is of the utmost importance. That includes bathing water and drinking water. Chlorine kills bacteria, friendly and unfriendly, in the intestines. It can be absorbed through the skin. I recommend installing a shower filter to remove chlorine (see Appendix C). Avoid swimming in chlorinated water as well.

I especially recommend regular use of low-heat saunas.

DIABETES, TYPE I...see *Autoimmune Disease*
DIABETES, TYPE II...see *Blood Sugar Imbalances*
DIVERTICULITIS...see *Chronic Digestive Disease*
DYSPEPSIA...see *Functional Bowel Disorders*
ECZEMA...see *Skin Health*
ENDOMETRIOSIS...see *Female Health*
EPSTEIN BARR VIRUS...see *Viral Diseases*
ERECTILE DYSFUNCTION...see *Male Health*

FEMALE HEALTH

- Endometriosis
- Fibrocystic Breast Disease
- Menopause
- Osteoporosis
- Ovarian Cysts
- Premenstrual Syndrome (PMS)
- Uterine fibroids

Overview

One of the key issues for women's health is to maintain balanced estrogen levels. By improving their estrogen profile, women can markedly reduce their risk of one of the major causes of death, breast cancer. This can be done simply with the dietary measures detailed below—especially the use of RevivAll Female Vitality Formula and Super Seed, as well as avoiding exposure to environmental xenoestrogens.

Most of us know that estrogen is the hormone responsible for stimulating development of female characteristics, and that changes girls into women. There is nothing evil or bad about estrogen—as long as the estrogen to which your body is exposed is derived from the healthy functioning of your organs and glands.

The key here is the body's balance of estrogen. Different aspects of your diet, lifestyle, even medications prescribed by your doctor, the cosmetics you use, and consumption of alcohol all influence estrogen balance in your body.

The body produces different types of estrogen: estradiol, estrone, and estriol. Estrone and estriol are much weaker estrogens than estradiol. The body converts estradiol, the most potent estrogen, either to "good" estrogen (2-hydroxyestrone) which is weakly anti-estrogenic and reduces risk of breast cancer, or "bad" estrogen (16-alpha-hydroxyestrone) which is more long-lived and potent, stimulates breast cell proliferation, and is carcinogenic.[63] High levels of this bad estrogen are a "risk marker" or an indication of increased risk of breast cancer.[64,65,66]

Phytoestrogens and lignans are a group of naturally occurring chemicals derived from plants; they have a structure similar to estrogen, and form part of our diet. They also have potentially anticarcinogenic biological activity.

Thus, they appear to be an effective dietary means for reducing cancer risk by improving estrogen metabolism. Many studies associate higher levels of circulating phytoestrogens and lignans with overall improved women's health and improved estrogen profiles.

And just how should women go about raising their blood levels of the lignans? That answer comes to us from a very recent report in the February 2002 issue of the *European Journal of Clinical Nutrition*.[67]

The purpose of this study was to investigate the effects of flaxseed supplementation as a part of daily diet on serum lipids, fatty acids and plasma enterolactone. Eighty volunteers participated in this clinical nutrition study, which was carried out in a controlled, double-blind manner. There was a significant increase in serum alpha-linolenic acid, eicosapentaenoic acid and docosahexaenoic acid, the major omega-3 fatty acids found in flaxseed. Serum enterolactone concentration was doubled during flaxseed supplementation.

"In this study we were able to show that, by adding ground flaxseed and flaxseed oil to one or two daily meals, it is possible to obtain significant effects on serum levels of enterolactone and alpha-linolenic acid," the researchers said.

This leads us to our next dramatic finding—that by raising levels of alpha-linolenic, eicosapentaenoic and docosahexaenoic acids women are further protecting themselves against breast cancer (as well as heart disease and arthritis).

Experimental studies have indicated that omega-3 fatty acids, including alpha-linolenic, eicosapentaenoic and docosahexaenoic acids, inhibit mammary tumor growth and metastasis. To clinically evaluate whether omega-3 fatty acids protect against breast cancer, researchers, reporting in the 2002 issue of the *International Journal of Cancer*, examined the fatty acid composition in adipose tissue from 241 patients with invasive, non-metastatic breast carcinoma and from 88 patients with benign breast disease, in a case-control study in Tours, central France.[68] Women with the highest levels of alpha-linolenic acid had a 61 percent reduced risk of breast cancer compared to women with the lowest levels. In a similar way, women with the highest levels of docosahexaenoic acid had a reduced risk of 69 percent, compared to women with the lowest levels. "In conclusion, our data based on fatty acids levels in breast adipose tissue suggest a protective effect of n-3 fatty acids on breast cancer risk and support the hypothesis that the balance between n-3 and n-6 fatty acids plays a role in breast cancer," the researchers said.

It is clear that by reducing levels of "bad" estrogen that women's risk of breast cancer is reduced. The most effective and safe way of doing so is with diet—including more flax, fish, high omega-3 eggs and fermented foods.

Measure Your "Good" & "Bad" Estrogen

An ELISA method for measuring 2- and 16-alpha-hydroxylated estrogen (OHE) metabolites in urine is available and the ratio of urinary 2-OHE/16-alpha-OHE (2/16-alpha ratio) is a useful biomarker for estrogen-related cancer risk. Contact Great Smokies Diagnostic Laboratory, 63 Zillicoa Street, Asheville, NC 28801. Their toll-free phone number is (800) 522-4762.

Diet

Choose mainly foods from the "Super" and "Healthy" categories until optimal health is achieved for at least three months (or if experiencing symptoms such as painful PMS, hot flashes, bone loss, low libido, or low energy, until symptoms are gone for at least three months.) Once symptoms are greatly improved, you may gradually add foods from the "Neutral" or "Dangerous" categories if desired. To attain and maintain vibrant health, I recommend consuming foods from the "Super" and "Healthy" categories as the main part of a healthy diet.

Therapeutic Foods

These therapeutic foods will help you get well. Appendix A lists sources where you can obtain these foods.

- *Cultured goat's milk dairy products:* Consume 8 to 32 ounces of the highest quality cultured dairy products from goat's milk. I recommend a 30 hour fermented yogurt called Probiogurt (see resource

section). Try to find yogurt that does not contain the organism *Streptococcus thermophilus*, a bacterial microbe that has been known to make immune-system disorders worse.

- *Grass-fed red meat:* Red meat from grass-fed cattle, buffalo, and lamb is very healthy and can be eaten a few times per week. This meat is a great source of protein, minerals, vitamin B_{12}, vitamins A and D, omega-3 fats, and CLA.
- *Omega-3 eggs:* Consume as many as two eggs high in omega-3 fatty acids each day. These eggs contain DHA, vitamins E and B_{12}, and antioxidants including lutein.
- *Extra virgin coconut oil:* This oil is perhaps the healthiest of the widely available oils. I recommend cooking almost exclusively with extra virgin coconut oil. Consume as much as two to three tablespoons per day of the oil in cooking, smoothies, or right off the spoon. It contains large amounts of lauric acid, a potent antimicrobial and one of the chief fatty acids in breast milk.
- *Ocean-caught fish:* This type of fish is perhaps the healthiest of all protein sources. Salmon, sardines, mackerel, herring and albacore tuna are high in the omega-3 fatty acids EPA and DHA. Ocean-caught fish can be consumed every day to enhance digestive and immune system health.
- *Cod liver oil:* Take one to three teaspoons of Olde World Icelandic Cod Liver Oil each day. The amount consumed should be based upon the amount of sunlight you receive. People in colder climates generally need to consume larger amounts. Cod liver oil is a fantastic source of the omega-3 fats DHA and EPA, as well as vitamins A and D.
- *Vegetable juice:* Consume vegetable juices that are low in carbohydrates, such as celery and green juices mixed with a small amount of higher carbohydrate veggies such as carrot or beet. Mix in some form of healthy fat with each glass of the juice. One to three teaspoons of cultured goat's milk, extra virgin coconut oil, canned or fresh coconut milk and cream, or flaxseed oil enhances absorption of minerals and prevents spikes in blood sugar.
- *Fermented vegetables:* Consume a few tablespoons of fermented vegetables such as sauerkraut with each meal to aid in digestion. Fermented vegetables are an excellent source of naturally occurring probiotics and enzymes.
- *Stocks:* It is a great idea to consume stocks on a regular basis, especially when you have a cold or flu. Stocks made from the bones of chicken, fish, lamb and beef contain minerals, gelatin, cartilage, collagen, and electrolytes from the vegetables. Stocks are an excellent source of proteins, especially collagen. They help to heal the gut lining and reduce inflammation.

Supplements

Take these health supplements to alleviate symptoms and get well. Appendix B explains where to obtain these supplements.

- *Perfect Food:* Take one to two tablespoons twice daily with eight ounces water or fresh vegetable juice.
- *RevivAll Female Vitality Formula:* Take six caplets twice a day, morning and evening, on an empty stomach at least 30 minutes away from food for 30 days. Decrease to three caplets twice per day for

60 days. Once health is greatly improved, you may reduce intake to a maintenance level of four caplets once per day first thing in the morning. RevivAll Female may be taken with other food supplements.

- **Clear Energy**: Take six caplets per day with meals for a total of 100 days. Thereafter, take three caplets per day with meals. Do not consume Clear Energy after 6:00 p.m.
- **Springs of Life:** Consume at least eight, eight-ounce glasses per day of purified water mixed with 12 drops of Springs of Life living water concentrate.
- **Super Seed:** Consume one, two-tablespoon serving twice per day, morning and evening, with eight or more ounces of purified water.
- **Goatein:** The only protein powder on the market made from organically produced goat's milk. This protein powder is partially pre-digested, low temperature dried and is usually well tolerated by those with food allergies and digestive problems. Take one to four tablespoons per day mixed in water, juice, smoothies, yogurt or can be used in baking.

Additional Therapies

For people who have or may have imbalanced intestinal flora or a weak immune system, avoiding contact with chlorinated water is of the utmost importance. That includes bathing water and drinking water. Chlorine kills bacteria, friendly and unfriendly, in the intestines. It can be absorbed through the skin. I recommend installing a shower filter to remove chlorine (see Appendix C). Avoid swimming in chlorinated water as well.

FIBROCYSTIC BREAST DISEASE...see *Female Health*
FLU...see *Cold and Flu*, see also *Viral Diseases*

FOOD ALLERGIES/CHEMICAL SENSITIVITIES
Overview

Food allergies and chemical sensitivities are conditions marked by our modern lifestyles. Food allergies may be life-threatening and debilitating or simply result in uncomfortable symptoms ranging from intestinal discomfort to faintness and rapid heartbeat (as in the case of persons sensitive to monosodium glutamate [MSG]). It is not uncommon to find chronic diseases linked with long-standing food allergies. In many cases we find that helping to restore proper digestion and a healthy intestinal lining are key to improving food allergies and intolerances.

Diet

Choose mainly foods from the "Super" and "Healthy" categories until optimal health is achieved for at least three months. If you have known allergies to certain foods, it is best to limit those for at least the first few months on the program: People who follow this program can often return to eating foods to which they were previously allergic once the gastrointestinal and immune systems are functioning properly. Once symptoms are greatly improved, you may gradually add foods from the "Neutral" or "Dangerous" categories if desired. Because people with food allergies/chemical sensitivities appear to have a predisposed weakness in their immune systems, I strongly recommend that they adhere to a diet of foods in the "Super" and "Healthy" categories for the rest of their lives.

Therapeutic Foods

These therapeutic foods will help you get well. Appendix A lists sources where you can obtain these foods.

- *Cultured goat's milk dairy products:* Consume 8 to 32 ounces of the highest quality cultured dairy products from goat's milk. I recommend a 30 hour fermented yogurt called Probiogurt (see resource section). Try to find yogurt that does not contain the organism *Streptococcus thermophilus*, a bacterial microbe that has been known to make immune-system disorders worse.
- *Grass-fed red meat:* Red meat from grass-fed cattle, buffalo, and lamb is very healthy and can be eaten a few times per week. This meat is a great source of protein, minerals, vitamin B_{12}, vitamins A and D, omega-3 fats, and CLA.
- *Omega-3 eggs:* Consume as many as two eggs high in omega-3 fatty acids each day. These eggs contain DHA, vitamins E and B_{12}, and antioxidants including lutein.
- *Extra virgin coconut oil:* This oil is perhaps the healthiest of the widely available oils. I recommend cooking almost exclusively with extra virgin coconut oil. Consume as much as two to four tablespoons per day of the oil in cooking, smoothies, or right off the spoon. It contains large amounts of lauric acid, a potent antimicrobial and one of the chief fatty acids in breast milk.
- *Ocean-caught fish:* This type of fish is perhaps the healthiest of all protein sources. Salmon, sardines, mackerel, herring and albacore tuna are high in the omega-3 fatty acids EPA and DHA. Ocean-caught fish can be consumed every day to enhance digestive and immune system health.
- *Cod liver oil:* Take one to three teaspoons of Olde World Icelandic Cod Liver Oil each day. The amount consumed should be based upon the amount of sunlight you receive. People in colder climates generally need to consume larger amounts. Cod liver oil is a fantastic source of the omega-3 fats DHA and EPA, as well as vitamins A and D.
- *Vegetable juice:* Consume vegetable juices that are low in carbohydrates, such as celery and green juices mixed with a small amount of higher carbohydrate veggies such as carrot or beet. Mix in some form of healthy fat with each glass of the juice. One to three teaspoons of cultured goat's milk, extra virgin coconut oil, canned or fresh coconut milk and cream, or flaxseed oil enhances absorption of minerals and prevents spikes in blood sugar.
- *Fermented vegetables:* Consume a few tablespoons of fermented vegetables such as sauerkraut with each meal to aid in digestion. Fermented vegetables are an excellent source of naturally occurring probiotics and enzymes.

- **Stocks:** It is a great idea to consume stocks on a regular basis, especially when you have a cold or flu. Stocks made from the bones of chicken, fish, lamb and beef contain minerals, gelatin, cartilage, collagen, and electrolytes from the vegetables. Stocks are an excellent source of proteins, especially collagen. They help to heal the gut lining and reduce inflammation.

Supplements

Take these health supplements to alleviate symptoms and get well. Appendix B explains where to obtain these supplements.

- **Primal Defense:** Start with one caplet per day on an empty stomach, 30 minutes before or one hour after meals. Increase usage by adding one additional caplet per day (i.e., one caplet the first day, two the second day, three the third day and so on). Once your dosage is up to 12 caplets per day, stay on that amount for a minimum of three months and then begin to gradually decrease to a maintenance dosage of between three to six caplets per day. Primal Defense is best taken first thing in the morning and right before bedtime with eight ounces pure water. Primal Defense may be taken with other nutritional supplements, but should be taken one hour apart from medications. If you experience symptoms of detoxification (i.e., increased elimination, loose stools, constipation, excess gas, flu-like symptoms or fever), reduce the dosage and work up slowly to 12 per day.
- **FYI:** Take four caplets three times per day on an empty stomach for one to four weeks, followed by six caplets per day for three to six months, and then reduce to a maintenance level of three caplets per day. If a relapse or "flare-up" occurs, take 12 caplets per day for at least one week or until symptoms are under control.
- **Omega-Zyme:** Take one to three caplets with each meal or snack.
- **Perfect Food:** Take one to two tablespoons twice daily with eight ounces of water or fresh vegetable juice.
- **Springs of Life:** Consume at least eight, eight-ounce glasses per day of purified water mixed with 12 drops of Springs of Life living water concentrate.
- **Super Seed:** Consume one serving twice per day, morning and evening, with eight or more ounces of purified water.
- **Goatein:** The only protein powder on the market made from organically produced goat's milk. This protein powder is partially pre-digested, low temperature dried and is usually well tolerated by those with food allergies and digestive problems. Take one to four tablespoons per day mixed in water, juice, smoothies, yogurt or can be used in baking.

Additional Therapies

For people who have or may have imbalanced intestinal flora or a weak immune system, avoiding contact with chlorinated water is of the utmost importance. That includes bathing water and drinking water. Chlorine kills bacteria, friendly and unfriendly, in the intestines. It can be absorbed through the skin. I recommend installing a shower filter to remove chlorine (see Appendix C). Avoid swimming in chlorinated water as well.

FUNCTIONAL BOWEL DISORDERS
- Chronic Constipation
- Chronic Diarrhea
- Dyspepsia
- Irritable Bowel Syndrome
- Lactose Intolerance
- Leaky Gut Syndrome

Overview

Functional gastrointestinal (GI) disorders affect millions of people of all ages—men, women, and children. They are the most commonly presented gastrointestinal illnesses seen by physicians in primary care or gastroenterology. Irritable bowel syndrome (IBS) and dyspepsia are the most common, notes the International Foundation for Functional Gastrointestinal Disorders.

As the international foundation further notes, "A functional disorder does not show any evidence of an organic or physical disease, and the cause of a functional GI disorder doesn't show up in a blood test or an x-ray. The disorders are diagnosed based on symptoms, and often require tests to rule out the likelihood of another disease."

It is now apparent that functional disorders increase morbidity and diminish the patient's quality of life. The social and economic costs of gastrointestinal disorders are enormous. The symptoms of these disorders can cause discomfort, ranging from inconvenience to deep personal distress. For those with severe symptoms the disorders can be debilitating, leaving them unable to fully participate in life and work.

SPECIAL REPORT
Pesticide Residues, One of the Factors Causing Functional Bowel Disorders

The causes and mechanisms involved in functional bowel disorders are numerous, subject to controversy and often hypothetical. However, research now suggests that pesticide residues in food might be one cause resulting in such disorders. Researchers showed that animals ingesting daily low doses of a pesticide exhibited morphological and functional alterations associated with these disorders.[69]

The team put forward the hypothesis that food contaminants could cause inflammation of the digestive mucosa associated with alterations in painful sensitivity. It showed that the chronic ingestion (three weeks) of a low dose of a pesticide, diquat, in rats resulted in morphological alterations to the digestive mucosa similar to those described in patients affected by functional bowel disorders. Moreover, chronic ingestion resulted in painful hypersensitivity to gastric distension, which mainly characterises functional bowel disorders. The doses used corresponded to those tolerated in agricultural products by the French and American authorities.

Diet

Choose mainly foods from the "Super" and "Healthy" categories until optimal health is achieved for at least three months. If you have known allergies to certain foods, it is best to limit those for at least the first few months on the program. People who follow this program can often return to eating foods to which they were previously allergic once the gastrointestinal and immune systems are functioning properly. Once symptoms are greatly improved, you may gradually add foods from the "Neutral" or "Dangerous" categories if desired. Because people with functional bowel disorders appear to have a predisposed weakness in their gastrointestinal tract, I strongly recommend that they adhere to a diet of foods in the "Super" and "Healthy" categories for the rest of their lives.

Therapeutic Foods

These therapeutic foods will help you get well. Appendix A lists sources where you can obtain these foods.

- *Cultured goat's milk dairy products:* Consume 8 to 32 ounces of Probiogurt, the highest quality cultured dairy product from goat's milk. Try to find yogurt that does not contain the organism *Streptococcus thermophilus*, a bacterial microbe that has been known to make immune-system disorders worse.
- *Grass-fed red meat:* Red meat from grass-fed cattle, buffalo, and lamb is very healthy and can be eaten a few times per week. This meat is a great source of protein, minerals, vitamin B_{12}, vitamins A and D, omega-3 fats, and CLA.
- *Omega-3 eggs:* Consume as many as two eggs high in omega-3 fatty acids each day. These eggs contain DHA, vitamins E and B_{12}, and antioxidants including lutein.
- *Extra virgin coconut oil:* This oil is perhaps the healthiest of the widely available oils. I recommend cooking almost exclusively with extra virgin coconut oil. Consume as much as two to four tablespoons per day of the oil in cooking, smoothies, or right off the spoon. It contains large amounts of lauric acid, a potent antimicrobial and one of the chief fatty acids in breast milk.
- *Ocean-caught fish:* This type of fish is perhaps the healthiest of all protein sources. Salmon, sardines, mackerel, herring and albacore tuna are high in the omega-3 fatty acids EPA and DHA. Ocean-caught fish can be consumed every day to enhance digestive and immune system health.
- *Cod liver oil*: Take one to three teaspoons of Olde World Icelandic Cod Liver Oil each day. The amount consumed should be based upon the amount of sunlight you receive. People in colder climates generally need to consume larger amounts. Cod liver oil is a fantastic source of the omega-3 fats DHA and EPA, as well as vitamins A and D.
- *Vegetable juice:* Consume vegetable juices that are low in carbohydrates, such as celery and green juices mixed with a small amount of higher carbohydrate veggies such as carrot or beet. Mix in some form of healthy fat with each glass of the juice. One to three teaspoons of cultured goat's milk, extra virgin coconut oil, canned or fresh coconut milk and cream, or flaxseed oil enhances absorption of minerals and prevents spikes in blood sugar.

- *Fermented vegetables:* Consume a few tablespoons of fermented vegetables such as sauerkraut with each meal to aid in digestion. Fermented vegetables are an excellent source of naturally occurring probiotics and enzymes.
- *Stocks:* It is a great idea to consume stocks on a regular basis, especially when you have a cold or flu. Stocks made from the bones of chicken, fish, lamb and beef contain minerals, gelatin, cartilage, collagen, and electrolytes from the vegetables. Stocks are an excellent source of proteins, especially collagen. They help to heal the gut lining and reduce inflammation.

Supplements

Take these health supplements to alleviate symptoms and get well. Appendix B explains where to obtain these supplements.

- *Primal Defense:* Start with one caplet per day on an empty stomach, 30 minutes before or one hour after meals. Increase usage by adding one additional caplet per day (i.e., one caplet the first day, two the second day, three the third day and so on). Once your dosage is up to 12 caplets per day, stay on that amount for a minimum of three months and then begin to gradually decrease to a maintenance dosage of between three to six caplets per day. Primal Defense is best taken first thing in the morning and right before bedtime with eight ounces pure water. Primal Defense may be taken with other nutritional supplements, but should be taken one hour apart from medications. If you experience symptoms of detoxification (i.e., increased elimination, loose stools, constipation, excess gas, flu-like symptoms or fever), reduce the dosage and work up slowly to 12 per day.
- *Omega-Zyme:* Take one to three caplets with each meal or snack.
- *Perfect Food:* Take one to two tablespoons twice daily with eight ounces water or fresh vegetable juice.
- *Springs of Life:* Consume at least eight, eight-ounce glasses per day of purified water mixed with 12 drops of Springs of Life living water concentrate.
- *Super Seed:* Consume one serving twice per day, morning and evening, with eight or more ounces of purified water.
- *Goatein:* The only protein powder on the market made from organically produced goat's milk. This protein powder is partially pre-digested, low temperature dried and is usually well tolerated by those with food allergies and digestive problems. Take one to four tablespoons per day mixed in water, juice, smoothies, yogurt or can be used in baking.

Additional Therapies

For people who have or may have imbalanced intestinal flora or a weak immune system, avoiding contact with chlorinated water is of the utmost importance. That includes bathing water and drinking water. Chlorine kills bacteria, friendly and unfriendly, in the intestines. It can be absorbed through the skin. I recommend installing a shower filter to remove chlorine (see Appendix C). Avoid swimming in chlorinated water as well.

GENERAL HEALTH MAINTENANCE

In today's world it is crucial to prevent disease before it starts. By following the principals outlined in this book you can improve your health and make great strides in preventing future diseases.

Diet

Follow the diet prescribed in Chapters 9 to 11 diligently for 90 days. I strongly recommend that people adhere to a diet of foods in the "Super" and "Healthy" categories for the rest of their lives.

Therapeutic Foods

These therapeutic foods will help you stay well. Appendix A lists sources where you can obtain these foods.

- *Cultured goat's milk dairy products:* Consume 8 to 32 ounces of the highest quality cultured dairy products from goat's milk. I recommend a 30 hour fermented yogurt called Probiogurt (see resource section). Try to find yogurt that does not contain the organism Streptococcus thermophilus, a bacterial microbe that has been known to make immune-system disorders worse.
- *Grass-fed red meat:* Red meat from grass-fed cattle, buffalo, and lamb is very healthy and can be eaten a few times per week. This meat is a great source of protein, minerals, vitamin B_{12}, vitamins A and D, omega-3 fats, and CLA.
- *Omega-3 eggs:* Consume as many as two eggs high in omega-3 fatty acids each day. These eggs contain DHA, vitamins E and B_{12}, and antioxidants including lutein.
- *Extra virgin coconut oil:* This oil is perhaps the healthiest of the widely available oils. I recommend cooking almost exclusively with extra virgin coconut oil. Consume as much as two to four tablespoons per day of the oil in cooking, smoothies, or right off the spoon. It contains large amounts of lauric acid, a potent antimicrobial and one of the chief fatty acids in breast milk.
- *Ocean-caught fish:* This type of fish is perhaps the healthiest of all protein sources. Salmon, sardines, mackerel, herring and albacore tuna are high in the omega-3 fatty acids EPA and DHA. Ocean-caught fish can be consumed every day to enhance digestive and immune system health.
- *Cod liver oil:* Take one to three teaspoons of Olde World Icelandic Cod Liver Oil each day. The amount consumed should be based upon the amount of sunlight you receive. People in colder climates generally need to consume larger amounts. Cod liver oil is a fantastic source of the omega-3 fats DHA and EPA, as well as vitamins A and D.
- *Berries:* The daily consumption of berries including blueberries, strawberries, blackberries and raspberries can provide the body with antioxidants which can neutralize harmful toxins that can damage the body. Berries supply rich sources of dietary fiber to enhance elimination.
- *Vegetable juice:* Consume vegetable juices that are low in carbohydrates, such as celery and green juices mixed with a small amount of higher carbohydrate veggies such as carrot or beet. Mix in some form of healthy fat with each glass of the juice. One to three teaspoons of cultured goat's milk, extra

virgin coconut oil, canned or fresh coconut milk and cream, or flaxseed oil enhances absorption of minerals and prevents spikes in blood sugar.

- *Fermented vegetables:* Consume a few tablespoons of fermented vegetables such as sauerkraut with each meal to aid in digestion. Fermented vegetables are an excellent source of naturally occurring probiotics and enzymes.
- *Stocks:* It is a great idea to consume stocks on a regular basis, especially when you have a cold or flu. Stocks made from the bones of chicken, fish, lamb and beef contain minerals, gelatin, cartilage, collagen, and electrolytes from the vegetables. Stocks are an excellent source of proteins, especially collagen. They help to heal the gut lining and reduce inflammation.

Supplements

Take these health supplements to alleviate symptoms and get well. Appendix B explains where to obtain these supplements.

- *Primal Defense:* Start with one caplet per day on an empty stomach, 30 minutes before or one hour after meals. Increase usage by adding one additional caplet per day (i.e., one caplet the first day, two the second day, three the third day and so on). Once your dosage is up to six to twelve caplets per day, stay on that amount for a minimum of three months and then begin to gradually decrease to a maintenance dosage of between three to six caplets per day. Primal Defense is best taken first thing in the morning and right before bedtime with eight ounces pure water. Primal Defense may be taken with other nutritional supplements, but should be taken one hour apart from medications. If you experience symptoms of detoxification (i.e., increased elimination, loose stools, constipation, excess gas, flu-like symptoms or fever), reduce the dosage and work up slowly to 12 per day.
- *Omega-Zyme:* Take one to three caplets with each meal or snack.
- *Perfect Food:* Take one to two tablespoons twice daily with eight ounces water or fresh vegetable juice.
- *Springs of Life:* Consume at least eight, eight-ounce glasses per day of purified water mixed with 12 drops of Springs of Life living water concentrate.
- *Super Seed:* Consume one serving twice per day, morning and evening, with eight or more ounces of purified water.
- *Goatein:* The only protein powder on the market made from organically produced goat's milk. This protein powder is partially pre-digested, low temperature dried and is usually well tolerated by those with food allergies and digestive problems. Take one to four tablespoons per day mixed in water, juice, smoothies, yogurt or can be used in baking.

Additional Therapies

In order to maintain health and prevent disease, avoiding contact with chlorinated water is of the utmost importance. That includes bathing water and drinking water. Chlorine kills bacteria, friendly and unfriendly, in the intestines. It can be absorbed through the skin. I recommend installing a shower filter to remove chlorine (see Appendix C). Avoid swimming in chlorinated water as well.

GASTROESOPHAGEAL REFLUX DISEASE (GERD)
Overview

When the acidic juices of the stomach splash upward into the esophagus, the result is heartburn. Normally, a ring of muscles called the esophageal sphincter prevents stomach acid from entering the esophagus. But if the muscles relax or open under pressure from acidic juices in the stomach, heartburn may result. Everyone gets heartburn from time to time, but severe, persistent heartburn that occurs two or more times per week is called gastroesophageal reflux disease, or GERD. Chronic GERD has the potential to scar and damage the lining of the esophagus. It can also lead to a condition called Barrett's esophagus, which carries the risk of developing esophageal cancer.

Heartburn has many different causes. Heartburn may be caused by overeating, stress, wearing clothes that fit too tightly, and lying down soon after eating. Alcohol, nicotine, and caffeine relax the esophageal sphincter and allow stomach acid to enter the esophagus. Certain kinds of spicy food can also cause heartburn in some people. Poor digestion is another major contributor to GERD.

Diet

Choose mainly foods from the "Super" and "Healthy" categories until optimal health is achieved for at least three months. Once symptoms are greatly improved, you may gradually add foods from the "Neutral" or "Dangerous" categories if desired. Because people with GERD appear to have a predisposed weakness in their gastrointestinal tract, I strongly recommend that they adhere to a diet of foods in the "Super" and "Healthy" categories for the rest of their lives.

Therapeutic Foods

These therapeutic foods will help you get well. Appendix A lists sources where you can obtain these foods.

- *Cultured goat's milk dairy products:* Consume 8 to 32 ounces of Probiogurt, the highest quality cultured dairy product from goat's milk. Try to find yogurt that does not contain the organism *Streptococcus thermophilus*, a bacterial microbe that has been known to make immune-system disorders worse.
- *Grass-fed red meat:* Red meat from grass-fed cattle, buffalo, and lamb is very healthy and can be eaten a few times per week. This meat is a great source of protein, minerals, vitamin B_{12}, vitamins A and D, omega-3 fats, and CLA.
- *Omega-3 eggs:* Consume as many as two eggs high in omega-3 fatty acids each day. These eggs contain DHA, vitamins E and B12, and antioxidants including lutein.
- *Extra virgin coconut oil:* This oil is perhaps the healthiest of the widely available oils. I recommend cooking almost exclusively with extra virgin coconut oil. Consume as much as two to four table-

spoons per day of the oil in cooking, smoothies, or right off the spoon. It contains large amounts of lauric acid, a potent antimicrobial and one of the chief fatty acids in breast milk.

- *Ocean-caught fish:* This type of fish is perhaps the healthiest of all protein sources. Salmon, sardines, mackerel, herring and albacore tuna are high in the omega-3 fatty acids EPA and DHA. Ocean-caught fish can be consumed every day to enhance digestive and immune system health.
- *Cod liver oil:* Take one to three teaspoons of Olde World Icelandic Cod Liver Oil each day. The amount consumed should be based upon the amount of sunlight you receive. People in colder climates generally need to consume larger amounts. Cod liver oil is a fantastic source of the omega-3 fats DHA and EPA, as well as vitamins A and D.
- *Vegetable juice:* Consume vegetable juices that are low in carbohydrates, such as celery and green juices mixed with a small amount of higher carbohydrate veggies such as carrot or beet. Mix in some form of healthy fat with each glass of the juice. One to three teaspoons of cultured goat's milk, extra virgin coconut oil, canned or fresh coconut milk and cream, or flaxseed oil enhances absorption of minerals and prevents spikes in blood sugar.
- *Fermented vegetables:* Consume a few tablespoons of fermented vegetables such as sauerkraut with each meal to aid in digestion. Fermented vegetables are an excellent source of naturally occurring probiotics and enzymes.
- *Stocks:* It is a great idea to consume stocks on a regular basis, especially when you have a cold or flu. Stocks made from the bones of chicken, fish, lamb and beef contain minerals, gelatin, cartilage, collagen, and electrolytes from the vegetables. Stocks are an excellent source of proteins, especially collagen. They help to heal the gut lining and reduce inflammation.

Supplements

Take these health supplements to alleviate symptoms and get well. Appendix B explains where to obtain these supplements.

- *Primal Defense:* Start with one caplet per day on an empty stomach, 30 minutes before or one hour after meals. Increase usage by adding one additional caplet per day (i.e., one caplet the first day, two the second day, three the third day and so on). Once your dosage is up to 12 caplets per day, stay on that amount for a minimum of three months and then begin to gradually decrease to a maintenance dosage of between three to six caplets per day. Primal Defense is best taken first thing in the morning and right before bedtime with eight ounces pure water. Primal Defense may be taken with other nutritional supplements, but should be taken one hour apart from medications. If you experience symptoms of detoxification (i.e., increased elimination, loose stools, constipation, excess gas, flu-like symptoms or fever), reduce the dosage and work up slowly to 12 per day.
- *Omega-Zyme:* Take one to three caplets with each meal or snack.
- *Acid Defense:* Take one to two tablespoons mixed in water upon rising and before bed. This supplement can be taken to relive symptoms of pain during an episode of heartburn.

- *Perfect Food:* Take one to two tablespoons twice daily with eight ounces water or fresh vegetable juice.
- *Springs of Life:* Consume at least eight, eight-ounce glasses per day of purified water mixed with 12 drops of Springs of Life living water concentrate.
- *Super Seed:* Consume one serving twice per day, morning and evening, with eight or more ounces of purified water.
- *Goatein:* The only protein powder on the market made from organically produced goat's milk. This protein powder is partially pre-digested, low temperature dried and is usually well tolerated by those with food allergies and digestive problems. Take one to four tablespoons per day mixed in water, juice, smoothies, yogurt or can be used in baking.

Additional Therapies

For people who have or may have imbalanced intestinal flora or a weak immune system, avoiding contact with chlorinated water is of the utmost importance. That includes bathing water and drinking water. Chlorine kills bacteria, friendly and unfriendly, in the intestines. It can be absorbed through the skin. I recommend installing a shower filter to remove chlorine (see Appendix C). Avoid swimming in chlorinated water as well.

GOUT…see *Joint Disorders*
GRAVE'S DISEASE…see *Autoimmune Disease*
HEARTBURN…see *Gastroesophageal Reflux Disease (GERD)*
HEAVY METAL POISONING…see *Detoxification*
HEPATITIS…see *Viral Diseases*
HERPES…see *Viral Diseases*
HYPOGLYCEMIA…see *Blood Sugar Imbalances*

IMMUNE HEALTH (OPTIMAL)

By now readers certainly are aware of my strongly held belief that immune health and gastrointestinal health are inexorably intertwined. Whether we are presently enjoying super health or suffering from illness, our immune system is of paramount importance to our well-being. If you are healthy, your immune system is charged with the important mission of maintaining your equilibrium. If you are ill, your immune system is charged with helping you to become well. No matter what your level of health, your immune system will play a role. That is why taking care of your immune health is so important to your overall health.

Diet

For general health it is best to consume a majority of your diet from the "Super" and "Healthy" categories.

Therapeutic Foods

These therapeutic foods will help you stay well. Appendix A lists sources where you can obtain these foods.

- *Cultured goat's milk dairy products:* Consume 8 to 32 ounces of the highest quality cultured dairy products from goat's milk. I recommend a 30 hour fermented yogurt called Probiogurt (see resource section). Try to find yogurt that does not contain the organism *Streptococcus thermophilus,* a bacterial microbe that has been known to make immune-system disorders worse.

- *Grass-fed red meat:* Red meat from grass-fed cattle, buffalo, and lamb is very healthy and can be eaten a few times per week. This meat is a great source of protein, minerals, vitamin B_{12}, vitamins A and D, omega-3 fats, and CLA.

- *Omega-3 eggs*: Consume as many as two eggs high in omega-3 fatty acids each day. These eggs contain DHA, vitamins E and B_{12}, and antioxidants including lutein.

- *Extra virgin coconut oil:* This oil is perhaps the healthiest of the widely available oils. I recommend cooking almost exclusively with extra virgin coconut oil. Consume as much as two to four tablespoons per day of the oil in cooking, smoothies, or right off the spoon. It contains large amounts of lauric acid, a potent antimicrobial and one of the chief fatty acids in breast milk.

- *Ocean-caught fish:* This type of fish is perhaps the healthiest of all protein sources. Salmon, sardines, mackerel, herring and albacore tuna are high in the omega-3 fatty acids EPA and DHA. Ocean-caught fish can be consumed every day to enhance digestive and immune system health.

- *Cod liver oil:* Take one to three teaspoons of Olde World Icelandic Cod Liver Oil each day. The amount consumed should be based upon the amount of sunlight you receive. People in colder climates generally need to consume larger amounts. Cod liver oil is a fantastic source of the omega-3 fats DHA and EPA, as well as vitamins A and D.

- *Vegetable juice:* Consume vegetable juices that are low in carbohydrates, such as celery and green juices mixed with a small amount of higher carbohydrate veggies such as carrot or beet. Mix in some form of healthy fat with each glass of the juice. One to three teaspoons of cultured goat's milk, extra virgin coconut oil, canned or fresh coconut milk and cream, or flaxseed oil enhances absorption of minerals and prevents spikes in blood sugar.

- *Fermented vegetables:* Consume a few tablespoons of fermented vegetables such as sauerkraut with each meal to aid in digestion. Fermented vegetables are an excellent source of naturally occurring probiotics and enzymes.

- *Stocks:* It is a great idea to consume stocks on a regular basis, especially when you have a cold or flu. Stocks made from the bones of chicken, fish, lamb and beef contain minerals, gelatin, cartilage, collagen, and electrolytes from the vegetables. Stocks are an excellent source of proteins, especially collagen. They help to heal the gut lining and reduce inflammation.

Supplements

Take these health supplements to maintain immune health. Appendix B explains where to obtain these supplements.

- *Primal Defense:* Take three to six caplets per day on an empty stomach.
- *Omega-Zyme:* Take one to three caplets with each meal or snack.
- *RevivAll Classic™:* Take two to four caplets per day on an empty stomach. RevivAll Classic may be taken with other whole food supplements such as Perfect Food and Primal Defense.
- *Perfect Food:* Take one to two tablespoons once or twice daily with eight ounces of water or fresh vegetable juice.
- *Springs of Life:* Consume at least eight, eight-ounce glasses per day of purified water mixed with 12 drops of Springs of Life living water concentrate.
- *Goatein:* The only protein powder on the market made from organically produced goat's milk. This protein powder is partially pre-digested, low temperature dried and is usually well tolerated by those with food allergies and digestive problems. Take one to four tablespoons per day mixed in water, juice, smoothies, yogurt or can be used in baking.
- *Super Seed:* Consume one serving twice per day, morning and evening, mixed in eight ounces puri-fied water.

Additional Therapies

For people who want to maintain balanced intestinal flora and a strong immune system, avoiding contact with chlorinated water is of the utmost importance. That includes bathing water and drinking water. Chlorine kills bacteria, friendly and unfriendly, in the intestines. It can be absorbed through the skin. I recommend installing a shower filter to remove chlorine (see Appendix C). Avoid swimming in chlorinated water as well.

INFLAMMATORY CONDITIONS

Inflammation is an underlying cause of many illnesses, including heart disease and stroke, as well as cancer, and autoimmune conditions such as rheumatoid arthritis and asthma, to name but a few. The entire program detailed in this book will help to maintain normal levels of inflammation. To determine inflammatory levels, ask your doctor to perform a relatively inexpensive and noninvasive high-sensitivity C-reactive protein test.

Diet

Follow the diet prescribed in Chapters 9 to 11 diligently for 6 to 12 months. After symptoms are completely gone for at least three months, you may gradually add foods from the "Neutral" or "Dangerous" categories, if you desire. Because people suffering from chronic inflammation appear to have a predisposed weakness in their immune systems, I strongly recommend that they adhere to a diet of foods in the "Super" and "Healthy" categories for the rest of their lives.

Therapeutic Foods

These therapeutic foods will help you get well. Appendix A lists sources where you can obtain these foods.

- *Cultured goat's milk dairy products:* Consume 8 to 32 ounces of the highest quality cultured dairy products from goat's milk. I recommend a 30 hour fermented yogurt called Probiogurt (see resource section). Try to find yogurt that does not contain the organism *Streptococcus thermophilus*, a bacterial microbe that has been known to make immune-system disorders worse.

- *Grass-fed red meat:* Red meat from grass-fed cattle, buffalo, and lamb is very healthy and can be eaten a few times per week. This meat is a great source of protein, minerals, vitamin B_{12}, vitamins A and D, omega-3 fats, and CLA.

- *Omega-3 eggs:* Consume as many as two eggs high in omega-3 fatty acids each day. These eggs contain DHA, vitamins E and B_{12}, and antioxidants including lutein.

- *Extra virgin coconut oil:* This oil is perhaps the healthiest of the widely available oils. I recommend cooking almost exclusively with extra virgin coconut oil. Consume as much as two to four tablespoons per day of the oil in cooking, smoothies, or right off the spoon. It contains large amounts of lauric acid, a potent antimicrobial and one of the chief fatty acids in breast milk.

- *Ocean-caught fish:* This type of fish is perhaps the healthiest of all protein sources. Salmon, sardines, mackerel, herring and albacore tuna are high in the omega-3 fatty acids EPA and DHA. Ocean-caught fish can be consumed every day to enhance digestive and immune system health.

- *Cod liver oil:* Take one to three teaspoons of Olde World Icelandic Cod Liver Oil each day. The amount consumed should be based upon the amount of sunlight you receive. People in colder climates generally need to consume larger amounts. Cod liver oil is a fantastic source of the omega-3 fats DHA and EPA, as well as vitamins A and D.

- *Vegetable juice:* Consume vegetable juices that are low in carbohydrates, such as celery and green juices mixed with a small amount of higher carbohydrate veggies such as carrot or beet. Mix in some form of healthy fat with each glass of the juice. One to three teaspoons of cultured goat's milk, extra virgin coconut oil, canned or fresh coconut milk and cream, or flaxseed oil enhances absorption of minerals and prevents spikes in blood sugar.

- *Fermented vegetables:* Consume a few tablespoons of fermented vegetables such as sauerkraut with each meal to aid in digestion. Fermented vegetables are an excellent source of naturally occurring probiotics and enzymes.

- *Stocks:* It is a great idea to consume stocks on a regular basis, especially when you have a cold or flu. Stocks made from the bones of chicken, fish, lamb and beef contain minerals, gelatin, cartilage, collagen, and electrolytes from the vegetables. Stocks are an excellent source of proteins, especially collagen. They help to heal the gut lining and reduce inflammation.

Supplements

Take these health supplements to alleviate symptoms and get well. Appendix B explains where to obtain these supplements.

- *Primal Defense:* Start with one caplet per day on an empty stomach, 30 minutes before or one hour after meals. Increase usage by adding one additional caplet per day (i.e., one caplet the first day, two the second day, three the third day and so on). Once your dosage is up to 12 caplets per day, stay on that amount for a minimum of three months and then begin to gradually decrease to a maintenance dosage of between three to six caplets per day. Primal Defense is best taken first thing in the morning and right before bedtime with eight ounces pure water. Primal Defense may be taken with other nutritional supplements, but should be taken one hour apart from medications. If you experience symptoms of detoxification (i.e., increased elimination, loose stools, constipation, excess gas, flu-like symptoms or fever), reduce the dosage and work up slowly to 12 per day.

- *Omega-Zyme:* Take one to three caplets with each meal or snack.

- *FYI:* Take four caplets three times per day on an empty stomach for one to four weeks, followed by six caplets per day for three to six months, and then reduce to a maintenance level of three caplets per day. If a relapse or "flare-up" occurs, take 12 caplets per day for at least one week or until symptoms are under control.

- *Perfect Food:* Consume two tablespoons once or twice per day with eight ounces water or vegetable juice.

- *RevivAll Classic:* Take three caplets twice per day on an empty stomach until symptoms are greatly reduced. Once symptoms are improved, consume two caplets daily for maintenance.

- *Springs of Life:* Consume at least eight, eight-ounce glasses per day of purified water mixed with 12 drops of Springs of Life living water concentrate.

- *Super Seed:* Consume one serving twice per day, morning and evening, with eight ounces purified water.

- *Goatein:* The only protein powder on the market made from organically produced goat's milk. This protein powder is partially pre-digested, low temperature dried and is usually well tolerated by those with food allergies and digestive problems. Take one to four tablespoons per day mixed in water, juice, smoothies, yogurt or can be used in baking.

Additional Therapies

For people who have or may have an imbalanced immune system, avoiding contact with chlorinated water is of the utmost importance. That includes bathing water and drinking water. Chlorine kills bacteria, friendly and unfriendly, in the intestines. It can be absorbed through the skin. I recommend installing a shower filter to remove chlorine (see Appendix C). Avoid swimming in chlorinated water as well.

INSOMNIA…see *Sleep Disorders*
IRRITABLE BOWEL SYNDROME …see *Functional Bowel Disorders*

JOINT DISORDERS

- Ankylosing Spondylitis
- Gout
- Osteoarthritis
- Rheumatoid Arthritis

Overview

Arthritis and related conditions affect nearly 43 million Americans, or about one of every six people, making it one of the most prevalent diseases in the United States. By 2020, as the baby boom generation ages, an estimated 60 million Americans will be affected by arthritis.

Arthritis is the leading cause of disability in the United States and although cost-effective interventions are available to reduce the burden of arthritis, they are currently underused.

Ankylosing Spondylitis

Ankylosing spondylitis (spinal arthritis) causes immobility of the back, and often the shoulders and neck. It affects more than 300,000 people—usually men.

Gout

Gout is usually associated with lifestyle and diet; gout affects some one million persons—usually men. Gout is caused by the buildup of acidic crystals, which lodge in the joints. Painful gout attacks often are first felt in the big toe.

Osteoarthritis

The most common form of arthritis is osteoarthritis, which is a mechanical disease that results from cartilage deterioration and trauma. Under the age of 45, osteoarthritis is more common in men. However, after age 45 it is ten times more common in women than men.[70] Forty million Americans have some form of osteoarthritis from mild to severe, including 80 percent of people over age 50. Some 20 million Americans suffer from disabling osteoarthritis. This number is likely to increase by three or four times over the next several decades.[71]

Rheumatoid Arthritis

Rheumatoid arthritis is an inflammatory- and immune-mediated disease. Rheumatoid arthritis, also known simply as RA, affects about 2.1 million people—usually women.

Rheumatoid arthritis is a chronic disease of the joints characterized by alternating periods of active inflammation and absence of symptoms, both of variable duration.[72] Some of the symptoms include a sense of utter fatigue and weakness, and running a very slight fever. The joints may become just a little stiff at first, but a few weeks later they become much stiffer and swollen. The stiffness and swelling may start in the small joints like the fingers and wrists but progress to larger joints and afflict both the joints and bodily organs. This is a systemic disease. It affects the body inside and outside. Interestingly, symmetrical joints such as the hands, wrists and ankles, are often hit first with an attack. The joints may even be "hot" to the touch. About one third of rheumatoid arthritis patients get luckier than most, and only a single joint area or two are affected; but for most, the pain will be spread throughout the entire body.

The usual age at which it strikes is in the 20 to 40 age group.[73] In terms of gender differentiation, rheumatoid arthritis is most likely to strike women aged 36 to 50, according to the National Rheumatism Foundation. The next major target is men 45 to 60. Some children and teenagers suffer various forms of rheumatoid arthritis.

Diet

Follow the diet prescribed in Chapters 9 to 11 diligently for 6 to 12 months. After symptoms are completely gone for at least three months, you may gradually add foods from the "Neutral" or "Dangerous" categories, if you desire. Because people with chronic joint disorders appear to have a pre-disposed weakness in their immune systems, I strongly recommend that they adhere to a diet of foods in the "Super" and "Healthy" categories for the rest of their lives.

Therapeutic Foods

These therapeutic foods will help you get well. Appendix A lists sources where you can obtain these foods.

- *Cultured goat's milk dairy products:* Consume 8 to 32 ounces of the highest quality cultured dairy products from goat's milk. I recommend a 30 hour fermented yogurt called Probiogurt (see resource section). Try to find yogurt that does not contain the organism *Streptococcus thermophilus*, a bacterial microbe that has been known to make immune-system disorders worse.
- *Grass-fed red meat*: Red meat from grass-fed cattle, buffalo, and lamb is very healthy and can be eaten a few times per week. This meat is a great source of protein, minerals, vitamin B_{12}, vitamins A and D, omega-3 fats, and CLA.
- *Omega-3 eggs:* Consume as many as two eggs high in omega-3 fatty acids each day. These eggs contain DHA, vitamins E and B_{12}, and antioxidants including lutein.
- *Extra virgin coconut oil:* This oil is perhaps the healthiest of the widely available oils. I recommend cooking almost exclusively with extra virgin coconut oil. Consume as much as two to four tablespoons per day of the oil in cooking, smoothies, or right off the spoon. It contains large amounts of lauric acid, a potent antimicrobial and one of the chief fatty acids in breast milk.
- *Ocean-caught fish:* This type of fish is perhaps the healthiest of all protein sources. Salmon, sardines, mackerel, herring and albacore tuna are high in the omega-3 fatty acids EPA and DHA. Ocean-caught fish can be consumed every day to enhance digestive and immune system health and is particularly beneficial for inflammatory types of arthritis.
- *Cod liver oil:* Take one to three teaspoons of Olde World Icelandic Cod Liver Oil each day. The amount consumed should be based upon the amount of sunlight you receive. People in colder climates generally need to consume larger amounts. Cod liver oil is a fantastic source of the omega-3 fats DHA and EPA, as well as vitamins A and D.

- *Vegetable juice:* Consume vegetable juices that are low in carbohydrates, such as celery and green juices mixed with a small amount of higher carbohydrate veggies such as carrot or beet. Mix in some form of healthy fat with each glass of the juice. One to three teaspoons of cultured goat's milk, extra virgin coconut oil, canned or fresh coconut milk and cream, or flaxseed oil enhances absorption of minerals and prevents spikes in blood sugar.
- *Fermented vegetables:* Consume a few tablespoons of fermented vegetables such as sauerkraut with each meal to aid in digestion. Fermented vegetables are an excellent source of naturally occurring probiotics and enzymes.
- *Stocks:* It is a great idea to consume stocks on a regular basis, especially when you have a cold or flu. Stocks made from the bones of chicken, fish, lamb and beef contain minerals, gelatin, cartilage, collagen, and electrolytes from the vegetables. Stocks are an excellent source of proteins, especially collagen. They help to heal the gut lining and reduce inflammation.

Supplements

Take these health supplements to alleviate symptoms and get well. Appendix B explains where to obtain these supplements.

- **Primal Defense:** Start with one caplet per day on an empty stomach, 30 minutes before or one hour after meals. Increase usage by adding one additional caplet per day (i.e., one caplet the first day, two the second day, three the third day and so on). Once your dosage is up to 12 caplets per day, stay on that amount for a minimum of three months and then begin to gradually decrease to a maintenance dosage of between three to six caplets per day. Primal Defense is best taken first thing in the morning and right before bedtime with eight ounces pure water. Primal Defense may be taken with other nutritional supplements, but should be taken one hour apart from medications. If you experience symptoms of detoxification (i.e., increased elimination, loose stools, constipation, excess gas, flu-like symptoms or fever), reduce the dosage and work up slowly to 12 per day.
- **Omega-Zyme:** Take one to three caplets with each meal or snack.
- **FYI:** Take four caplets three times per day on an empty stomach for one to four weeks, followed by six caplets per day for three to six months, and then reduce to a maintenance level of three caplets per day. If a relapse or "flare-up" occurs, take 12 caplets per day for at least one week or until symptoms are under control (see also Chapter 5).
- **Perfect Food:** Consume two tablespoons once or twice per day with eight ounces water or vegetable juice.
- **Springs of Life:** Consume at least eight, eight-ounce glasses per day of purified water mixed with 12 drops of Springs of Life living water concentrate.
- **Super Seed:** Consume one serving twice per day, morning and evening, with eight ounces purified water.
- **Goatein:** The only protein powder on the market made from organically produced goat's milk. This protein powder is partially pre-digested, low temperature dried and is usually well tolerated by those

with food allergies and digestive problems. Take one to four tablespoons per day mixed in water, juice, smoothies, yogurt or can be used in baking.

Additional Therapies

For people who have or may have an imbalanced immune system, avoiding contact with chlorinated water is of the utmost importance. That includes bathing water and drinking water. Chlorine kills bacteria, friendly and unfriendly, in the intestines. It can be absorbed through the skin. I recommend installing a shower filter to remove chlorine (see Appendix C). Avoid swimming in chlorinated water as well.

We've known for hundreds of years that fish oils play a role in arthritis. British doctors used to give their patients cod liver oil to alleviate rheumatism. In particular, seafood rich in omega-3 fatty acids may prove to be extremely beneficial for anyone suffering inflammatory types of arthritis, especially rheumatoid arthritis. Three or more servings weekly of select seafood dishes could do more for your arthritis than any medical drug or surgery.

Salmon, tuna, sardines, herring, anchovies and mackerel are rich sources of omega-3 fatty acids. These fatty acids, found in such limited amounts in most people's diets today, suppress production of substances such as cytokines and leukotrienes that are produced by white blood cells and are responsible for the inflammation accompanying arthritis.[74] Eating these fats is likely to reduce the body's overall inflammation levels, thin the blood and reduce your risk for heart attack and stroke, as well as arthritis.

LACTOSE INTOLERANCE…see *Functional Bowel Disorders*
LEAKY GUT SYNDROME…see *Functional Bowel Disorders*
LOW BACK PAIN…see *Inflammatory Conditions*
LUPUS…see *Autoimmune Disease*

MALE HEALTH
- Benign Prostatic Hypertrophy   •   Prostatitis
- Erectile Dysfunction

Benign Prostatic Hypertrophy (BPH)

A combination of connective tissue, gland, and muscle, the prostate provides the power that propels the semen through the urethra and out the penis. The prostate plays a key role in men's sexuality, providing more than 90 percent of his ejaculate, including the enzyme-filled fluid called semen required for fertilization of the ovum.[75] So you can see why the health of the prostate is key for maintaining lifetime potency and virility.

The prostate needs male hormones to function. The main male hormone is testosterone, which is made mainly by the testes.

Yet as men age, the prostate can become enlarged. This enlargement, in turn, can be the source of much suffering and embarrassment. Indeed, prostate enlargement, which your doctor may call benign prostatic hypertrophy or hyperplasia (or BPH), is the most common prostate disorder.

Men who have an enlarged prostate commonly begin producing a toxic form of testosterone called dihydrotestosterone (DHT). (Interestingly, DHT is also linked to hair loss. In the case of the prostate, excess production of DHT is closely linked with enlarged prostate tissue.)

Symptoms include difficulty starting and stopping urination, frequent nighttime trips to the bathroom, and the unsettling feeling that, although you've tried, voiding simply isn't complete.[76] These all result when the prostate squeezes and pinches off the urethra, and the bladder outlet becomes obstructed.[77]

By age 60 at least half of all men are suffering from symptoms of an enlarged prostate.[78] For some men, there may be only a minor discomfort and the symptoms can be stoically shrugged off as simply a condition of aging. Other men, for whom the symptoms are more severe, however, require medical help.*

Erectile Dysfunction

Impotence is a consistent inability to sustain an erection sufficient for sexual intercourse. Medical professionals often use the term "erectile dysfunction" or ED to describe this disorder and to differentiate it from other problems that interfere with sexual intercourse, such as lack of sexual desire and problems with ejaculation and orgasm.

Impotence can be a total inability to achieve erection, an inconsistent ability to do so, or a tendency to sustain only brief erections. These variations make defining impotence and estimating its incidence difficult. Experts believe impotence affects between 10 and 15 million American men. In 1985, the National Ambulatory Medical Care Survey counted 525,000 doctor-office visits for erectile dysfunction. But this is probably a significant underestimate of the extent of the problem, since many men are too embarrassed to seek help and because the population is rapidly aging.

What is the truth about men's impotency? Some experts suggest 90 percent of cases of erectile dysfunction in men over age 50 are due to physical factors, such as a health condition like diabetes or heart and circulatory disease, injury, or drug side effects.[79] Any disorder that impairs blood flow in the penis has the potential to cause impotence. This is buttressed by the Massachusetts Male Aging Study which found that both psychological and organic factors affect the burdensome problems of aging, particularly men's potency.[80] Incidence rises with age: about 5 percent of men at the age of 40 and between 15 and 25 percent of men at the age of 65 experience impotence.

As men age, their sexual function is impaired by the same types of atherosclerotic processes that cause heart disease. That is why for so many men erectile dysfunction should be taken very seriously. It is often an early warning sign of heart disease.

* However, be aware that some cases of BPH are actually prostatitis. For this reason, men should use a supplement such as RevivALL Male Vitality Formula, which addresses both BPH and prostatitis.

Like the arteries to the heart, when the vessels leading to the sexual organs clog up with plaque, blood flow is impaired. This makes achieving an erection difficult and also leads to poor sensation.[81]

Natural remedies may require "longer to bring about a result," says Thomas Kurzel, N.D. However, he adds that, "botanical medicines offer many of the same therapeutic benefits as drug therapies without the sometime severe side effects."

Prostatitis

The prostate gland and seminal vesicle (the male appendages) form a unit embryologically, anatomically and functionally. The prostate, an organ which is well supplied with blood and normally undergoes periods of congestion, is the central point of this organ system, and is liable to be afflicted with acute or chronic infections. Approximately 30 percent of males between the age of 25 and 40 years with prostate complaints have true prostatitis and 30 percent a genitoanal syndrome, the remainder having other pathological prostatic conditions. Because of the similarity of symptoms, it is difficult even for experts to differentiate the various clinical syndromes.

Aside from the typical complex of complaints, acute prostatitis is often accompanied by fever and chills. In addition to analgesics, therapy includes high-dosed chemotherapy with antibiotics. Should the inflammation not be brought under control, a prostatic abscess or other condition may develop. In spite of specific chemotherapy, acute prostatitis regardless of the causative agent may develop into a chronic inflammation.

Chronic prostatitis, on the other hand, proceeds blandly and without fever. It is often the residual condition following acute prostatitis, although it may also ascend along the ducts or spread via the blood.

That is why the healing protocols (below and especially use of RevivALL Male Vitality Formula) are so important, since they can permanently resolve the problem by attacking the problem at the root cause, which is often inadequate immune and endocrine system function.

Diet

Choose mainly foods from the "Super" and "Healthy" categories until optimal health is achieved for at least three months (or if experiencing symptoms, i.e., BPH, low libido, low energy, until symptoms are gone for at least three months). Once symptoms are greatly improved, you may gradually add foods from the "Neutral" or "Dangerous" categories if desired. To attain and maintain vibrant health, I recommend consuming foods from the "Super" and "Healthy" categories as the main part of a healthy diet.

Therapeutic Foods

These therapeutic foods will help you get well. Appendix A lists sources where you can obtain these foods.

- **Cultured goat's milk dairy products:** Consume 8 to 32 ounces of the highest quality cultured dairy products from goat's milk. I recommend a 30 hour fermented yogurt called Probiogurt (see resource section). Try to find yogurt that does not contain the organism *Streptococcus thermophilus,* a bacterial microbe that has been known to make immune-system disorders worse.

- *Grass-fed red meat:* Red meat from grass-fed cattle, buffalo, and lamb is very healthy and can be eaten a few times per week. This meat is a great source of protein, minerals, vitamin B_{12}, vitamins A and D, omega-3 fats, and CLA.
- *Omega-3 eggs:* Consume as many as two eggs high in omega-3 fatty acids each day. These eggs contain DHA, vitamins E and B_{12}, and antioxidants including lutein.
- *Extra virgin coconut oil:* This oil is perhaps the healthiest of the widely available oils. I recommend cooking almost exclusively with extra virgin coconut oil. Consume as much as two to four tablespoons per day of the oil in cooking, smoothies, or right off the spoon. It contains large amounts of lauric acid, a potent antimicrobial and one of the chief fatty acids in breast milk.
- *Ocean-caught fish:* This type of fish is perhaps the healthiest of all protein sources. Salmon, sardines, mackerel, herring and albacore tuna are high in the omega-3 fatty acids EPA and DHA. Ocean-caught fish can be consumed every day to enhance digestive and immune system health.
- *Cod liver oil:* Take one to three teaspoons of Olde World Icelandic Cod Liver Oil each day. The amount consumed should be based upon the amount of sunlight you receive. People in colder climates generally need to consume larger amounts. Cod liver oil is a fantastic source of the omega-3 fats DHA and EPA, as well as vitamins A and D.
- *Vegetable juice:* Consume vegetable juices that are low in carbohydrates, such as celery and green juices mixed with a small amount of higher carbohydrate veggies such as carrot or beet. Mix in some form of healthy fat with each glass of the juice. One to three teaspoons of cultured goat's milk, extra virgin coconut oil, canned or fresh coconut milk and cream, or flaxseed oil enhances absorption of minerals and prevents spikes in blood sugar.
- *Fermented vegetables:* Consume a few tablespoons of fermented vegetables such as sauerkraut with each meal to aid in digestion. Fermented vegetables are an excellent source of naturally occurring probiotics and enzymes.
- *Stocks:* It is a great idea to consume stocks on a regular basis, especially when you have a cold or flu. Stocks made from the bones of chicken, fish, lamb and beef contain minerals, gelatin, cartilage, collagen, and electrolytes from the vegetables. Stocks are an excellent source of proteins, especially collagen. They help to heal the gut lining and reduce inflammation.

Supplements

Take these health supplements to alleviate symptoms and get well. Appendix B explains where to obtain these supplements.

- *Perfect Food:* Take one to two tablespoons twice daily with eight ounces water or fresh vegetable juice.
- *Clear Energy:* Take six caplets per day with meals for a total of 100 days. Thereafter, take three caplets per day with meals. Do not consume Clear Energy after 6:00 p.m.

SPECIAL REPORT: Flower Pollen for Men's Health

Flower pollen concentrate has been used in the treatment of chronic prostatitis for nearly 30 years with favorable results. The beneficial effect of such extracts on patients suffering from age-related prostate conditions was first established in Sweden in 1960 by Dr. Ask Upmark of Lund University. Many clinical studies since have confirmed that men enjoy stronger urine stream with complete, decisive voiding when flower pollen extract is used.

In 1989, researchers reported that they gave pollen extract to 15 patients, ranging in age from 23 to 63 years.[82] These men had either chronic prostatitis or prostatodynia (a more generalized type of chronic pelvic pain). The men used the flower pollen for one to eighteen months. During this time, seven patients became symptom-free, six significantly improved and two failed to respond. Two patients had a recurrence of symptoms after cessation of treatment, which cleared up after recommencing treatment. Researchers concluded that the pollen extract was "effective in the treatment of chronic prostatitis and prostatodynia." Its precise mode of action is not known, although experimental studies suggest that it has anti-inflammatory and antiandrogenic properties.

Another study was published in *The Prostate* in 2001. These researchers note that flower pollen "can work as a potent anti-inflammatory agent against chronic prostatitis."[83]

While the majority of research studies have focused on pollen concentrate's effect on prostatitis, other studies show it protects the liver from chemical toxins and has anticancer potential, including reducing risk of prostate cancer.

- *RevivAll Male Vitality Formula:* Take three RevivAll Male caplets twice a day, morning and evening, on an empty stomach at least 30 minutes away from food for 30 days. Decrease to two caplets twice per day for 60 days. Once health is greatly improved, you may reduce intake to a maintenance level of two caplets once per day first thing in the morning. RevivAll Male may be taken with other food supplements. RevivAll contains flower pollen extract (see below).
- *Springs of Life:* Consume at least eight, eight-ounce glasses per day of purified water mixed with 12 drops of Springs of Life living water concentrate.
- *Super Seed:* Consume one serving twice per day, morning and evening, with eight ounces purified water.
- *Goatein:* The only protein powder on the market made from organically produced goat's milk. This protein powder is partially pre-digested, low temperature dried and is usually well tolerated by those with food allergies and digestive problems. Take one to four tablespoons per day mixed in water, juice, smoothies, yogurt or can be used in baking.

MEMORY LOSS…see *Brain Health*
MENOPAUSE…see *Female Health*

MENTAL DISORDERS

- Addiction
- Agoraphobia
- Anxiety
- Depression Disorders
- Violent, Impulsive Behavior
- Postpartum Depression
- Schizophrenia

Overview

Mental disorders are common in the United States and internationally. An estimated 22.1 percent of Americans ages 18 and older—about one in five adults—suffer from a diagnosable mental disorder in a given year, notes the National Institute for Mental Health. When applied to the 1998 U.S. Census residential population estimate, this figure translates to 44.3 million people. In addition, four of the ten leading causes of disability in the United States and other developed countries are mental disorders— major depression, bipolar disorder, schizophrenia, and obsessive-compulsive disorder. Many people suffer from more than one mental disorder at a given time.

Addiction

Many people view drug abuse and addiction as strictly a social problem. Parents, teens, older adults, and other members of the community tend to characterize people who take drugs as morally weak or as having criminal tendencies. They believe that drug abusers and addicts should be able to stop taking drugs if they are willing to change their behavior.

These myths have not only stereotyped those with drug-related problems, but also their families, their communities, and the health care professionals who work with them. Drug abuse and addiction comprise a public health problem that affects many people and has wide-ranging social consequences.

Addiction does begin with drug abuse when an individual makes a conscious choice to use drugs, but addiction is not just "a lot of drug use." Recent scientific research provides overwhelming evidence that not only do drugs interfere with normal brain functioning creating powerful feelings of pleasure, but they also have long-term effects on brain metabolism and activity. At some point, changes occur in the brain that can turn drug abuse into addiction, a chronic, relapsing illness. Those addicted to drugs suffer from a compulsive drug craving and usage and cannot quit by themselves.

Holistic treatment can have a profound effect not only on drug abusers, but on society as a whole by significantly improving social and psychological functioning, decreasing related criminality and violence, and reducing the spread of AIDS. It can also dramatically reduce the costs to society of drug abuse.

Anxiety

Anxiety disorders include panic disorder, obsessive-compulsive disorder, post-traumatic stress disorder, generalized anxiety disorder, and phobias (social phobia, agoraphobia, and specific phobia).

- Approximately 19.1 million American adults ages 18 to 54, or about 13.3 percent of people in this age group in a given year, have an anxiety disorder.
- Anxiety disorders frequently co-occur with depressive disorders, eating disorders, or substance abuse.
- Many people have more than one anxiety disorder.
- Women are more likely than men to have an anxiety disorder. Approximately twice as many women as men suffer from panic disorder, post-traumatic stress disorder, generalized anxiety disorder, agoraphobia, and specific phobia, though about equal numbers of women and men have obsessive-compulsive disorder and social phobia.

Agoraphobia

Agoraphobia involves intense fear and avoidance of any place or situation where escape might be difficult or help unavailable in the event of developing sudden panic-like symptoms. Approximately 3.2 million American adults ages 18 to 54, or about 2.2 percent of people in this age group in a given year, have agoraphobia.

Depression

Depressive disorders encompass major depressive disorder, dysthymic disorder, and bipolar disorder. Bipolar disorder is included because people with this illness have depressive episodes as well as manic episodes.

- Approximately 18.8 million American adults, or about 9.5 percent of the U.S. population age 18 and older in a given year, have a depressive disorder.
- Nearly twice as many women (12.0 percent) as men (6.6 percent) are affected by a depressive disorder each year. These figures translate to 12.4 million women and 6.4 million men in the United States.
- Depressive disorders may be appearing earlier in life in people born in recent decades compared to the past.
- Depressive disorders often co-occur with anxiety disorders and substance abuse.

Postpartum Depression

Having a baby is a joyous time for most women. After childbirth, though, many mothers feel sad, afraid, angry or anxious. Most new mothers have these feelings in a mild form called postpartum blues. Sometimes these feelings are called "baby blues." Postpartum blues almost always go away in a few days.

About 10 percent of new mothers have a greater problem called postpartum depression. Postpartum depression lasts longer and is more intense. It often requires counseling and treatment. Postpartum depression can occur after any birth, not just the first.

Schizophrenia

- Approximately 2.2 million American adults, or about 1.1 percent of the population age 18 and older in a given year, have schizophrenia.

- Schizophrenia affects men and women with equal frequency.
- Schizophrenia often first appears earlier in men, usually in their late teens or early twenties, than in women, who are generally affected in their twenties or early thirties.

Violent, Impulsive Behavior

Spousal abuse, criminal activity and other examples of violent, impulsive behavior can be linked to alcohol abuse, environmental pollution (especially industrial chemicals such as some pesticides and heavy metals), and genetics.

Diet

Follow the diet prescribed in Chapters 9 through 11 diligently for 6 to 12 months. After symptoms are completely gone for at least three months, you may gradually add foods from the "Neutral" or "Dangerous" categories, if you desire. Because people with mental disorders appear to have derangements of the neurogastroimmunomodulatory network, I strongly recommend that they adhere to a diet of foods in the "Super" and "Healthy" categories for the rest of their lives.

Therapeutic Foods

These therapeutic foods will help you get well. Appendix A lists sources where you can obtain these foods.

- *Cultured goat's milk dairy products:* Consume 8 to 32 ounces of the highest quality cultured dairy products from goat's milk. I recommend a 30 hour fermented yogurt called Probiogurt (see resource section). Try to find yogurt that does not contain the organism *Streptococcus thermophilus*, a bacterial microbe that has been known to make immune-system disorders worse.
- *Grass-fed red meat:* Red meat from grass-fed cattle, buffalo, and lamb is very healthy and can be eaten a few times per week. This meat is a great source of protein, minerals, vitamin B_{12}, vitamins A and D, omega-3 fats, and CLA.
- *Omega-3 eggs:* Consume as many as one to three eggs high in omega-3 fatty acids each day. These eggs contain DHA, vitamins E and B_{12}, and antioxidants including lutein.
- *Extra virgin coconut oil:* This oil is perhaps the healthiest of the widely available oils. I recommend cooking almost exclusively with extra virgin coconut oil. Consume as much as two to four tablespoons per day of the oil in cooking, smoothies, or right off the spoon. It contains large amounts of lauric acid, a potent antimicrobial and one of the chief fatty acids found in breast milk.
- *Ocean-caught fish:* This type of fish is perhaps the healthiest of all protein sources. Salmon, sardines, mackerel, herring and albacore tuna are high in the omega-3 fatty acids EPA and DHA. Ocean-caught fish can be consumed every day to enhance digestive and immune system health.
- *Cod liver oil:* Take one to three teaspoons of Olde World Icelandic Cod Liver Oil each day. The amount consumed should be based upon the amount of sunlight you receive. People in colder climates gener-

ally need to consume larger amounts. Cod liver oil is a fantastic source of the omega-3 fats DHA and EPA, as well as fat-soluble vitamins A and D.

- *Vegetable juice:* Consume vegetable juices that are low in carbohydrates, such as celery and green juices mixed with a small amount of higher carbohydrate veggies such as carrot or beet. Mix in some form of healthy fat with each glass of the juice. One to three teaspoons of cultured goat's milk, extra virgin coconut oil, canned or fresh coconut milk and cream, or flaxseed oil enhances absorption of minerals and prevents spikes in blood sugar.
- *Fermented vegetables:* Consume a few tablespoons of fermented vegetables such as sauerkraut with each meal to aid in digestion. Fermented vegetables are an excellent source of naturally occurring probiotics and enzymes.
- *Stocks:* It is a great idea to consume stocks on a regular basis, especially when you have a cold or flu. Stocks made from the bones of chicken, fish, lamb and beef contain minerals, gelatin, cartilage, collagen, and electrolytes from the vegetables. Stocks are an excellent source of proteins, especially collagen. They help to heal the gut lining and reduce inflammation.

Supplements

Take these health supplements to alleviate symptoms and get well. Appendix B explains where to obtain these supplements.

- *Primal Defense:* Start with one caplet per day on an empty stomach, 30 minutes before or one hour after meals. Increase usage by adding one additional caplet per day (i.e., one caplet the first day, two the second day, three the third day and so on). Once your dosage is up to 12 caplets per day, stay on that amount for a minimum of three months and then begin to gradually decrease to a maintenance dosage of between three to six caplets per day. Primal Defense is best taken first thing in the morning and right before bedtime with eight ounces pure water. Primal Defense may be taken with other nutritional supplements, but should be taken one hour apart from medications. If you experience symptoms of detoxification (i.e., increased elimination, loose stools, constipation, excess gas, flu-like symptoms or fever), reduce the dosage and work up slowly to 12 per day.
- *Omega-Zyme:* Take one to three caplets with each meal or snack.
- *Perfect Food :* Take one to two tablespoons twice daily with eight ounces water or fresh vegetable juice.
- *Springs of Life:* Consume at least eight, eight-ounce glasses per day of purified water mixed with 12 drops of Springs of Life living water concentrate.
- *Goatein:* The only protein powder on the market made from organically produced goat's milk. This protein powder is partially pre-digested, low temperature dried and is usually well tolerated by those with food allergies and digestive problems. Take one to four tablespoons per day mixed in water, juice, smoothies, yogurt or can be used in baking.

Additional Therapies

For people who have or may have imbalanced immune systems, avoiding contact with chlorinated water is of the utmost importance. That includes bathing water and drinking water. Chlorine kills bacteria, friendly and unfriendly, in the intestines. It can be absorbed through the skin. I recommend installing a shower filter to remove chlorine (see Appendix C). Avoid swimming in chlorinated water as well.

SPECIAL REPORT: Importance of Omega-3 Fatty Acids

I strongly urge persons with mental disorders to increase their intake of both flaxseed and flax oil, as well as omega-3 fatty acid-rich seafood.

Dr. Donald O. Rudin must be given credit for launching the early research into the impact of omega-3 fatty acids on mental health. The former director of the Department of Molecular Biology at Eastern Pennsylvania Psychiatric Institute, Dr. Rudin began working with flaxseed oil in the early 1980s with patients at his clinic. At that time, he performed a clinical trial with 44 patients with various mental disorders. Providing from two to six tablespoons a day of flaxseed oil, he found the results to be astounding. Within two hours of providing some patients the flax oil he observed that their "mood is improved and depression is lifted."[84]

Omega-3 fats make up one of the two families of fats, the omega-3s and the omega-6s, that are absolutely essential to human life. Yet, Dr. Rudin knew that the dietary availability of omega-3 fatty acids had declined to only 20 percent of the level found in diets a century ago.

Even during the 1980s when his initial pilot study involving 44 patients took place and nutrition was on so many persons' minds, he observed, "Although we live in a time of nutrition consciousness, when everyone is enthusiastic about restoring nutrients to the diet, omega-3—until recently—was virtually ignored."

As a researcher with 35 years of experience, Dr. Rudin suspected that many modern diseases were signs of a new kind of malnutrition—an epidemic affecting Americans.

In other words, in his own way, Dr. Rudin was uncovering an unknown supernatural phenomenon—the key role that omega-3 fatty acids play in maintaining optimal mental health.

With so many patients at his clinic that simply could not be helped by medical drugs and procedures, the doctor wondered what would happen if the omega-3 fats were restored to their diets. Since Dr. Rudin worked in a clinical setting, he decided to set up a small but representative pilot study, using volunteers suffering from chronic ailments that were not being cured by current conventional treatments. He would add the missing omega-3 oils to their diets and see what happened...

One patient experienced dramatically improved moods. Dr. Rudin says, "Three days after starting on 6 tablespoons of [flaxseed oil] daily, she developed a marked sense of increased physical energy and unique exuberance." This finding was replicated in varying degree among most of the patients. By six to eight weeks, most of them were sleeping better, more energetic, and less anxious and depressed. Switching the patients to other types of fats (i.e., omega-6 fatty acids which are overly prevalent in the modern American diet) resulted in a return of their symptoms.

We now know that the omega-3 fatty acids truly can help most common mood disorders, including depression, postpartum depression, impulsive, violent behavior, and bipolar disorder.[85]

For most of us who seek to simply improve our mood and mental outlooks, we can safely increase our intake of fish and flax oil, since each provides a different set of omega-3 fatty acids.

MULTIPLE SCLEROSIS...see *Autoimmune Disease*
MYASTHENIA GRAVIS...see *Autoimmune Disease*

MYCOPLASMA INFECTIONS

Overview

Human mycoplasma infection is not new, but recognition by medical scientists and doctors has come relatively late. As a result, many persons with some of medical science's most difficult-to-treat chronic diseases have not received adequate medical treatment.

Mycoplasmas are small microorganisms without cell walls. The word mycoplasma itself is derived from the ancient Greek *mỹkēs* which is a combined linguistic form for "mushroom, fungus," and plasma, the non-cellular fluid portion of the blood. Thus, we see, mycoplasmas are blood fungi. They are also *pleomorphic*, meaning they have the ability to change shape and form during their life cycle and under varying conditions. This gives them a highly unique ability to evade even healthily functioning immune systems (more on this later).

Mycoplasmas are the smallest, simplest self-replicating organisms currently known, being built of a plasma membrane, ribosomes (organelles functioning as the site of protein manufacture), and a circular double-stranded DNA molecule without a distinct nuclear membrane.[86]

Mycoplasmas are the simplest organism capable of independent life with a minimal set of genes. The recent complete sequencing of the genome of the human pathogen *Mycoplasma genitalium* shows us that its genome is only 580 kb long and contains only 470 predicted coding sequences or genes (as compared with 1,727 in *Haemophilus influenzae* and about 4,000 in *E. coli*).

This drastic economization in genetic information must be associated with the parasitic mode of life of mycoplasmas. During their evolution, mycoplasmas lost their cell walls and many biosynthetic systems involved in synthesis of macromolecule building blocks. These instead were to be provided by their host. Thus, for example, *M. genitalium* carries only one gene involved in amino acid biosynthesis, and very few genes for vitamin and nucleic acid precursors; the lack of genes involved in fatty acid biosynthesis leads to dependence on the host's fatty acids. Nevertheless, these minimal organisms carry all the essential genes needed to maintain their parasitism, so that a significant number of mycoplasmal genes are devoted to adhesins (attachment organelles) and variable surface antigens directed towards evasion of the host immune system.

Unfortunately, diagnosis of mycoplasma infections is difficult. Culturing mycoplasmas is difficult and may take months to obtain results.

Polymerase chain reaction (PCR) techniques are becoming more widely available. With PCR, very small amounts of blood and blood cells, like white blood cells that have DNA, can be isolated, then amplified (polymerase chain reaction) to find the infections inside the blood of a patient.

Indeed, the major scientific and clinical roadblock has been that medical science has not known until quite recently how to confirm the presence of mycoplasma infection in humans. Because until recently, it was very difficult to find these types of infections, "that's why you didn't hear very much about it," says Dr. Garth L. Nicolson, chief scientific officer and research professor, professor of internal medicine and chief of the Institute for Molecular Medicine, Huntington Beach, California.[87] Dr. Nicolson is one of the foremost authorities in the world on the mycoplasmas and related infections.

Even though you have probably never heard of mycoplasmas, their parasitic existence in the human body may be key to prolongation of disabling chronic diseases. Among the most intractable medical conditions linked to mycoplasma infections are chronic fatigue syndrome; fibromyalgia; rheumatoid arthritis; respiratory maladies including chronic asthma; inflammatory bowel disease; heart disease; neurological disorders such as Parkinson's, Lou Gehrig's disease; and Gulf War illness.

Diet

Follow the diet prescribed in Chapters 9 to 11 diligently for 6 to 12 months. For the first 30 days it is best to limit or even restrict fruit and honey consumption. Make sure that if you do consume fruit it is the less sweet, high nutrient, high-fiber fruits such as berries, apples or grapefruit.

After symptoms are completely gone for at least six months, you may gradually add foods from the "Neutral" or "Dangerous" categories, if you desire. Because people with fungal and parasitic overgrowth appear to have a predisposed weakness in their intestinal tracts, I strongly recommend that they adhere to a diet of foods in the "Super" and "Healthy" categories for the rest of their lives.

Therapeutic Foods

These therapeutic foods will help you get well. Appendix A lists sources where you can obtain these foods.

- *Cultured goat's milk dairy products:* Consume 8 to 32 ounces of the highest quality cultured dairy products from goat's milk. I recommend a 30 hour fermented yogurt called Probiogurt (see resource section). Try to find yogurt that does not contain the organism *Streptococcus thermophilus*, a bacterial microbe that has been known to make immune-system disorders worse.
- *Grass-fed red meat:* Red meat from grass-fed cattle, buffalo, and lamb is very healthy and can be eaten a few times per week. This meat is a great source of protein, minerals, vitamin B_{12}, vitamins A and D, omega-3 fats, and CLA.
- *Omega-3 eggs:* Consume as many as two eggs high in omega-3 fatty acids each day. These eggs contain DHA, vitamins E and B_{12}, and antioxidants including lutein.
- *Extra virgin coconut oil:* This oil is perhaps the healthiest of the widely available oils. I recommend cooking almost exclusively with extra virgin coconut oil. Consume as much as four to six tablespoons of the oil in cooking, in smoothies, or right off the spoon. It contains large amounts of lauric acid, a potent antimicrobial and one of the chief fatty acids in breast milk.
- *Ocean-caught fish:* This type of fish is perhaps the healthiest of all protein sources. Salmon, sardines, mackerel, herring and albacore tuna are high in the omega-3 fatty acids EPA and DHA. Ocean-caught fish can be consumed every day to enhance digestive and immune system health.

- *Cod liver oil:* Take one to three teaspoons of Olde World Icelandic Cod Liver Oil each day. The amount consumed should be based upon the amount of sunlight you receive. People in colder climates generally need to consume larger amounts. Cod liver oil is a fantastic source of the omega-3 fats DHA and EPA, as well as vitamins A and D.
- *Vegetable juice:* Consume vegetable juices that are low in carbohydrates, such as celery and green juices mixed with a small amount of higher carbohydrate veggies such as carrot or beet. Mix in some form of healthy fat with each glass of the juice. One to three teaspoons of cultured goat's milk, extra virgin coconut oil, canned or fresh coconut milk and cream, or flaxseed oil enhances absorption of minerals and prevents spikes in blood sugar.
- *Fermented vegetables:* Consume a few tablespoons of fermented vegetables such as sauerkraut with each meal to aid in digestion. Fermented vegetables are an excellent source of naturally occurring probiotics and enzymes.
- *Stocks:* It is a great idea to consume stocks on a regular basis, especially when you have a cold or flu. Stocks made from the bones of chicken, fish, lamb and beef contain minerals, gelatin, cartilage, collagen, and electrolytes from the vegetables. Stocks are an excellent source of proteins, especially collagen. They help to heal the gut lining and reduce inflammation.

Supplements

Take these health supplements to alleviate symptoms and get well. Appendix B explains where to obtain these supplements.

- *Fungal Defense:* Follow the 14-day protocol as directed on the label.
- *Primal Defense:* Following the 14-day Fungal Defense protocol, take 12 caplets of Primal Defense per day; stay on that amount for a minimum of three months or when tests for abnormal microbes come back negative. Then begin to gradually decrease to a maintenance dosage of between three to six caplets per day. Primal Defense is best taken first thing in the morning and right before bedtime with eight ounces pure water. Primal Defense may be taken with other nutritional supplements, but should be taken one hour apart from medications. If you experience symptoms of detoxification (i.e., increased elimination, loose stools, constipation, excess gas, flu-like symptoms or fever), reduce the dosage and work up slowly to 12 per day.
- *Perfect Food:* Take one to two tablespoons twice daily with eight ounces water or fresh vegetable juice. You may take Perfect Food together with Primal Defense. Best taken on an empty stomach away from food.
- *Omega-Zyme:* Take one to three caplets with each meal or snack.
- *Springs of Life:* Consume at least eight, eight-ounce glasses per day of purified water mixed with 12 drops of Springs of Life living water concentrate.
- *Super Seed:* Consume one serving twice per day, morning and evening, with eight or more ounces of purified water. (Consuming a fiber supplement is essential during the first two weeks of the program. Thereafter, consume fiber as needed.)

- *Goatein:* The only protein powder on the market made from organically produced goat's milk. This protein powder is partially pre-digested, low temperature dried and is usually well tolerated by those with food allergies and digestive problems. Take one to four tablespoons per day mixed in water, juice, smoothies, yogurt or can be used in baking.

Additional Therapies

For people who have or may have imbalanced intestinal flora, avoiding contact with chlorinated water is of the utmost importance. That includes bathing water and drinking water. Chlorine kills bacteria, friendly and unfriendly, in the intestines. It can be absorbed through the skin. I recommend installing a shower filter to remove chlorine (see Appendix C). Avoid swimming in chlorinated water as well.

OSTEOARTHRITIS…see *Joint Disorders*
OSTEOPOROSIS…see *Female Health*
OVARIAN CYSTS…see *Female Health*
PARKINSON'S DISEASE…see *Brain Health*
PERVASIVE DEVELOPMENTAL DISORDERS… see *Children's Health*
POSTPARTUM DEPRESSION…see *Mental Disorders*
PREMENSTRUAL SYNDROME…see *Female Health*
PROSTATITIS…see *Male Health*
PSORIASIS…see *Skin Health*
RHEUMATOID ARTHRITIS…see *Joint Disorders and Autoimmune Disease*
SCHIZOPHRENIA…see *Mental Disorders*
SCLERODERMA…see *Autoimmune Disease*
SEASONAL ALLERGIES…see *Upper Respiratory Health*
SHINGLES…see *Viral Diseases*
SINUSITIS…see *Upper Respiratory Health*

SKIN HEALTH
- Acne
- Atopic Dermatitis (Dermatitis, Eczema)
- Psoriasis

Overview

It is my experience that people suffering from acne, dermatitis and psoriasis frequently suffer from imbalanced immune system and intestinal flora. Once these imbalances are corrected by eating the proper foods and rebalancing the digestive tract with HSOs, the symptoms of even the most serious skin disorders have greatly improved.

Acne

Acne is a disorder resulting from the action of hormones on the skin's oil glands (sebaceous glands), which leads to plugged pores and outbreaks of lesions commonly called pimples or zits. Acne lesions usually occur on the face, neck, back, chest, and shoulders. Nearly 17 million people in the United States have acne, making it the most common skin disease. Although acne is not a serious health threat, severe acne can lead to disfiguring, permanent scarring, which can be upsetting to people who are affected by the disorder.

The exact cause of acne is unknown, but doctors believe it results from several related factors. One important factor is an increase in hormones called androgens (male sex hormones). These increase in both boys and girls during puberty and cause the sebaceous glands to enlarge and make more sebum. Hormonal changes related to pregnancy or starting or stopping birth control pills can also cause acne.

Another factor is heredity or genetics. Researchers believe that the tendency to develop acne can be inherited from parents. For example, studies have shown that many school-age boys with acne have a family history of the disorder. Certain drugs, including androgens and lithium, are known to cause acne. Greasy cosmetics may alter the cells of the follicles and make them stick together, producing a plug.

Many nutrition researchers believe that the outer appearance of the skin is directly related to the health of the digestive tract and immune system. An imbalance in intestinal flora and increased gut permeability (leaky gut syndrome) are almost always found in those suffering from acne. By following the diet and supplement recommendations in this book the symptoms of acne should greatly improve.

Atopic Dermatitis (Eczema)

Atopic dermatitis is a chronic (long-lasting) disease that affects the skin. The word "dermatitis" means inflammation of the skin. "Atopic" refers to a group of diseases that are hereditary (that is, run in families) and often occur together, including asthma, allergies such as hay fever, and atopic dermatitis. In atopic dermatitis, the skin becomes extremely itchy and inflamed, causing redness, swelling, cracking, weeping, crusting, and scaling. Atopic dermatitis most often affects infants and young children, but it can continue into adulthood or first show up later in life. In most cases, there are periods of time when the disease is worse, called exacerbations or flares, followed by periods when the skin improves or clears up entirely, called remissions. Many children with atopic dermatitis will experience a permanent remission of the disease when they get older, although their skin often remains dry and easily irritated. Environmental factors can bring on symptoms of atopic dermatitis at any time in the lives of individuals who have inherited the atopic disease trait.

Atopic dermatitis is often referred to as "eczema," which is a general term for the many types of dermatitis. Atopic dermatitis is the most common of the many types of eczema.

Psoriasis

Psoriasis is a chronic (long-lasting) skin disease characterized by scaling and inflammation. Scaling occurs when cells in the outer layer of the skin reproduce faster than normal and pile up on the skin's surface.

Psoriasis affects between one and two percent of the United States population, or about 5.5 million people. Although the disease occurs in all age groups and about equally in men and women, it primarily affects adults. People with psoriasis may suffer discomfort, including pain and itching, restricted motion in their joints, and emotional distress.

In its most typical form, psoriasis results in patches of thick, red skin covered with silvery scales. These patches, which are sometimes referred to as plaques, usually itch and may burn. The skin at the joints may crack. Psoriasis most often occurs on the elbows, knees, scalp, lower back, face, palms, and soles of the feet but it can affect any skin site. The disease may also affect the fingernails, the toenails, and the soft tissues inside the mouth and genitalia. About 15 percent of people with psoriasis have joint inflammation that produces arthritis symptoms. This condition is called psoriatic arthritis.

Recent research indicates that psoriasis is likely a disorder of the immune system. This system includes a type of white blood cell, called a T cell, that normally helps protect the body against infection and disease. Scientists now think that, in psoriasis, an abnormal immune system causes activity by T cells in the skin. These T cells trigger the inflammation and excessive skin cell reproduction seen in people with psoriasis.

In about one-third of the cases, psoriasis is inherited. Researchers are studying large families affected by psoriasis to identify a gene or genes that cause the disease. (Genes govern every bodily function and determine the inherited traits passed from parent to child.)

People with psoriasis may notice that there are times when their skin worsens, then improves. Conditions that may cause flare-ups include changes in climate, infections, stress, and dry skin. Also, certain medicines, most notably beta-blockers, which are used to treat high blood pressure, and lithium or drugs used to treat depression, may trigger an outbreak or worsen the disease.

Diet

Follow the diet prescribed in Chapters 9 to 11 diligently for 6 to 12 months. After symptoms are completely gone for at least three months, you may gradually add foods from the "Neutral" or "Dangerous" categories, if you desire. Because people with chronic skin problems appear to have a predisposed immuno-gastrointestinal weakness that presents as skin problems, I strongly recommend that they adhere to a diet of foods in the "Super" and "Healthy" categories for the rest of their lives.

Therapeutic Foods

These therapeutic foods will help you get well. Appendix A lists sources where you can obtain these foods.

- ***Cultured goat's milk dairy products:*** Consume 8 to 32 ounces of the highest quality cultured dairy products from goat's milk. I recommend a 30 hour fermented yogurt called Probiogurt (see resource section). Try to find yogurt that does not contain the organism *Streptococcus thermophilus*, a bacterial microbe that has been known to make immune-system disorders worse.

- **Grass-fed red meat:** Red meat from grass-fed cattle, buffalo, and lamb is very healthy and can be eaten a few times per week. This meat is a great source of protein, minerals, vitamin B_{12}, vitamins A and D, omega-3 fats, and CLA.
- **Omega-3 eggs:** Consume as many as two eggs high in omega-3 fatty acids each day. These eggs contain DHA, vitamins E and B_{12}, and antioxidants including lutein.
- **Extra virgin coconut oil:** This oil is perhaps the healthiest of the widely available oils. I recommend cooking almost exclusively with extra virgin coconut oil. Consume as much as two to four tablespoons per day of the oil in cooking, smoothies, or right off the spoon. It contains large amounts of lauric acid, a potent antimicrobial and one of the chief fatty acids in breast milk.
- **Ocean-caught fish:** This type of fish is perhaps the healthiest of all protein sources. Salmon, sardines, mackerel, herring and albacore tuna are high in the omega-3 fatty acids EPA and DHA. Ocean-caught fish can be consumed every day to enhance digestive and immune system health.
- **Cod liver oil:** Take one to three teaspoons of Olde World Icelandic Cod Liver Oil each day. The amount consumed should be based upon the amount of sunlight you receive. People in colder climates generally need to consume larger amounts. Cod liver oil is a fantastic source of the omega-3 fats DHA and EPA, as well as vitamins A and D.
- **Vegetable juice:** Consume vegetable juices that are low in carbohydrates, such as celery and green juices mixed with a small amount of higher carbohydrate veggies such as carrot or beet. Mix in some form of healthy fat with each glass of the juice. One to three teaspoons of cultured goat's milk, extra virgin coconut oil, canned or fresh coconut milk and cream, or flaxseed oil enhances absorption of minerals and prevents spikes in blood sugar.
- **Fermented vegetables:** Consume a few tablespoons of fermented vegetables such as sauerkraut with each meal to aid in digestion. Fermented vegetables are an excellent source of naturally occurring probiotics and enzymes.
- **Stocks:** It is a great idea to consume stocks on a regular basis, especially when you have a cold or flu. Stocks made from the bones of chicken, fish, lamb and beef contain minerals, gelatin, cartilage, collagen, and electrolytes from the vegetables. Stocks are an excellent source of proteins, especially collagen. They help to heal the gut lining and reduce inflammation.

Supplements

Take these health supplements to alleviate symptoms and get well. Appendix B explains where to obtain these supplements.

- **Primal Defense:** Start with one caplet per day on an empty stomach, 30 minutes before or one hour after meals. Increase usage by adding one additional caplet per day (i.e., one caplet the first day, two the second day, three the third day and so on). Once your dosage is up to 12 caplets per day, stay on that amount for a minimum of three months and then begin to gradually decrease to a maintenance dosage of between three to six caplets per day. Primal Defense is best taken first thing in the morning and right before bedtime with eight ounces pure water. Primal Defense may be taken with other nutritional supplements, but should be taken one hour apart from medications. If you experience symptoms of detoxification (i.e., increased elimination, loose stools, constipation, excess gas, flu-like symptoms or fever), reduce the dosage and work up slowly to 12 per day.

- *Omega-Zyme:* Take one to three caplets with each meal or snack.
- *RM-10:* Take nine caplets per day in three divided doses for 30 to 120 days on an empty stomach. Thereafter, consume a maintenance dosage of two to five caplets per day.
- *FYI:* Take four caplets three times per day on an empty stomach for 30 days, followed by six caplets per day for three to six months, and then reduce to a maintenance level of three caplets per day. If a relapse or "flare-up" occurs, take 12 caplets per day for at least one week or until symptoms are under control.
- *Perfect Food:* Take one to two tablespoons twice daily with eight ounces water or fresh vegetable juice.
- *Springs of Life:* Consume at least eight, eight-ounce glasses per day of purified water mixed with 12 drops of Springs of Life living water concentrate.
- *Super Seed:* Consume one serving twice per day, morning and evening, with eight ounces purified water.
- *Goatein:* The only protein powder on the market made from organically produced goat's milk. This protein powder is partially pre-digested, low temperature dried and is usually well tolerated by those with food allergies and digestive problems. Take one to four tablespoons per day mixed in water, juice, smoothies, yogurt or can be used in baking.

Additional Therapies

All skin conditions will benefit from healthy intestinal flora. For people who have or may have imbalanced intestinal flora, avoiding contact with chlorinated water is of the utmost importance. That includes bathing water and drinking water. Chlorine kills bacteria, friendly and unfriendly, in the intestines. It can be absorbed through the skin. I recommend installing a shower filter to remove chlorine (see Appendix C) and to improve your skin health. Avoid swimming in chlorinated water as well.

Using extra virgin extra virgin coconut oil topically can be great for skin problems of any kind. Rub a small amount on the affected area daily. Be sure not to over-apply as the oil may rub off onto clothing or furniture.

SLEEP DISORDERS

Overview

"Some 35% of Americans complain of occasional difficulties with sleeping, and about half this number report the problem as serious," note Peter J. Hauri, Ph.D., and Mary S. Esther, M.D., in a June 1990 report in *Mayo Clinic Proceedings*. Across the Atlantic, F. Hohagen and co-investigators note, in a 1993 report in the *European Archives of Psychiatry and Clinical Neuroscience*, results of their study, of some 2,512 patients, that demonstrate that insomnia is a common health problem in Europe as well. They note, "Every fifth person aged 18-65 years who consulted the general physician for health problems suffered from a sleep problem severe enough to cause impairment of daytime functioning and only half of the patients did not complain of any sleep problem at all."

Eight hours is often cited in lay discussions as an ideal amount of sleep to get every night. Yet, medical sleep experts note that individual requirements vary widely, and that no two people's sleep needs are necessarily alike. Hauri and Esther define insomnia as the "chronic inability to obtain the amount of sleep needed for [personal] optimal functioning and well-being."

The quality of one's sleeping hours is also important, note German E. Berrios and Colin M. Shapiro in the March 27, 1993 *British Medical Journal* (*BMJ*). Deep refreshing sleep is a great restorer of both physical and emotional health, they say. Berrios and Shapiro add in their BMJ report: "About a third of people who go to see their general practitioners and about two thirds of those who see psychiatrists complain that they are dissatisfied with the restorative quality of their sleep…. Patients often blame the quality of their sleep for any recently developed feelings of fatigue, depression, irritability, tension, sleepiness, lack of concentration, drowsiness, or muscular aches."

The causes of chronic insomnia and poor sleep vary widely. Hauri and Esther say that more than half of all cases of insomnia are related to psychiatric problems such as depression, anxiety, or stress. Meanwhile, in the April 24, 1993 *BMJ*, Chris Idzikowski and Colin M. Shapiro note that a wide range of drugs affect sleep, including appetite suppressants, steroids, blood pressure drugs like reserpine, and thyroid hormones.

Another cause of insomnia includes one's sleep environment. "Changes in the temperature or light in the bedroom, environmental noises and smells, and the quality of the mattress and pillows may lead to disruptions of the initiation or maintenance of sleep," say Berrios and Shapiro. "Using the bedroom for cooking, eating, studying, or watching television (as in a one room flat) may also cause insomnia in those whose sleep is fragile."

The use of alcohol and illegal drugs can also impair one's sleep quality, say Hauri and Esther. Finally, organic causes of poor sleep and insomnia, such as the chronic pain of rheumatoid arthritis, can cause an overall decrease in sleep efficiency, they say.

Advancing age itself also is associated with declining sleep quality. It's a fact that most people sleep less at a single stretch than they did when they were younger, observes the 1992 *Johns Hopkins Medical Handbook*. "People in their sixties and older awaken for a few seconds an astounding 150 times a night," says the handbook. "By contrast, young adults awaken briefly about five times. Even though transient awakenings usually go unremembered in the morning, they may create the subjective impression of fitful nights." Many older people believe that because they are more advanced in years they should not need as much sleep as when they were younger, and they cannot understand why they no longer feel rested in the morning. But if they think they can get by with less sleep or a reduced quality of sleep, they are possibly harboring an illusion potentially dangerous to their health. "It's a myth that we need less sleep as we grow older," reports the 1992 Johns Hopkins Medical Handbook.

Indeed, for all people, especially the elderly, getting a good night's sleep is essential to optimal health. In 1990, C.P. Pollak and co-investigators reported in the *Journal of Community Health* that in their study of some 1,855 elderly people, insomnia was a greater hazard and led to far greater mortality than risks associated with age, daily living problems, other areas of poor health, and low income. A five-year epidemiologic study on the use of conventional hypnotic drugs and mortality in more than 1,000 elderly people found a significant increase in mortality among individuals using some form of hypnotic medication for sleep but not for those taking the same kind of drugs for other reasons, note R. Rumble and K. Morgan in a 1992 report in the *Journal of the American Geriatric Society*.

Diet

It is interesting to note that sleep disorders are frequently associated with gastrointestinal conditions. Thus, by enhancing your gastrointestinal health, you will also be supporting healthful sleep. Follow the diet prescribed in Chapters 9 to 11 diligently for three to six months. After symptoms are completely gone for at least three months, you may gradually add foods from the "Neutral" or "Dangerous" categories, if you desire.

Therapeutic Foods

These therapeutic foods will help you get well. Appendix A lists sources where you can obtain these foods.

- *Cultured goat's milk dairy products:* Consume 8 to 32 ounces of the highest quality cultured dairy products from goat's milk. I recommend a 30 hour fermented yogurt called Probiogurt (see resource section). Try to find yogurt that does not contain the organism *Streptococcus thermophilus*, a bacterial microbe that has been known to make immune-system disorders worse.
- *Grass-fed red meat:* Red meat from grass-fed cattle, buffalo, and lamb is very healthy and can be eaten a few times per week. This meat is a great source of protein, minerals, vitamin B_{12}, vitamins A and D, omega-3 fats, and CLA.
- *Omega-3 eggs:* Consume as many as two eggs high in omega-3 fatty acids each day. These eggs contain DHA, vitamins E and B_{12}, and antioxidants including lutein.
- *Extra virgin coconut oil:* This oil is perhaps the healthiest of the widely available oils. I recommend cooking almost exclusively with extra virgin coconut oil. Consume as much as two to four tablespoons per day of the oil in cooking, smoothies, or right off the spoon. It contains large amounts of lauric acid, a potent antimicrobial and one of the chief fatty acids in breast milk.
- *Ocean-caught fish:* This type of fish is perhaps the healthiest of all protein sources. Salmon, sardines, mackerel, herring and albacore tuna are high in the omega-3 fatty acids EPA and DHA. Ocean-caught fish can be consumed every day to enhance digestive and immune system health.
- *Cod liver oil:* Take one to three teaspoons of Olde World Icelandic Cod Liver Oil each day. The amount consumed should be based upon the amount of sunlight you receive. People in colder climates gener-

ally need to consume larger amounts. Cod liver oil is a fantastic source of the omega-3 fats DHA and EPA, as well as vitamins A and D.

- *Vegetable juice:* Consume vegetable juices that are low in carbohydrates, such as celery and green juices mixed with a small amount of higher carbohydrate veggies such as carrot or beet. Mix in some form of healthy fat with each glass of the juice. One to three teaspoons of cultured goat's milk, extra virgin coconut oil, canned or fresh coconut milk and cream, or flaxseed oil enhances absorption of minerals and prevents spikes in blood sugar.
- *Fermented vegetables:* Consume a few tablespoons of fermented vegetables such as sauerkraut with each meal to aid in digestion. Fermented vegetables are an excellent source of naturally occurring probiotics and enzymes.
- *Stocks:* It is a great idea to consume stocks on a regular basis, especially when you have a cold or flu. Stocks made from the bones of chicken, fish, lamb and beef contain minerals, gelatin, cartilage, collagen, and electrolytes from the vegetables. Stocks are an excellent source of proteins, especially collagen. They help to heal the gut lining and reduce inflammation.

Supplements

Take these health supplements to alleviate symptoms and get well. Appendix B explains where to obtain these supplements.

- *RM-10:* Consume three caplets of RM-10 three times per day on an empty stomach for 10 days (for a total of nine caplets daily), followed by five caplets per day for 80 days. Once symptoms are gone, consume two to four caplets daily for maintenance.
- *Omega-Zyme:* Take one to three caplets with each meal or snack.
- *Perfect Food:* Take two tablespoons once or twice daily with eight ounces water or fresh vegetable juice.
- *Springs of Life:* Consume at least eight, eight-ounce glasses per day of purified water mixed with 12 drops of Springs of Life living water concentrate.
- *Super Seed:* Consume one serving twice per day, morning and evening, with eight ounces purified water.
- *Goatein:* The only protein powder on the market made from organically produced goat's milk. This protein powder is partially pre-digested, low temperature dried and is usually well tolerated by those with food allergies and digestive problems. Take one to four tablespoons per day mixed in water, juice, smoothies, yogurt or can be used in baking.

Additional Therapies

For people who have or may have imbalanced intestinal flora, avoiding contact with chlorinated water is of the utmost importance. That includes bathing water and drinking water. Chlorine kills bacteria, friendly and unfriendly, in the intestines. It can be absorbed through the skin. I recommend installing a shower filter to remove chlorine (see Appendix C). Avoid swimming in chlorinated water as well.

Relaxation therapy can be extraordinarily helpful. Some insomniacs are unable to recognize that they are insensitive to the internal state of their body. They are unable to realize they are tense, even though their fingers may be drumming the table and their feet may be tapping nervously. Learning relaxation skills helps most patients with insomnia to sleep better. Techniques used to teach relaxation skills include abdominal breathing and progressive muscle relaxation (tensing and then relaxing individual muscle groups).

Other ways to induce sleep include exercise in the late afternoon or early evening or eating a light bedtime snack consisting of a food high in the amino acid tryptophan and calcium (e.g., goat's milk yogurt, cream, or soft cheese).

Restoring the health of the gut and immune system has an amazing balancing effect on the body. This restored level of balance usually brings about improved sleeping patterns, even in those with insomnia. There is little or no evidence that people eating a more primitive diet suffered from sleeping disorders. Therefore adopting the age-old principles of primitive health can go a long way towards reversing sleeping disorders.

SPORTS INJURIES...see *Inflammatory Conditions*

STRESS

Overview

Stress can be a killer. It's a medical fact. Neuropsychologist Kenneth R. Pelletier, of the University of California School of Medicine, notes that stress-related psychological and physiological disorders have become the number one social and health problem in America over the last decade. He goes on to point out that stress-induced disorders have long since replaced epidemics of infectious disease as the major medical problem of the modern era.[88]

Look at your friends. The stressed ones—the ones who are always rushed and under the gun—are the ones who always seem to be at greater risk for high blood pressure, insomnia, migraines, impotency, asthma, hay fever, arthritis, ulcers, alcoholism, and drug addiction.

Stress is a killer. The belief that stress, depression and hopelessness contribute to susceptibility to disease dates to 200 A.D. when Galen, the Greek physician, commented that cancer seems to afflict melancholy women more frequently than the happy.[89] Yet, for most people, these influences on cancer susceptibility are generally unappreciated.[90]

There is substantial evidence of a relation between the mind and survival in breast cancer patients.[91] A number of studies have found that passive, emotionally suppressed breast cancer patients have worse prognoses.[92,93] In 1995, the *British Medical Journal* reported that the risk of breast cancer was increased by as much as fourfold following severely stressful events in the preceding five years.[94] Others have emphasized the mind's role in relation to the susceptibility to cancer and to survival from cancer. "Mounting evidence suggests that active expression of emotions is related to cancer incidence and prognosis....

Research suggests that people's response to challenge may affect whether and how they develop cancer."[95]

Heart disease, another major killer of men and women, has been shown to have a strong link to stress and depression. Studies such as those of psychologist John Barefoot, of the Duke University Medical Center, have conclusively proven that depression plays a role in the development of heart disease. In the Barefoot study, which began in 1964, those people with the highest scores for despair, low self-esteem, difficulties concentrating and low motivation had a 70 percent higher risk of suffering a heart attack and 60 percent higher risk of death overall compared to men and women with low scores.

Feeling stressed has real implications for health, causing increased heart rate, constricted blood vessels, and high blood pressure. Ominously, those who took part in the Barefoot study were, for the most part, suffering from what is known as subclinical depression, which is often precipitated by prolonged chronic, low-level stress which at first seems acceptable but over time becomes cumulatively devastating to health.

This is the type of stress that most of us go through. Unfortunately, prolonged stress, when we feel helpless to change, turns into depression and also anger. In other words, stress brews all of the dark, dangerous emotions and attitudes, and hopelessness. It's a dangerous matrix of emotions with outside triggers. It becomes a trap due to *conditioning* when we are unable to break dangerous behavioral and thought patterns.

These signals of desperation are not taken seriously by patients themselves or their doctors and they are usually not treated comprehensively with a program for turning on the body's own healing powers. The irony is that this type of "subclinical" stress is the kind we all need to beat, and the kind that outsmarts too many people. What's more, patients are treated for stress frequently with tranquilizing and other symptom-masking drugs. This doesn't promote healing or insight into the condition.

Steps for Stress

There may be many reasons for feeling helpless. Yet, trying to avoid constant suppression of aggression is important.[96] Dealing with problems directly by voicing concerns and taking constructive action is essential to dealing effectively with stress. Feeling free to ask questions, voice concerns, and question authority are examples of active responses.

Being able to see the larger picture and the orderly beauty of Nature is calming and relaxing. For both sexes, they need a way to work out their problems while alone and yet not lonely. This can come from walks in Nature or a regular program of exercise. By getting your mind off your problems on a conscious level, it has a chance to go to work on those problems unconsciously and get you the answer you need, but you must be willing to *let go* to accomplish this.

Exercise is important.

Exercise may be as formal as a running track or it may be as spontaneous as gardening and walking a country road.

It is important that we discard this sense of time urgency that makes life so stressful. When we are operating with time urgency we never get to know what we really need deep within and this can contribute to prolonged stress.

The Fighting or Warrior Spirit

Develop a warrior or fighting spirit. A warrior or fighting spirit is based on confidence that positive steps can be taken in response to any stressful situation. Fighting spirit is also based on a sense of hope for the future. It is the opposite of helplessness and hopelessness.

All sorts of self-enhancing projects can help people to fight off stress. If you love gardening, set aside time each day to do so. Don't deny yourself. If you love playing guitar, play the guitar everyday. If you love playing with your grandchildren or children, play with them. Get involved in these types of self-enhancing projects. Everyone has **something** that they love doing. It might be riding horses.

It's important to exercise daily. It's a great stress reliever and helps people to lose weight by readjusting their metabolism naturally. Studies have shown that people who exercise tend to eat healthier. Their bodies don't seem to crave the same amount of sugar as do bodies of people who are sedentary. They end up eating fruits, vegetables, high quality proteins, fats and high-fiber foods with copious amounts of liquid, especially filtered water, because that is what their bodies crave. Exercise is the best defense against stress. It seems to tune up all aspects of health function and even makes the body more resistant to environmental carcinogens and other toxins.

Stress Triggers

To deal effectively with stress, conduct a personal appraisal of your own stress triggers. It is also important to recognize that stress triggers are often overlapping, fueling each other. Financial difficulties can create relationship difficulties. Illness can become financially devastating and test any relationship. Experts have found five areas that seem to produce the greatest stress.

Physical—Air, noise, and light pollution can create extreme stress, turning homes and workplaces into pressure chambers. Overcrowding in urban living situations also creates stress. Loss of health is a catalyst for many other stresses, particularly financial, relationship, and job.

Job-related—Deadline pressures on the job, the constant sense of competition in work, an individual's poor relationship with a difficult boss, and not working at a job that is meaningful or enjoyable are all major stresses. When we lose our major job, major stresses occur. University of Michigan researcher Sidney Cobb studied one hundred auto paint factory workers starting from six weeks before their jobs were to be terminated, following them for two years. Incidence of hypertension, peptic ulcers, arthritis, and psychosomatic disorders all increased. Moreover, three wives were hospitalized with rare peptic ulcers.

Financial—Money difficulties are a prime cause of divorce, domestic violence, and worry.

Relationship—A difficult time with a relative, mate, child, or friend can create unyielding stress. A death in the family or loss of a relationship can also be stressful.

Social change—Marriage, pregnancy, job changes or moving can also become excessively stressful if focused into too short of a period. One of the first modern scientists to document the stress of social change was Adolph Meyer, a professor of psychiatry at Johns Hopkins University. By keeping "life charts," he found that illnesses tended to occur at times when clusters of major events occurred in people's lives within a fairly short period of time.

Diet

To avoid and reverse the damaging effects of stress on the body it is best to consume mainly foods from the "Super" and "Healthy" categories.

Therapeutic Foods

These therapeutic foods will help you get well. Appendix A lists sources where you can obtain these foods.

- *Cultured goat's milk dairy products:* Consume 8 to 32 ounces of the highest quality cultured dairy products from goat's milk. I recommend a 30 hour fermented yogurt called Probiogurt (see resource section). Try to find yogurt that does not contain the organism *Streptococcus thermophilus*, a bacterial microbe that has been known to make immune-system disorders worse.
- *Grass-fed red meat:* Red meat from grass-fed cattle, buffalo, and lamb is very healthy and can be eaten a few times per week. This meat is a great source of protein, minerals, vitamin B_{12}, vitamins A and D, omega-3 fats, and CLA.
- *Omega-3 eggs:* Consume as many as two eggs high in omega-3 fatty acids each day. These eggs contain DHA, vitamins E and B_{12}, and antioxidants including lutein.
- *Extra virgin coconut oil:* This oil is perhaps the healthiest of the widely available oils. I recommend cooking almost exclusively with extra virgin coconut oil. Consume as much as two to four tablespoons per day of the oil in cooking, smoothies, or right off the spoon. It contains large amounts of lauric acid, a potent antimicrobial and one of the chief fatty acids in breast milk.
- *Ocean-caught fish:* This type of fish is perhaps the healthiest of all protein sources. Salmon, sardines, mackerel, herring and albacore tuna are high in the omega-3 fatty acids EPA and DHA. Ocean-caught fish can be consumed every day to enhance digestive and immune system health.
- *Cod liver oil:* Take one to three teaspoons of Olde World Icelandic Cod Liver Oil each day. The amount consumed should be based upon the amount of sunlight you receive. People in colder climates generally need to consume larger amounts. Cod liver oil is a fantastic source of the omega-3 fats DHA and EPA, as well as vitamins A and D.
- *Vegetable juice:* Consume vegetable juices that are low in carbohydrates, such as celery and green juices mixed with a small amount of higher carbohydrate veggies such as carrot or beet. Mix in some form of healthy fat with each glass of the juice. One to three teaspoons of cultured goat's milk, extra virgin coconut oil, canned or fresh coconut milk and cream, or flaxseed oil enhances absorption of minerals and prevents spikes in blood sugar.
- *Fermented vegetables:* Consume a few tablespoons of fermented vegetables such as sauerkraut with each meal to aid in digestion. Fermented vegetables are an excellent source of naturally occurring probiotics and enzymes.

- **Stocks:** It is a great idea to consume stocks on a regular basis, especially when you have a cold or flu. Stocks made from the bones of chicken, fish, lamb and beef contain minerals, gelatin, cartilage, collagen, and electrolytes from the vegetables. Stocks are an excellent source of proteins, especially collagen. They help to heal the gut lining and reduce inflammation.

Supplements

Take these health supplements to alleviate symptoms and get well. Appendix B explains where to obtain these supplements.

- **Clear Energy:** Take six caplets of this stress-fighting formula daily with meals for 100 days. After the 100-day initial program, you may reduce the dosage to three caplets per day with meals.
- **Primal Defense:** Start with one caplet per day on an empty stomach, 30 minutes before or one hour after meals. Increase usage by adding one additional caplet per day (i.e., one caplet the first day, two the second day, three the third day and so on). Once your dosage is up to 12 caplets per day, stay on that amount for a minimum of three months and then begin to gradually decrease to a maintenance dosage of between three to six caplets per day. Primal Defense is best taken first thing in the morning and right before bedtime with eight ounces pure water. Primal Defense may be taken with other nutritional supplements, but should be taken one hour apart from medications. If you experience symptoms of detoxification (i.e., increased elimination, loose stools, constipation, excess gas, flu-like symptoms or fever), reduce the dosage and work up slowly to 12 per day.
- **Omega-Zyme:** Take one to three caplets with each meal or snack.
- **Perfect Food:** Take one to two tablespoons twice daily with eight ounces water or fresh vegetable juice.
- **Springs of Life:** Consume at least eight, eight-ounce glasses per day of purified water mixed with 12 drops of Springs of Life living water concentrate.
- **Super Seed:** Consume one serving twice per day, morning and evening, with eight ounces purified water.
- **Goatein:** The only protein powder on the market made from organically produced goat's milk. This protein powder is partially pre-digested, low temperature dried and is usually well tolerated by those with food allergies and digestive problems. Take one to four tablespoons per day mixed in water, juice, smoothies, yogurt or can be used in baking.

Additional Therapies

Stress levels will benefit from healthy intestinal flora. For people who have or may have imbalanced intestinal flora, avoiding contact with chlorinated water is of the utmost importance. That includes bathing water and drinking water. Chlorine kills bacteria, friendly and unfriendly, in the intestines. It can be absorbed through the skin. I recommend installing a shower filter to remove chlorine (see Appendix C). Avoid swimming in chlorinated water as well.

SYNDROME X...see *Blood Sugar Imbalances*
TRIGLYCERIDES (ELEVATED)...see *Cardiovascular Health*
ULCERATIVE COLITIS...see *Chronic Digestive Disease*
ULCERS...see *Chronic Digestive Disease*

UPPER RESPIRATORY HEALTH
- Asthma
- Seasonal Allergies
- Sinusitis

Overview

Asthma

Asthma is the leading chronic illness of childhood, is responsible for substantial infant morbidity, and has a significant impact on use of health resources, say researchers from the Department of Pediatrics, University of Washington, and the Center for Health Studies, Group Health Cooperative, Seattle.[97]

Other researchers note that asthma prevalence in children has increased 58 percent since 1980 and that mortality has increased by 78 percent.[98] Interestingly, the burden of the disease is most acute in urban areas and among racial and ethnic minority populations; hospitalization and morbidity rates for nonwhites are more than twice those for whites.

Although studies illustrating causal effects between outdoor air pollution and asthma prevalence are scant, air pollution appears to significantly worsen symptoms among children already with the disease. Decreased lung function, bronchial inflammation and other asthma symptoms such as recurrent wheezing, breathlessness, chest tightness and coughing have been associated with exposure to particulates, ozone, smoke, sulfur dioxide, and nitric oxide.

Research in the past decade has revealed the importance of inflammation of the airways in asthma and successful clinical therapies aimed at reducing chronic inflammation. Asthma is associated with the body's production of pro-inflammatory fatty compounds called leukotrienes, secreted by the immune system's white blood cells (leukocytes) as a reaction to common environmental allergens and pollutants including house dust mites, animal dander, cockroaches, fungal spores, pollens, and industrial airborne contaminants.

Ordinarily, white blood cells defend the body against infecting organisms and foreign agents, both in the tissues and in the bloodstream itself. But in persons with asthma, the white blood cells tend to produce excess amounts of pro-inflammatory leukotrienes.

One way to counter the body's excess production of leukotrienes is to enhance intake of omega-3 fatty acids. The omega-3 fatty acids cause the body to produce more of the less inflammatory 5-series leukotrienes. This shift is directly related to relief from asthma symptoms, notes an expert.[99]

Seafood is a rich source of omega-3 fatty acids, and it has been shown that children who eat fish more than once a week have only one-third the risk of asthma compared with children who do not eat fish regularly.[100] However, it is sometimes difficult to convince children to consume those seafood dishes highest in omega-3 fatty acids (e.g., salmon and mackerel). Flaxseed oil, also a rich source of omega-3 fatty acids on the other hand, can be blended into tasty smoothies, yogurt or veggie juice.

Please also keep in mind children need to get "dirty," that they need to be exposed to the germs and microbes naturally present in the soil and brought home by older brothers or sisters or friends. These incidental exposures help to educate the immune system and enable it to mature so that it doesn't over-react to every little antigen or allergen present in the environment. Your child will not benefit from being kept in an overly sterile environment; rather, such seclusion could well lead to imbalances in the immune system's Th1/Th2 cells (see Chapter 3). So forgo the excess use of sterilants around the home as well.

Allergies (Seasonal)

The same principles detailed above for asthma apply to seasonal allergies. See also homeostatic soil organisms (Chapter 3).

Sinusitis

Closely related in occurrence to bronchitis, chronic tracheobronchial inflammations are often found concomitantly with chronic sinusitis. Sinusitis usually develops by continuous spreading of rhinitis, but may also arise following injury. Local factors such as conchal hyperplasia, septal deviation and nasal polyps may be contributory.

Increasing exposure to environmental pollutants as well as the ever more frequent prevalence of congenital IgA deficiency are thought to be responsible for the growing incidence of chronic inflammations of the nasal sinuses.

Chronic sinusitis is difficult to treat. Today, operative therapy with curettage of the mucosa is often considered inadequate, as it is generally limited to correction of the airway blockage and, if necessary, fenestration of the respective sinus. Medical therapy includes the prescription of secretolytics and locally applied decongestants. Furthermore, a number of antibiotics are available, although they rarely attain effective concentrations in the mucosa or bone of the nasal sinuses.

Healing of the chronic inflammation is seldom possible with the usual conservative measures. Surgical irritation with instillation of antibiotics and corticosteroids entails the risk of sensitization of the mucous membranes. Corticosteroids additionally interfere with the defensive mechanisms which are already somewhat impaired.

The goal, once again, is to support the normal inflammatory process and the natural eliminative functions while stimulating the immune system. With this in mind, natural strategies to moderate inflammatory reactions within the body are quite helpful.

Diet

Follow the diet prescribed in Chapters 9 to 11 diligently for 6 to 12 months. After symptoms are completely gone for at least three months, you may gradually add foods from the "Neutral" or

"Dangerous" categories, if you desire. Because people with upper respiratory disorders appear to have a predisposed weakness in their intestinal tracts, I strongly recommend that they adhere to a diet of foods in the "Super" and "Healthy" categories for the rest of their lives.

Therapeutic Foods

These therapeutic foods will help you get well. Appendix A lists sources where you can obtain these foods.

- *Cultured goat's milk dairy products:* Consume 8 to 32 ounces of the highest quality cultured dairy products from goat's milk. I recommend a 30 hour fermented yogurt called Probiogurt (see resource section). Try to find yogurt that does not contain the organism *Streptococcus thermophilus*, a bacterial microbe that has been known to make immune-system disorders worse.
- *Grass-fed red meat:* Red meat from grass-fed cattle, buffalo, and lamb is very healthy and can be eaten a few times per week. This meat is a great source of protein, minerals, vitamin B_{12}, vitamins A and D, omega-3 fats, and CLA.
- *Omega-3 eggs:* Consume as many as two eggs high in omega-3 fatty acids each day. These eggs contain DHA, vitamins E and B_{12}, and antioxidants including lutein.
- *Extra virgin coconut oil:* This oil is perhaps the healthiest of the widely available oils. I recommend cooking almost exclusively with extra virgin coconut oil. Consume as much as two to four tablespoons per day of the oil in cooking, smoothies, or right off the spoon. It contains large amounts of lauric acid, a potent antimicrobial and one of the chief fatty acids in breast milk.
- *Ocean-caught fish:* This type of fish is perhaps the healthiest of all protein sources. Salmon, sardines, mackerel, herring and albacore tuna are high in the omega-3 fatty acids EPA and DHA. Ocean-caught fish can be consumed every day to enhance digestive and immune system health.
- *Cod liver oil:* Take one to three teaspoons of Olde World Icelandic Cod Liver Oil each day. The amount consumed should be based upon the amount of sunlight you receive. People in colder climates generally need to consume larger amounts. Cod liver oil is a fantastic source of the omega-3 fats DHA and EPA, as well as vitamins A and D.
- *Vegetable juice:* Consume vegetable juices that are low in carbohydrates, such as celery and green juices mixed with a small amount of higher carbohydrate veggies such as carrot or beet. Mix in some form of healthy fat with each glass of the juice. One to three teaspoons of cultured goat's milk, extra virgin coconut oil, canned or fresh coconut milk and cream, or flaxseed oil enhances absorption of minerals and prevents spikes in blood sugar.
- *Fermented vegetables:* Consume a few tablespoons of fermented vegetables such as sauerkraut with each meal to aid in digestion. Fermented vegetables are an excellent source of naturally occurring probiotics and enzymes.
- *Stocks:* It is a great idea to consume stocks on a regular basis, especially when you have a cold or flu. Stocks made from the bones of chicken, fish, lamb and beef contain minerals, gelatin, cartilage, col-

lagen, and electrolytes from the vegetables. Stocks are an excellent source of proteins, especially collagen. They help to heal the gut lining and reduce inflammation.

Supplements

Take these health supplements to alleviate symptoms and get well. Appendix B explains where to obtain these supplements.

- *Primal Defense:* Start with one caplet per day on an empty stomach, 30 minutes before or one hour after meals. Increase usage by adding one additional caplet per day (i.e., one caplet the first day, two the second day, three the third day and so on). Once your dosage is up to 12 caplets per day, stay on that amount for a minimum of three months and then begin to gradually decrease to a maintenance dosage of between three to six caplets per day. Primal Defense is best taken first thing in the morning and right before bedtime with eight ounces pure water. Primal Defense may be taken with other nutritional supplements, but should be taken one hour apart from medications. If you experience symptoms of detoxification (i.e., increased elimination, loose stools, constipation, excess gas, flu-like symptoms or fever), reduce the dosage and work up slowly to 12 per day.
- *Omega-Zyme:* Take one to three caplets with each meal or snack.
- *RM-10:* Take nine caplets per day of RM-10 in three divided doses for 30 to 120 days on an empty stomach. Thereafter consume a maintenance dosage of two to five caplets per day.
- *FYI:* Take four caplets three times per day on an empty stomach for 30 days followed by six caplets per day for three to six months, and then reduce to a maintenance level of three caplets per day. If a relapse or "flare-up" occurs, take 12 caplets per day for at least one week or until symptoms are under control.
- *Perfect Food:* Take one to two tablespoons twice daily with eight ounces water or fresh vegetable juice.
- *Springs of Life:* Consume at least eight, eight-ounce glasses per day of purified water mixed with 12 drops of Springs of Life living water concentrate.
- *Super Seed:* Consume one serving twice per day, morning and evening, with eight ounces purified water.
- *Goatein:* The only protein powder on the market made from organically produced goat's milk. This protein powder is partially pre-digested, low temperature dried and is usually well tolerated by those with food allergies and digestive problems. Take one to four tablespoons per day mixed in water, juice, smoothies, yogurt or can be used in baking.

Additional Therapies

For people who have or may have imbalanced intestinal flora, avoiding contact with chlorinated water is of the utmost importance. That includes bathing water and drinking water. Chlorine kills bacteria, friendly and unfriendly, in the intestines. It can be absorbed through the skin. I recommend installing a shower filter to remove chlorine (see Appendix C). Avoid swimming in chlorinated water as well.

URINARY TRACT INFECTIONS

Overview

A urinary tract infection (UTI) is an infection anywhere in the urinary tract. Your urinary tract includes the organs that collect and store urine and release it from your body. They are the kidneys, ureters, bladder, and urethra.

Usually, a UTI (also known as cystitis) is caused by bacteria that can also live in the digestive tract, in the vagina, or around the urethra, which is at the entrance to the urinary tract. Most often these bacteria enter the urethra and travel to the bladder and kidneys. Usually, your body removes the bacteria, and you have no symptoms. However, some people seem to be prone to infection, including women and older people. People with UTIs as well as cystitis have improved greatly by following the diet, supplement and lifestyle program outlined in this book.

Diet

Follow the diet prescribed in Chapters 9 to 11 diligently for 6 to 12 months. After symptoms are completely gone for at least three months, you may gradually add foods from the "Neutral" or "Dangerous" categories, if you desire. Because people with recurrent bladder infections appear to have a predisposed weakness in their urinary tracts, we strongly recommend that they adhere to a diet of foods in the "Super" and "Healthy" categories for the rest of their lives. Please note that maintaining a healthy gastrointestinal flora is critical to reducing your risk of UTIs and their recurrence.

Therapeutic Foods

These therapeutic foods will help you get well. Appendix A lists sources where you can obtain these foods.

- *Cultured goat's milk dairy products:* Consume 8 to 32 ounces of the highest quality cultured dairy products from goat's milk. I recommend a 30 hour fermented yogurt called Probiogurt (see resource section). Try to find yogurt that does not contain the organism Streptococcus thermophilus, a bacterial microbe that has been known to make immune-system disorders worse.
- *Grass-fed red meat:* Red meat from grass-fed cattle, buffalo, and lamb is very healthy and can be eaten a few times per week. This meat is a great source of protein, minerals, vitamin B_{12}, vitamins A and D, omega-3 fats, and CLA.
- *Omega-3 eggs:* Consume as many as two eggs high in omega-3 fatty acids each day. These eggs contain DHA, vitamins E and B_{12}, and antioxidants including lutein.
- *Extra virgin coconut oil:* This oil is perhaps the healthiest of the widely available oils. I recommend cooking almost exclusively with extra virgin coconut oil. Consume as much as two to four tablespoons per day of the oil in cooking, smoothies, or right off the spoon. It contains large amounts of lauric acid, a potent antimicrobial and one of the chief fatty acids in breast milk.
- *Ocean-caught fish:* This type of fish is perhaps the healthiest of all protein sources. Salmon, sardines, mackerel, herring and albacore tuna are high in the omega-3 fatty acids EPA and DHA. Ocean-caught

fish can be consumed every day to enhance digestive and immune system health.

- *Cod liver oil:* Take one to three teaspoons of Olde World Icelandic Cod Liver Oil each day. The amount consumed should be based upon the amount of sunlight you receive. People in colder climates generally need to consume larger amounts. Cod liver oil is a fantastic source of the omega-3 fats DHA and EPA, as well as vitamins A and D.
- *Vegetable juice:* Consume vegetable juices that are low in carbohydrates, such as celery and green juices mixed with a small amount of higher carbohydrate veggies such as carrot or beet. Mix in some form of healthy fat with each glass of the juice. One to three teaspoons of cultured goat's milk, extra virgin coconut oil, canned or fresh coconut milk and cream, or flaxseed oil enhances absorption of minerals and prevents spikes in blood sugar.
- *Fermented vegetables:* Consume a few tablespoons of fermented vegetables such as sauerkraut with each meal to aid in digestion. Fermented vegetables are an excellent source of naturally occurring probiotics and enzymes.
- *Berries:* Berries, especially blueberries and cranberries, are extremely important for those suffering from recurrent bladder infections as they are able to inhibit bacteria from sticking to the wall of the bladder. These berries are some of the best sources of antioxidants found in any foods.
- *Stocks:* It is a great idea to consume stocks on a regular basis, especially when you have a cold or flu. Stocks made from the bones of chicken, fish, lamb and beef contain minerals, gelatin, cartilage, collagen, and electrolytes from the vegetables. Stocks are an excellent source of proteins, especially collagen. They help to heal the gut lining and reduce inflammation.

Supplements

Take these health supplements to alleviate symptoms and get well. Appendix B explains where to obtain these supplements.

- *Primal Defense:* Start with one caplet per day on an empty stomach, 30 minutes before or one hour after meals. Increase usage by adding one additional caplet per day (i.e., one caplet the first day, two the second day, three the third day and so on). Once your dosage is up to 12 caplets per day, stay on that amount for a minimum of three months and then begin to gradually decrease to a maintenance dosage of between three to six caplets per day. Primal Defense is best taken first thing in the morning and right before bedtime with eight ounces pure water. Primal Defense may be taken with other nutritional supplements, but should be taken one hour apart from medications. If you experience symptoms of detoxification (i.e., increased elimination, loose stools, constipation, excess gas, flu-like symptoms or fever), reduce the dosage and work up slowly to 12 per day.
- *Omega-Zyme:* Take one to three caplets with each meal or snack.
- *FYI:* Take four caplets three times per day on an empty stomach for one to four weeks, followed by six caplets per day for three to six months, and then reduce to a maintenance level of three caplets per day. If a relapse or "flare-up" occurs, take 12 caplets per day for at least one week or until symptoms are under control.

- *Perfect Food:* Take one to two tablespoons twice daily with eight ounces water or fresh vegetable juice.
- *Springs of Life:* Consume at least eight, eight-ounce glasses per day of purified water mixed with 12 drops of Springs of Life living water concentrate.
- *Super Seed:* Consume one serving twice per day, morning and evening, with eight ounces purified water.
- *Goatein:* The only protein powder on the market made from organically produced goat's milk. This protein powder is partially pre-digested, low temperature dried and is usually well tolerated by those with food allergies and digestive problems. Take one to four tablespoons per day mixed in water, juice, smoothies, yogurt or can be used in baking.

Additional Therapies

For people who have or may have imbalanced intestinal flora, avoiding contact with chlorinated water is of the utmost importance. That includes bathing water and drinking water. Chlorine kills bacteria, friendly and unfriendly, in the intestines. It can be absorbed through the skin. I recommend installing a shower filter to remove chlorine (see Appendix C). Avoid swimming in chlorinated water as well.

Changing some of your daily habits may help you avoid UTIs.

- Drink lots of fluid to flush the bacteria from your system. Water is best. Try for six to eight glasses a day.
- Urinate frequently and go when you first feel the urge. Bacteria can grow when urine stays too long in the bladder.
- Urinate shortly after sex. This can flush away bacteria that might have entered your urethra during sex.
- After using the toilet, always wipe from front to back, especially after a bowel movement.
- Wear cotton underwear and loose-fitting clothes so that air can keep the area dry. Avoid tight-fitting jeans and nylon underwear, which trap moisture and can help bacteria grow.
- For women, using a diaphragm or spermicide for birth control can lead to UTIs by increasing bacteria growth. If you have trouble with UTIs, consider modifying your birth control method. Unlubricated condoms or spermicidal condoms increase irritation and foster bacterial symptoms. Consider switching to lubricated condoms without spermicide, or use a nonspermicidal lubricant.

UTERINE FIBROIDS...see *Female Health*
VAGINITIS...see *Female Health*
VIOLENT, IMPULSIVE BEHAVIOR...see *Mental Disorders*

VIRAL DISEASES

- Colds
- Epstein Barr Virus
- Flu
- Hepatitis
- Herpes Simplex
- Shingles

Overview

Viruses are the smallest of parasites; they are completely dependent on cells (bacterial, plant, or animal) to reproduce. Viruses are composed of an outer cover of protein and sometimes lipid, and a nucleic acid core of RNA or DNA. In many cases, this core penetrates susceptible cells and initiates the infection.

Viruses range from 0.02 to 0.3 µ; too small for light microscopy but visible using electron microscopy. Viruses can be identified by biophysical and biochemical methods. Like most other parasites, viruses stimulate host antibody production.

Several hundred different viruses infect humans. Because many have been only recently recognized, their clinical effects are not fully understood. Many viruses infect hosts without producing symptoms; nevertheless, because of their wide and sometimes universal prevalence, they create important medical and public health problems.

Viruses that primarily infect humans are spread mainly via respiratory and enteric excretions. These viruses are found worldwide, but their spread is limited by inborn resistance, prior immunizing infections or vaccines, sanitary and other public health control measures, and prophylactic antiviral drugs.

Zoonotic viruses pursue their biologic cycles chiefly in animals; humans are secondary or accidental hosts. These viruses are limited to areas and environments able to support their nonhuman natural cycles of infection (vertebrates or arthropods or both).

Some viruses have oncogenic properties. Human T-cell lymphotropic virus type 1 (a retrovirus) is associated with human leukemia and lymphoma. Epstein-Barr virus has been associated with malignancies such as nasopharyngeal carcinoma, Burkitt's lymphoma, Hodgkin's disease, and lymphomas in immunosuppressed organ transplant recipients. Kaposi's sarcoma-associated virus is associated with Kaposi's sarcoma, primary effusion lymphomas, and Castleman's disease (a lymphoproliferative disorder).

Slow viral diseases are characterized by prolonged incubations and cause some chronic degenerative diseases, including subacute sclerosing panencephalitis (measles virus), progressive rubella panencephalitis, progressive multifocal leukoencephalopathy (JC virus), and Creutzfeldt-Jakob disease (a prion disease).

Latency—a quiescent infection by a virus—permits recurrent infection despite immune responses and facilitates person-to-person spread. Herpes viruses exhibit latency.

Only a few viral diseases can be diagnosed clinically or epidemiologically (e.g., by well-known viral syndromes). Diagnosis usually requires testing. Serologic examination during acute and convalescent stages is sensitive and specific but slow; more rapid diagnosis can sometimes be made using culture, polymerase chain reaction, or viral antigen tests. Histopathology can sometimes be helpful.

Conventional medicine utilizes vaccines for active immunity against influenza, measles, mumps, poliomyelitis, rabies, rubella, hepatitis A, hepatitis B, varicella, and yellow fever. An effective adenovirus vaccine is available but is used only in high-risk groups, such as military recruits. Immunoglobulins are also available for passive immune prophylaxis.

Therapeutic or prophylactic drugs against some viruses are available: amantadine or rimantadine for influenza A; acyclovir, valacyclovir, and famciclovir for herpes simplex or varicella-zoster infections; ganciclovir, foscarnet, and cidofovir for cytomegalovirus infections; and reverse transcriptase inhibitors, protease inhibitors, and others for HIV. Currently, the use of interferon is limited to hepatitis B and C and human papillomavirus.

Exciting research has shown that two microorganisms found in the soil B. *Subtilis* and B. *Lichenformis* produce surfactants that are capable of destroying lipid-enveloped viruses such HHV-6, other members of the herpes family, and many other types of viruses. HSOs are believed to stimulate the body to produce up to 16 types of alpha-interferon, all of which are capable of reducing the viral load of the body.

Diet

Follow the diet prescribed in Chapters 9 to 11 diligently for 6 to 12 months. After symptoms are completely gone for at least three months, you may gradually add foods from the "Neutral" or "Dangerous" categories, if you desire. Because people with chronic viral diseases appear to have a predisposed weakness in their immune systems, we strongly recommend that they adhere to a diet of foods in the "Super" and "Healthy" categories for the rest of their lives.

Therapeutic Foods

These therapeutic foods will help you get well. Appendix A lists sources where you can obtain these foods.

- *Cultured goat's milk dairy products:* Consume 8 to 32 ounces of the highest quality cultured dairy products from goat's milk. I recommend a 30 hour fermented yogurt called Probiogurt (see resource section). Try to find yogurt that does not contain the organism *Streptococcus thermophilus*, a bacterial microbe that has been known to make immune-system disorders worse.
- *Grass-fed red meat:* Red meat from grass-fed cattle, buffalo, and lamb is very healthy and can be eaten a few times per week. This meat is a great source of protein, minerals, vitamin B_{12}, vitamins A and D, omega-3 fats, and CLA.
- *Omega-3 eggs:* Consume as many as two eggs high in omega-3 fatty acids each day. These eggs contain DHA, vitamins E and B_{12}, and antioxidants including lutein.
- *Extra virgin coconut oil:* This oil is perhaps the healthiest of the widely available oils. I recommend cooking almost exclusively with extra virgin coconut oil. Consume as much as two to four tablespoons per day of the oil in cooking, smoothies, or right off the spoon. It contains large amounts of lauric acid, a potent antimicrobial and one of the chief fatty acids in breast milk.
- *Ocean-caught fish:* This type of fish is perhaps the healthiest of all protein sources. Salmon, sardines, mackerel, herring and albacore tuna are high in the omega-3 fatty acids EPA and DHA. Ocean-caught fish can be consumed every day to enhance digestive and immune system health.
- *Cod liver oil:* Take one to three teaspoons of Olde World Icelandic Cod Liver Oil each day. The amount consumed should be based upon the amount of sunlight you receive. People in colder climates gener-

ally need to consume larger amounts. Cod liver oil is a fantastic source of the omega-3 fats DHA and EPA, as well as vitamins A and D.

- *Vegetable juice:* Consume vegetable juices that are low in carbohydrates, such as celery and green juices mixed with a small amount of higher carbohydrate veggies such as carrot or beet. Mix in some form of healthy fat with each glass of the juice. One to three teaspoons of cultured goat's milk, extra virgin coconut oil, canned or fresh coconut milk and cream, or flaxseed oil enhances absorption of minerals and prevents spikes in blood sugar.
- *Fermented vegetables:* Consume a few tablespoons of fermented vegetables such as sauerkraut with each meal to aid in digestion. Fermented vegetables are an excellent source of naturally occurring probiotics and enzymes.
- *Stocks:* It is a great idea to consume stocks on a regular basis, especially when you have a cold or flu. Stocks made from the bones of chicken, fish, lamb and beef contain minerals, gelatin, cartilage, collagen, and electrolytes from the vegetables. Stocks are an excellent source of proteins, especially collagen. They help to heal the gut lining and reduce inflammation.

Supplements

Take these health supplements to alleviate symptoms and get well. Appendix B explains where to obtain these supplements.

- *Primal Defense:* Start with one caplet per day on an empty stomach, 30 minutes before or one hour after meals. Increase usage by adding one additional caplet per day (i.e., one caplet the first day, two the second day, three the third day and so on). Once your dosage is up to 12 caplets per day, stay on that amount for a minimum of three months and then begin to gradually decrease to a maintenance dosage of between three to six caplets per day. Primal Defense is best taken first thing in the morning and right before bedtime with eight ounces pure water. Primal Defense may be taken with other nutritional supplements, but should be taken one hour apart from medications. If you experience symptoms of detoxification (i.e., increased elimination, loose stools, constipation, excess gas, flu-like symptoms or fever), reduce the dosage and work up slowly to 12 per day.
- *Omega-Zyme:* Take one to three caplets with each meal or snack.
- *RM-10:* Take nine caplets per day in three divided doses for 120 days on an empty stomach. Thereafter consume a maintenance dosage of two to five caplets per day.
- *FYI:* Take four caplets three times per day on an empty stomach for 30 days, followed by six caplets per day for three to six months, and then reduce to a maintenance level of three caplets per day. If a relapse or "flare-up" occurs, take 12 caplets per day for at least one week or until symptoms are under control.
- *Perfect Food:* Take one to two tablespoons twice daily with eight ounces water or fresh vegetable juice.

- *Springs of Life:* Consume at least eight, eight-ounce glasses per day of purified water mixed with 12 drops of Springs of Life living water concentrate.
- *Super Seed:* Consume one serving twice per day, morning and evening, with eight ounces purified water.
- *Goatein:* The only protein powder on the market made from organically produced goat's milk. This protein powder is partially pre-digested, low temperature dried and is usually well tolerated by those with food allergies and digestive problems. Take one to four tablespoons per day mixed in water, juice, smoothies, yogurt or can be used in baking.

Additional Therapies

For people who have or may have an imbalanced immune system, avoiding contact with chlorinated water is of the utmost importance. That includes bathing water and drinking water. Chlorine kills bacteria, friendly and unfriendly, in the intestines. It can be absorbed through the skin. I recommend installing a shower filter to remove chlorine (see Appendix C). Avoid swimming in chlorinated water as well.

WEIGHT MANAGEMENT

Overview

Health professionals define "overweight" as an excess amount of body weight that includes muscle, bone, fat, and water. Obesity specifically refers to an excess amount of body weight greater than 30 percent over one's ideal weight. Some people, such as bodybuilders or other athletes with a lot of muscle, can be overweight without being obese. Everyone needs a certain amount of body fat for stored energy, heat insulation, shock absorption, and other functions. As a rule, women have more body fat than men.

Health care providers are concerned not only with how much fat a person has, but also where the fat is located on the body. Women typically collect fat in their hips and buttocks, giving them a "pear" shape. Men usually build up fat around their bellies, giving them more of an "apple" shape. Of course some men are pear-shaped and some women become apple-shaped, especially after menopause. If you carry fat mainly around your waist, you are more likely to develop obesity-related health problems. Women with a waist measurement of more than 35 inches or men with a waist measurement of more than 40 inches have a higher health risk because of their fat distribution.

Obesity is more than a cosmetic problem; it is a health hazard. Approximately 280,000 adult deaths in the United States each year are related to obesity. Several serious medical conditions have been linked to obesity, including adult-onset diabetes, heart disease, high blood pressure, and stroke. Obesity is also linked to higher rates of certain types of cancer. Obese men are more likely than non-obese men to die from cancer of the colon, rectum, or prostate. Obese women are more likely than non-obese women to die from cancer of the gallbladder, breast, uterus, cervix, or ovaries.

Other diseases and health problems linked to obesity include:
- Gallbladder disease and gallstones.

- Liver disease.
- Osteoarthritis, a disease in which the joints deteriorate. This is possibly the result of excess weight on the joints.
- Gout, another disease affecting the joints.
- Pulmonary (breathing) problems, including sleep apnea in which a person can stop breathing for a short time during sleep.
- Reproductive problems in women, including menstrual irregularities and infertility.

Health care providers generally agree that the more obese a person is, the more likely he or she is to develop health problems.

Emotional suffering may be one of the most painful parts of obesity. American society emphasizes physical appearance and often equates attractiveness with slimness, especially for women. Such messages make overweight people feel unattractive.

By following the diet, lifestyle and supplement programs outlined in this book, people who are overweight and even obese can greatly improve their health and lose excess body fat without being deprived of essential nutrients or the foods they enjoy.

Diet

Follow the diet prescribed in Chapters 9 to 11 diligently for 6 to 12 months. People with weight problems should be careful to avoid or limit high-carbohydrate foods as well as polyunsaturated fats such as corn, soy and safflower oil. People with metabolic disorders should participate in moderate exercise. Even if you choose mostly healthy foods, you should take care not to eat an excessive amount of calories. After you have reached your ideal weight, you may gradually add foods from the "Neutral" or "Dangerous" categories, if you desire. Because people with weight problems appear to have a predisposed weakness in their metabolism, I strongly recommend that they adhere to a diet of foods in the "Super" and "Healthy" categories for the rest of their lives.

Therapeutic Foods

These therapeutic foods will help you get well. Appendix A lists sources where you can obtain these foods.
- *Cultured goat's milk dairy products:* Consume four to eight ounces per day of the highest quality cultured dairy products from goat's milk. I recommend a 30 hour fermented yogurt called Probiogurt (see resource section). Try to find yogurt that does not contain the organism *Streptococcus thermophilus*, a bacterial microbe that has been known to make immune-system disorders worse.
- *Grass-fed red meat:* Red meat from grass-fed cattle, buffalo, and lamb is very healthy and can be eaten a few times per week. This meat is a great source of protein, minerals, vitamin B_{12}, vitamins A and D, omega-3 fats, and CLA.
- *Omega-3 eggs:* Consume as many as two eggs high in omega-3 fatty acids each day. These eggs contain DHA, vitamins E and B_{12}, and antioxidants including lutein.

- *Extra virgin coconut oil:* This oil is perhaps the healthiest of the widely available oils. I recommend cooking almost exclusively with extra virgin coconut oil. Consume as much as two to three tablespoons of the oil in cooking, in smoothies, or right off the spoon. It contains large amounts of lauric acid, a potent antimicrobial and one of the chief fatty acids in breast milk and also enhances thyroid function, which aids weight loss.
- *Ocean-caught fish:* This type of fish is perhaps the healthiest of all protein sources. Salmon, sardines, mackerel, herring and albacore tuna are high in the omega-3 fatty acids EPA and DHA. Ocean-caught fish can be consumed every day to enhance digestive and immune system health.
- *Cod liver oil:* Take one teaspoon of Olde World Icelandic Cod Liver Oil each day. The amount consumed should be based upon the amount of sunlight you receive. People in colder climates generally need to consume larger amounts. Cod liver oil is a fantastic source of the omega-3 fats DHA and EPA, as well as vitamins A and D.
- *Vegetable juice:* Consume vegetable juices that are low in carbohydrates, such as celery and green juices mixed with a small amount of higher carbohydrate veggies such as carrot or beet. Mix in some form of healthy fat with each glass of the juice. One to three teaspoons of cultured goat's milk, extra virgin coconut oil, canned or fresh coconut milk and cream, or flaxseed oil enhances absorption of minerals and prevents spikes in blood sugar.
- *Fermented vegetables:* Consume a few tablespoons of fermented vegetables such as sauerkraut with each meal to aid in digestion. Fermented vegetables are an excellent source of naturally occurring probiotics and enzymes.
- *Stocks:* It is a great idea to consume stocks on a regular basis, especially when you have a cold or flu. Stocks made from the bones of chicken, fish, lamb and beef contain minerals, gelatin, cartilage, collagen, and electrolytes from the vegetables. Stocks are an excellent source of proteins, especially collagen. They help to heal the gut lining and reduce inflammation.

Supplements

Take these health supplements to alleviate symptoms and get well. Appendix B explains where to obtain these supplements.

- *Zero Gravity™:* Take two caplets 30 minutes before each meal for a total of six caplets per day until desired weight is achieved. Thereafter take one caplet 30 minutes before each meal for maintenance.
- *Perfect Food:* Take one to two tablespoons twice daily with eight ounces water or fresh vegetable juice.
- *Springs of Life:* Consume at least eight, eight-ounce glasses per day of purified water mixed with 12 drops of Springs of Life living water concentrate.
- *Super Seed:* Consume one serving twice per day, morning and evening, with eight ounces purified water.
- *Goatein:* The only protein powder on the market made from organically produced goat's milk. This protein powder is partially pre-digested, low temperature dried and is usually well tolerated by those with food allergies and digestive problems. Take one to four tablespoons per day mixed in water, juice, smoothies, yogurt or can be used in baking.

SPECIAL CLINICAL REPORT

Lose Weight, Get Healthy with The Zero Gravity Weight-management Program

Experts say weight loss programs work best with a complete approach. That means it is vitally important to adhere to a whole foods diet rich in fresh fruits and vegetables and high quality proteins and healthy fats with a significant decrease in refined carbohydrates (bread, pasta, cereal, sugar soft drinks) and processed fats (margarine, shortening, refined cooking oils). It is also important to drink a minimum of eight glasses of water each day to flush out accumulated toxins and waste material.

The Zero Gravity program from Garden of Life combines three different whole food concentrates and a liquid concentrate to aid dieters. The program offers a natural, non-addictive weight management solution that contains no stimulants that could cause potentially harmful side effects such as rapid heart rate, anxiety, insomnia, and hypertension. The Zero Gravity program is based on ancient whole foods and beverages containing naturally occurring compounds—derived from whole fruit, sea vegetable extracts and tea infusions of roots, bark and leaves—that can contribute to healthy weight loss. Along the way, participants should see improved cholesterol profiles and lowered blood pressure.

Weight-loss Benefits of Grapefruit—One of the key ingredients in Zero Gravity is grapefruit, a wonderful dietary aid when consumed both as a whole food or nutritional supplement. I recommend one to two servings a day of grapefruit when dieting. In fact, a major weight loss center that's part of a prestigious East Coast University released the results of their study incorporating grapefruit. Though one cannot say grapefruit was responsible exclusively for their weight loss, participants in the study lost an average of 19 pounds in 13 weeks. They significantly lowered their cholesterol and blood pressure.

Whole organic grapefruit concentrate—including pectin, seeds and peel—is a key ingredient in Zero Gravity. Grapefruit is one of nature's richest sources of antioxidants, bioflavonoids, enzymes, and fiber. It is high in the soluble fiber pectin, which helps lower blood cholesterol. The whole organic grapefruit concentrate in one daily serving of Zero Gravity contains the key nutrients found in two to three normally eaten grapefruits. The complete combination of pectin, seeds and peel of the whole grapefruit actively inhibits enzymes in the intestinal tract that are responsible for the conversion of carbohydrates into storable fats. This action is naturally accomplished without disturbing the uptake of necessary micronutrients such as vitamin C, potassium and folic acid. Whole grapefruit decreases the risks of heart disease by reducing high cholesterol. The pectin in grapefruit has been shown to normalize blood sugar levels and prevent sugar spikes in diabetics by reducing carbohydrates that enter the bloodstream.

Blueberry Extract Aids Blood Sugar Balance—One of the major reasons for our late afternoon bingeing is that we experience blood sugar spikes. Residents of the Caucasian region of the former Soviet Union have traditionally taken medicinal teas infused with leaves of the blueberry plant, as a self treatment for blood sugar imbalances, diabetes and hypoglycemia. Blueberry leaf extract has been shown to reduce total cholesterol as well as non-desirable low density lipoprotein levels. In fact, a 1996 study from the Institute of Pharmacological Sciences, University of Milano, Italy, notes that blueberry leaf infusions are traditionally used as a folk medicine treatment of diabetes. In their study, plasma glucose levels were consistently found to drop by about 26 percent at different stages of diabetes. Unexpectedly and pleasantly, plasma triglycerides were decreased by 39 percent.[101]

Sea Vegetables & Detoxification—When we diet, our body's adipose (fatty) tissues release fat-soluble toxins such as dioxin into the bloodstream where they can initiate harmful biochemical reactions. The brown and green seaweed extracts in Zero Gravity have been harvested from the Canary Islands near Spain. These edible seaweeds contain large quantities of fucoidan fiber to absorb fat-soluble toxins that are released into the bloodstream during weight-loss periods. This was shown in a 2002 study from the *Journal of Agricultural and Food Chemistry* where researchers report "that the administration of seaweed…is efficient in preventing the absorption and reabsorption of dioxin from the gastrointestinal tract and might be useful in treatment of humans exposed to dioxin."[102] Brown seaweed also possesses a variety of compounds such as alginates that bind with toxins and escort them from the body. In particular, brown seaweed improves thyroid function, aids in detoxification, and balances blood sugar and cholesterol levels.

Making Yourself Fat-Proof—As most dieters will tell you, fat is stubborn stuff. For individuals genetically predisposed to obesity, this fact is particularly worrisome. But findings published in the December 2000 issue of the journal *Nature Genetics* could eventually help fight obesity. The key, researchers say, may be targeting a fat-protecting protein known as perilipin.

Earlier studies had suggested that perilipin was involved in lipid maintenance and energy metabolism, notes reporter Kate Wong of *ScientificAmerican.com*. Now, thanks to research by Lawrence Chan and co-investigators at the Baylor College of Medicine, we know that perilipin-free mice have about half as much body fat, more muscle and a consistently higher metabolic rate than mice with ample amounts of perilipin—despite eating 25 percent more food and leading sedentary lives. "Furthermore, fat cells in perilipin-free mice were half as large as those in the normal mice," the reporter says. "The researchers also examined the effects of perilipin in mice genetically programmed to be obese." There again the results were dramatic: the mice lacking perilipin grew up to be lean and healthy, in contrast to those that produced the protein.

"Perilipin works by coating the surface of fat storage droplets inside fat cells, protecting them from hormone-sensitive lipase, HSL, a fat-metabolizing enzyme," Chan notes on the *ScientificAmerican.com* website. Without perilipin, HSL burns the fat right away. "These results are very exciting because not only is perilipin active in humans, it is made almost exclusively by fat cells."

In many Traditional Chinese Medicine formulas mentioned in both the *Shanghan Lun* and *Jingui Yaolue* herbal texts, magnolia bark is frequently included in remedies used for digestive system disorders, abdominal bloating and discomfort. But now we know that magnolol, one of the active phytochemical constituents in magnolia bark, contains naturally occurring perilipin inhibitors, which might be yet another key factor in weight loss. Magnolol significantly reduces lipid droplets, which act as storage for fat triglycerides in adipose tissue. Thus, the natural perilipin inhibitor magnolol contained in Zero Gravity provides an important, necessary function in healthy weight management.

Better than Chitosan or Xenical®?—The combination of two Russian herbs, long used in Europe for weight loss, can truly help you to win the war against fat. One has safe fat-blocking properties. The other helps to eliminate excess fat.

Rhododendron caucasium—Xenical®, the brand name for orlistat, is a weight-management drug that was moderately successful in clinical trials, reducing fat absorption by 30 percent. It works by inhibiting lipase enzymes in the intestine, which are necessary to break down triglycerides into fatty acids that can then be absorbed from the gut. Unlike the medical fat-binding drug, *Rhododendron caucasium* won't bind with fat or remove essential fat-soluble vitamins. Rather, this alpine tea, traditionally enjoyed by the people of the Republic of Georgia in the former Soviet Union, contains high amounts of polyphenol antioxidants that specifically inhibit the action of the lipase enzyme, thus helping to safely prevent uptake of fat. In particular, the young spring leaves of rhododendron inhibit gastrointestinal lipase. The body requires lipase to break down dietary fat into small, absorbable particles. When gastrointestinal lipase is inhibited, about 15 to 20 percent more fat is passed through the digestive tract to be excreted without removing vital fat-soluble vitamins.

Rhodiola rosea—In Zero Gravity, rhododendron is combined with another herb, known as "arctic root," or *Rhodiola rosea*. Originally grown in the harsh Russian climate, rhodiola is a hardy root whose medicinal properties function as the quintessential adaptogen. Rhodiola is a powerful anti-stress, mood- and memory-enhancing herb. Nicknamed the "ginseng alternative," *Rhodiola rosea* is said to be more effective than St. John's wort, *Ginkgo biloba* and *Panax ginseng* as an all-around phytomedicine and together the pair are great for weight loss, notes plant biochemist Dr. Zakir Ramazanov, a professor of plant biochemistry and molecular biology who has authored more than 130 scientific articles and patents in the field of biotechnology, plant biochemistry, molecular biology, and natural phytoactive nutritional products.

Rhodiola contains the phytochemical rosavin, which helps weight loss by activating adipose lipase (also known as hormone-sensitive lipase). This enzyme is responsible for regulating stored fat, the most difficult kind of fat to eliminate or reduce. By activating adipose lipase, rhodiola helps to stimulate the release of fatty acids into the bloodstream.

When both rhododendron and rhodiola are combined, the results are fantastic. In a study, women who were 30 percent overweight (average weight 165 pounds), were treated with the combination for three months. During the first six week, their weight loss was minimal—about five to six percent—but by eight weeks had reached 14 percent for a total weight loss average. Waist size was reduced by an average of 11.5 percent. (Bust size, however, was reduced only about five percent, an important consideration for women who fear that losing weight will reduce their breast size.)

When the complete Zero Gravity program is utilized, the results can be highly gratifying. Daphne, a study participant, notes that over a period of two years she put on 50 pounds and tried all kinds of diets. She was usually able to lose weight but only briefly, gaining back what she lost as well as additional pounds. With Zero Gravity, "I've lost 15 pounds in the first 12 weeks."

But, really, your first goal must be to make positive changes in your life. This should include improved eating habits and exercise. Besides their direct weight-loss benefits, the whole food supplements help you to feel great. "My goal was to lose weight steadily with good food, healthy practices, and exercises for a strong cardiovascular system," notes Jenny, another participant in the Zero Gravity weight-loss study. "It included a change in my eating habits and adding Zero Gravity and Perfect Food to my regimen. Friends are beginning to say things like 'Jenny, your skin looks wonderful—you're looking good!' But even more than my appearance is how I feel—and after losing over 20 pounds in 12 weeks, I feel great!"

Part V–
Resources

Food Sources

I have successfully used the foods listed in this appendix in clinical practice and scientific research. The foods are listed in descending order based on their effectiveness according to clinical observations. Undoubtedly, many more products than are listed here meet the criteria for being put on the list. Where possible, I have included addresses, telephone numbers, fax numbers, and website addresses to help you obtain these foods. Many of the foods listed here are available in health food stores and grocery stores. Others can only be obtained by mail order. This list is not exhaustive. Substitutes for some of these foods exist.

RED MEAT

Eat Wild
Internet: www.eatwild.com
Explains the benefits of eating meat and dairy products from grass-fed, not grain-fed, animals. On the Suppliers page, you can find out how to purchase grass-fed meat and dairy products in your area.

White Egret Farm
15704 Webberville Rd., FM 969,
Austin, TX 78724
Tel: 512/276-7408 or 512/276-7505
Fax: 512/276-7489
Internet: www.whiteegretfarm.com
Offers unprocessed natural beef and goat products and natural free-range turkeys, as well as goat's milk yogurt and goat's milk cheese.

POULTRY

White Egret Farm
15704 Webberville Rd., FM 969,
Austin, TX 78724
Tel: 512/276-7408 or 512/276-7505
Fax: 512/276-7489
Internet: www.whiteegretfarm.com
Offers free-range turkey as well as unprocessed natural beef and goat products, goat's milk, and goat's cheese. No hormones or antibiotics are used.

Eat Wild
Internet: www.eatwild.com
Go to the Suppliers page, where you can find out how to purchase free-range poultry in your area.

Oaklyn Plantation
1312 Oaklyn Rd., Darlington, SC 29532
Tel: 843/395-0793
Fax: 843/395-0794
Internet: www.freerangechicken.com
Offers free-range chickens raised without antibiotics or growth hormones.

We also recommend poultry from these producers. It is available in many grocery and health food stores.
* Wellington Farms
* Rocky Junior
* Empire Kosher Chicken

CHICKEN FEET
(For Chicken Soup Recipe)

Oaklyn Plantation
1312 Oaklyn Rd., Darlington, SC 29532
Tel: 843/395-0793
Fax: 843/395-0794
Internet: www.freerangechicken.com
Offers free-range chickens raised without antibiotics or growth hormones. Use chicken feet in broth recipes.

FISH

Barlean's Fishery
4936 Lake Terrell Rd.,
Ferndale, WA 98248
Tel: 360/384-0485
Internet: www.barleans.com
Offers ecologically wild harvested salmon, a rich source of omega-3 fatty acids.

EcoFish, Inc.
78 Market St., Portsmouth, NH 03801
Tel: 603/430-0101
Fax: 603/430-9929
Internet: www.ecofish.com
Offers ocean-caught salmon, halibut, tuna, and other fish

Avalon
201 SW Second St., Corvallis, OR 97333
Tel: 541/752-7418
Internet: www.oregongourmet.com
Offers an assortment of smoked wild northwest salmon.

We also recommend fish from these producers. These products are available in many grocery and health food stores.
* Miramonte Alaskan Pink canned salmon

* Crown Prince Brisling Sardines with skin and bones
* Crown Prince Herring

EXTRA VIRGIN COCONUT OIL™
Garden of Life
770 Northpoint Pkwy,
West Palm Beach, FL 33407
Tel: 800/622-8986
Fax: 561/575-5488
Internet: www.gardenoflifeusa.com
Offers Extra Virgin Coconut Oil™, an unheated, organically produced oil produced using traditional fermentation methods. The oil contains 52 to 55 percent lauric acid

EGGS
Gold Circle Farms
Internet: www.goldcirclefarms.com
Offers DHA Omega-3 eggs. Gold Circle Farm eggs are available from many grocery and health food stores.

Locally produced eggs from free-range chickens are also acceptable.

GOAT'S MILK YOGURT
White Egret Farm
15704 Webberville Rd., FM 969,
Austin, TX 78724
Tel: 512/276-7408 or 512/276-7505
Fax: 512/276-7489
Internet: www.whiteegretfarm.com
Offers Probiogurt, a 30-hour yogurt that contains no Streptococcus thermophilus.

Although not as therapeutic, I also recommend goat's milk yogurt from Redwood Hills Farm. This yogurt is available in some grocery and health food stores.

GOAT'S MILK BUTTER
White Egret Farm
15704 Webberville Rd., FM 969,
Austin, TX 78724
Tel: 512/276-7408 or 512/276-7505
Fax: 512/276-7489
Internet: www.whiteegretfarm.com
Offers Pure Cultured Goat's Milk Butter

Mt. Sterling Cheese Cooperative
P.O. Box 103, Sterling, WI 54645
Tel: 608/734 3151
or 866/289-4628 (toll free)
Fax: 608/734-3810
Internet: www.buygoatcheese.com
Offers goat's cheese and goat's milk butter.

I also recommend Golden Fleece goat's milk butter. It is available in some grocery and health food stores.

FERMENTED VEGETABLES
Rejuvenative Foods
(Deer Garden Foods)
P.O. Box 8464, Santa Cruz, CA 95061
Tel: 800/805-7957
Internet: www.rejuvenative.com
Offers the highest quality raw fermented vegetables, including sauerkraut and kimchi. These foods are available in some grocery and health food stores or by internet or mail orders.

NUT AND SEED BUTTERS
Rejuvenative Foods
(Deer Garden Foods)
P.O. Box 8464, Santa Cruz, CA 95061
Tel: 800/805-7957
Internet: www.rejuvenative.com
Offers the highest quality raw organic nut and seed butters, include butters made from almond, sesame, pumpkin, cashew, and sunflower seeds. These foods are available in some grocery and health food stores or by internet or mail orders.

CULINARY OILS
(Suitable for Cooking)
Garden of Life
770 Northpoint Pkwy,
West Palm Beach, FL 33407
Tel: 800/622-8986
Fax: 561/575-5488
Internet: www.gardenoflifeusa.com
Offers Extra Virgin Coconut Oil™, an unheated, organically produced oil produced using traditional fermentation methods. The oil contains 52 to 55 percent lauric acid.

Purity Farms
14635 Westcreek Rd.,
Sedalia, CO 80135
Tel: 303/647-2368
Fax: 303/647-9875
Internet: www.purityfarms.com
Offers organic ghee, the traditional Indian clarified butter.

I also recommend organic virgin olive oil made by the following producer. These products are available in many grocery and health food stores.
* Bionaturae Organic Extra Virgin Olive Oil

COCONUT PRODUCTS
Thai Kitchen
Tel: 800/967-8424
or 510/268-0209 ex. 103
Internet: www.thaikitchen.com
Offers Thai Kitchen Pure Coconut Milk, as well as other coconut milk and coconut cream products.

Garden of Life
770 Northpoint Pkwy,
West Palm Beach, FL 33407
Tel: 800/622-8986
Fax: 561/575-5488
Internet: www.gardenoflifeusa.com
Offers Extra Virgin Coconut Oil™, an unheated, organically produced oil produced using traditional fermentation methods. The oil contains 52 to 55 percent lauric acid.

BREADS AND CEREALS
Nature's Path
7453 Progress Way, Delta,
BC, Canada V4G 1E8
Tel: 604/940-0505
Internet: www.naturespath.com
Offers many fine cereals and breads, including Manna Bread. These products are available in many grocery and health food stores.

Food for Life
2991 E. Doherty St., Corona, CA 91719
Tel: 800/797-5090 or 909/279-5090
Internet: www.food-for-life.com
Offers many fine sprouted breads and cereals, including Sprouted Bread (Red Label), Ezekial 4:9 Bread, Ezekial 4:9 Cereal, and sprouted tortillas. These products are available in many grocery and health food stores.

Pacific Bakery
P.O. Box 950, Oceanside, CA 92049
Tel: 760/757-6020
Internet: www.pacificbakery.com
Offers yeast-free baked goods, including yeast-free organic whole spelt and yeast-free organic whole kamut.

Sunnyvale Bakeries
(Martin Roth & Co.)
2410 Santa Clara St.,
Richmond, CA 94804
Tel: 510/527-7066
Fax: 510/527-0178
Offers sprouted organic breads.

OMEGA-3-RICH OILS
(Not for Cooking)
Garden of Life
770 Northpoint Pkwy,
West Palm Beach, FL 33407
Tel: 800/622-8986
Fax: 561/575-5488
Internet: www.gardenoflifeusa.com
Offers Olde World Icelandic Cod Liver Oil, which has an excellent flavor.

Barlean's Organic Oils
4936 Lake Terrell Rd.,
Ferndale, WA 98248
Tel: 360/384-0485
Internet: www.barleans.com
*Offers organic high-lignan flax seed oil.
This product is available at some grocery
stores and health food stores.*

Omega Nutrition
6515 Aldrich Rd.,
Bellingham, WA 98226
Tel: 800/661-3529 or 360/384-1238
Fax: 360/384-0700
Internet: www.omeganutrition.com
*Offers organic flax oil, olive oil, and my
personal favorite, organic garlic-chili-flax oil.*

HONEY
Really Raw Honey Company
3500 Boston Street, Suite 32,
Baltimore, MD 21224
Tel: 800/732-5729 or 410/675-7233
Fax: 410/675-7411
Internet: www.ReallyRawHoney.com
*Offers the finest enzyme-rich raw honey.
This product is also available in some grocery
and health food stores.*

Farm Style Raw Apitherapy Honey
Honey Gardens Apiaries
P.O. Box 189, Hinesburg, VT 05461
Tel: 802/985-5852 or 800/416-2083
Fax: 802/985-9039
Internet: www.honeygardens.com
/contact.htm
*Offers raw honey, propolis, and other bee
products. These products are available in
some grocery stores and health food stores.*

Manuka Honey USA
88878 Highway 101 N, P.O. Box 2474,
Florence, OR 97439
Tel: 541/902-0979 or 800/395-2196
Fax: 541/902-8825
Internet: www.manukahoneyusa.com
*Offers a variety of raw honey products. These
products are available in some grocery stores and
health food stores.*

SALT/SEASONINGS
The Grain and Salt Society
273 Fairway Dr., Asheville, NC 28805
Tel: 800/867-7258
Fax: 828/299-1640
Internet: www.celtic-seasalt.com
*Offers Celtic sea salt (course and fine) and
other health food products. These products
are available in some grocery stores and
health food stores.*

Rapunzel
Internet: www.rapunzel.com
*Offers a good selection of seasonings includ-
ing herbamare, a seasoning made with sea
salt and organic herbs. You can order these
products on the Internet or look for them in
health food and grocery stores.*

RealSalt
(Redmond RealSalt)
P.O. Box 219, Redmond, UT 84652
Tel: 800/367-7258
Fax: 435/529-7486
Internet: www.realsalt.com
*RealSalt is mined in central Utah.
This product is available in grocery
and health food stores.*

APPLE CIDER VINEGAR
Bragg Apple Cider Vinegar
Bragg Live Foods
P.O. Box 7, Santa Barbara, CA 93102
Tel: 800/446-1990
*Offers an apple cider vinegar made from
organically grown apples, as well as other
natural products. This product is available in
some grocery stores and health food stores.*

SNACKS
Jennie's Macaroons
*These cookies are made with only three
ingredients: coconut, honey, and egg
whites with a high amount of lauric acid.
This product is available is some grocery
stores and health food stores.*

Govinda's Raw Power
Raw Power Food
2651 Ariane Dr., San Diego, CA 92117
Tel: 800/900-0108
Fax: 619/270-0696
*Govinda's Raw Power is a healthy snack
made from germinated seeds and dried
fruit. It is available in some grocery stores
and health food stores.*

CONDIMENTS
Westbrae Natural Foods
(Distributed by Novelco Distribution)
264 South La Cienega Blvd., Suite 1193
Beverly Hills, CA 90211
Tel: 562/948-2872
Fax: 707/202-7129
Internet:
www.novelco.com/westbrae/index.htm
*Offers natural catsup and mustard.
These products are available in some
grocery stores and health food stores.*

Spectrum Organic Products
1304 South Point Blvd., Suite 280,
Petaluma, CA 94954
Tel: 707/778-8900
Fax: 707/765-8470
Internet: www.spectrumorganic.com
*Offers a healthy, organic Omega-3
mayonnaise using expeller pressed soy and
flax seed oils. This product is available in
some grocery and health food stores.*

Recommended Supplements

The nutritional supplements in Appendix B have been successfully used in clinical practice and scientific research. This list is not exhaustive. Undoubtedly, more products than are listed here meet the criteria of this book.

The supplements listed in this appendix can be purchased at your local health food store, pharmacy, distributor of healthcare products or from complimentary and alternative healthcare practitioners.

To purchase the recommended products in Canada please contact the following distributor:

Advantage Health Matters, (800) 338-6138

www.advantagehealthmatters.com

A note about the Garden of Life formulas below. I tried over 500 nutritional supplements to no avail during my bout with Crohn's disease. After realizing that the supplements I needed to overcome my disease were not available, I decided to develop these supplements myself in collaboration with some of the top research scientists worldwide.

Garden of Life products have been used successfully by hundreds of thousands of individuals suffering from digestive ailments and immune-system disorders. Thousands of medical doctors and health practitioners have dispensed Garden of Life supplements to their patients.

IMMUNE SYSTEM ENHANCEMENT

RM-10
Garden of Life
770 Northpoint Pkwy,
West Palm Beach, FL 33407
Tel: 800/622-8986
Fax: 561/575-5488
Internet: www.gardenoflifeusa.com
I developed RM-10 to save the life of my grandmother when she had cancer (see Chapter 4). With 10 medicinal mushrooms and properly harvested cat's claw and aloe vera, all potentiated with the Poten-Zyme process, this is probably the best all around immune support formula now available.

RevivAll Classic
Garden of Life
770 Northpoint Pkwy,
West Palm Beach, FL 33407
Tel: 800/622-8986
Fax: 561/575-5488
Internet: www.gardenoflifeusa.com
RevivAll Classic is a proprietary whole food blend containing naturally occurring phytosterols/sterolins, vitamins, minerals, amino acids and enzymes. Each caplet of RevivAll Classic contains organically grown imopotea (New Guinea sweet potato), garbanzo beans, soy beans, red lentils, azuki beans*, kidney beans, brown rice, sesame seed, flaxseed, sunflower seed, pumpkin seed and phytosterol blend.

PROBIOTICS
Primal Defense
Garden of Life
770 Northpoint Pkwy,
West Palm Beach, FL 33407
Tel: 800/622-8986
Fax: 561/575-5488
Internet: www.gardenoflifeusa.com
Primal Defense with homeostatic soil organisms is the key to your overall health. It contains soil organisms as old as the Earth itself and as necessary to our well-being as proteins or fats.

Continental Liquid Acidophilus (Plain)

Continental Culture Specialists, Inc.
Internet: www.continentalyogurt.com
Continental Culture Specialists produce liquid acidophilus that I recommend as a substitute for Probiogurt and can be used in recipes to make fermented foods on your own. Continental liquid acidophilus is available at health food stores nationwide.

ANTI-INFLAMMATORY
FYI

Garden of Life
770 Northpoint Pkwy,
West Palm Beach, FL 33407
Tel: 800/622-8986
Fax: 561/575-5488
Internet: www.gardenoflifeusa.com
FYI is detailed in Chapter 5. This formula attacks inflammation in seven different ways. Inflammation, as we now know, plays an important role in heart disease, cancer, and arthritis, to name only a few conditions.

DIGESTIVE ENZYMES
Omega-Zyme

Garden of Life
770 Northpoint Pkwy,
West Palm Beach, FL 33407
Tel: 800/622-8986
Fax: 561/575-5488
Internet: www.gardenoflifeusa.com
Omega-Zyme is the most comprehensive digestive enzyme formula now available. It is essential to have with you at all times, especially when traveling if your diet strays.

FIBER
Super Seed

Garden of Life
770 Northpoint Pkwy,
West Palm Beach, FL 33407
Tel: 800/622-8986
Fax: 561/575-5488
Internet: www.gardenoflifeusa.com
Super Seed is a certified organic blend of seeds, sprouted grains and legumes. These are abundant in mucilaginous soluble fiber, essential fatty acids and lignans. Again, such concentrates provide you with super nutritional whole foods that give your body the nutrients it truly requires.

GREEN SUPER FOODS
Perfect Food

Garden of Life
770 Northpoint Pkwy,
West Palm Beach, FL 33407
Tel: 800/622-8986
Fax: 561/575-5488
Internet: www.gardenoflifeusa.com
Perfect Food is a blend of super green foods— the most effective green food blend today— that provides us with important supplemental phytonutrients from young cereal grasses, sprouts and seeds. When consumed twice daily, Perfect Food will also aid in quenching appetite and providing the body with much needed minerals. By taking Perfect Food every day you'll never have to go without your five to ten servings of veggies. Once again, we use our Poten-Zyme process to liberate all of the nutrients in these foods.

UPPER GI SUPPORT (ACID REFLUX)
Acid Defense

Garden of Life
770 Northpoint Pkwy,
West Palm Beach, FL 33407
Tel: 800/622-8986
Fax: 561/575-5488
Internet: www.gardenoflifeusa.com

ESSENTIAL FATTY ACIDS
Garden of Life

770 Northpoint Pkwy,
West Palm Beach, FL 33407
Tel: 800/622-8986
Fax: 561/575-5488
Internet: www.gardenoflifeusa.com
Offers Olde World Icelandic Cod Liver Oil, which has an excellent flavor.

ANTI-FUNGAL/ CANDIDA PRODUCTS
Fungal Defense

Garden of Life
770 Northpoint Pkwy, West Palm Beach, FL 33407
Tel: 800/622-8986
Fax: 561/575-5488
Internet: www.gardenoflifeusa.com

STRUCTURED WATER
Springs of Life

Garden of Life
770 Northpoint Pkwy,
West Palm Beach, FL 33407
Tel: 800/622-8986
Fax: 561/575-5488
Internet: www.gardenoflifeusa.com
Springs of Life is a structured water supplement to be added to your water. We want every glass of purified or filtered water that you consume to be as health giving as possible, and Springs of Life helps every glass of water to be a healthful experience, returning to your body biologically active enzymes, minerals and trace elements. It naturally energizes and transforms water, returning it to the pristine quality that indigenous people drank hundreds of years ago.

GOAT'S MILK PROTEIN POWDER
Goatein

Garden of Life
770 Northpoint Pkwy,
West Palm Beach, FL 33407
Tel: 800/622-8986
Fax: 561/575-5488
Internet: www.gardenoflifeusa.com
Goatein is the only protein powder on the market made from organically produced goat's milk. This protein powder is partially pre-digested, low temperature dried and is usually well tolerated by those with food allergies and digestive problems. Goatein is a naturally rich source of essential amino acids and glutamine.

PRE-DIGESTED PROTEIN AND COLOSTRUM SUPPLEMENT
Goatein IG

Garden of Life
770 Northpoint Pkwy,
West Palm Beach, FL 33407
Tel: 800/622-8986
Fax: 561/575-5488
Internet: www.gardenoflifeusa.com
Goatenin IG is the only goat's milk protein-colostrum formula on the market today. It is high in immunoproteins. These building blocks of proteins are crucial for proper immune system function. Because Goatenin IG is processed without excessive heat or acids, it contains biologically active cystine, glycine, and glutamic acid in tri-peptide form. The combination of these three amino acids produces glutathione. Glutathione functions as a principal antioxidant, scavenging free radicals and environmental toxins such as lipid perox-

ides that can damage and destroy healthy cells. Goatenin IG also provides immune supportive agents called immunoglobulins, including IgA, IgD, IgE, IgG, and IgM. These antibodies naturally fight off bacteria, viruses, allergens and yeast.

Immunoglobulins (found in colostrum) are able to neutralize even the most harmful bacteria, viruses, and yeasts. Goatein IG contains a virtual army of immunoproteins, including proline-rich polypeptide, which supports and regulates the thymus gland, lactoferrin, a protein that transports essential iron to the red blood cells and prevents harmful bacteria from utilizing the iron they require to grow and flourish, and lactalbumins, which research indicates may be highly effective against numerous viruses.

One of the most important ingredients in colostrum is insulinlike growth factor-1 (IGF-1), which has been studied for its ability to stimulate healing, promote muscle growth and aid in the production of immune cells. It also helps to stabilize blood sugar levels, similar to the function of insulin, in addition to increasing the body's fat-burning potential.

MEN'S HEALTH FORMULA
RevivAll Male Vitality Formula
Garden of Life
770 Northpoint Pkwy,
West Palm Beach, FL 33407
Tel: 800/622-8986
Fax: 561/575-5488
Internet: www.gardenoflifeusa.com
I developed RevivAll Male Vitality Formula to aid men with typical male health problems such as prostate enlargement and prostatitis. Especially noteworthy is our use of New Guinea sweet potato, flower pollen concentrate and phytosterols, in addition to our whole food vitality blend consisting of predigested (via Poten-Zyme fermentation) garbanzo beans, red lentils, soy beans, flaxseed, sunflower, sesame and pumpkin seed, and azuki and kidney beans, barley, and brown rice. All ingredients are organically grown.

WOMEN'S HEALTH FORMULA
RevivAll Female Vitality Formula
Garden of Life
770 Northpoint Pkwy,
West Palm Beach, FL 33407
Tel: 800/622-8986
Fax: 561/575-5488
Internet: www.gardenoflifeusa.com
For many years, most of the research on health was done on men. Not until recently have science and research realized that women exhibit markedly different health symptoms and progression of diseases. Women have quite special needs due, in large part, to their unique and complex hormonal, physiological, chemical, and structural makeup. Garden of Life formulated RevivAll Female Vitality Formula, which is designed to address the specific and unique health challenges facing women today. As women age, their estrogen and progesterone levels drop significantly. This leads to an array of uncomfortable health problems including: hormonal imbalances, arthritic and joint pain, irregular periods, fibrocystic breasts, food and environmental allergies, menopausal symptoms, decreased sex drive, hot flashes, mood swings, lack of energy, weight gain, diabetes, weakened immune system, osteoporosis, increased risk of cancer, and depression. Consuming phytonutrient-rich whole foods such as those contained in RevivAll Female Vitality Formula is a great way to maintain optimal female health throughout your lifetime.

WEIGHT MANAGEMENT FORMULA
Zero Gravity
Garden of Life
770 Northpoint Pkwy,
West Palm Beach, FL 33407
Tel: 800/622-8986
Fax: 561/575-5488
Internet: www.gardenoflifeusa.com

ENERGY FORMULA/ ANTI-STRESS
Clear Energy
Garden of Life
770 Northpoint Pkwy,
West Palm Beach, FL 33407
Tel: 800/622-8986
Fax: 561/575-5488
Internet: www.gardenoflifeusa.com
Clear Energy is a super tonic formula based on adaptogens. What is an adaptogen? The response of the body's stress system—what we might call "reactivity"— depends on adaptation—the capacity of the organism (or a cell) to protect itself from stressors. In other words, adaptogens increase the capacity of the body's stress systems to respond to external signals without incurring long-term damage. The reactivity of host defense systems is maintained and damaging effects of various stressors decreased. Herbs with such qualities are important to protecting the body from stress and delivering us from the vagaries of stress-related exhaustion. Because much of our lack of energy today is stress-related, we also see that adaptogens promote a more energetic, clearer thinking you. One such up and coming adaptogen found in Clear Energy is Rhodiola rosea. Though well known in Russia, its recognition in America is quite limited. Writing in Alternative Medicine Reviews, an expert notes Rhodiola rosea is a popular plant in traditional medical systems in Eastern Europe and Asia with a reputation for stimulating the nervous system, decreasing depression, enhancing work performance, eliminating fatigue, and preventing high altitude sickness. Rhodiola rosea has been categorized as an adaptogen by Russian researchers due to its observed ability to increase resistance to a variety of chemical, biological, and physical stressors. Its claimed benefits include antidepressant, anticancer, cardioprotective, and central nervous system enhancement.

Besides Rhodiola rosea, Clear Energy also contains noted anti-stress adaptogens such as Siberian ginseng, American ginseng, Cordyceps sinensis, reishi, astragalas, and others. All of these herbs—combined with the Poten-Zyme fermentation process— work together as a super tonic. Take note of Clear Energy. It's a great formula.

ANTIOXIDANT FORMULA
Fruits of Life and **Radical Fruits**
Garden of Life
770 Northpoint Pkwy,
West Palm Beach, FL 33407
Tel: 800/622-8986
Fax: 561/575-5488
Internet: www.gardenoflifeusa.com
This delicious tasting antioxidant fruit blend contains certified organic low temperature dried concentrates of blueberry, raspberry, strawberry, blackberry, prunes and raisins— as well as a "live food" blend of biologically active alkalizing minerals, enzymes and probiotics from goat's milk. It is notable that Fruits of Life is the first and only product to contain the six top fruit antioxidant foods on the planet in one whole food concentrate, according to research at Tufts University.

Lifestyle Recommendations

I or my associates have successfully used the products listed in this appendix in clinical practice and scientific research. Undoubtedly, more products than can be listed here meet the criteria of this book. Where possible, I have listed addresses, telephone numbers, fax numbers, and website addresses to help you obtain these products.

Product	Where to Obtain
Blender	Vita-Mix—800/437-4654 www.vita-mix.com
Cookware	Stainless Steel, Waterless Cookware (Many fine brands available)
Sauna	Health Mate Sauna PLH Products, 800/946-6001 www.healthmatesauna.com/index.shtml
Steam Bath	Aromaspa—800/800-7222 www.aromaspa.com
Elimination Bench	Life Step—800/500-9395 www.prohealthsolutions.com
Skin Brush	Available at fine health food stores
Shower Filter	N.E.E.D.S.—800/634-1380 www.needs.com New Wave Enviro Products, Inc.—800/592-8371 Also available at fine health food stores.
Air Purifier	N.E.E.D.S.—800/634-1380 www.needs.com
Full Spectrum Lighting	www.naturallighting.com
Essential Oils	Many brands available at fine health food stores.
Produce Wash	Many brands available at fine health food stores.

APPENDIX D

Educational Materials

Appendix D lists websites, organizations, and books of interest to readers. You are also invited to peer into the last part of this book, "References." There, you will find the names of many more articles and books that pertain to gastrointestinal health.

WEB SITES

Optimal Wellness Center
A health Web site by Dr. Joseph Mercola. Includes an archive of doctor Mercola's weekly health newsletters.
Internet: www.mercola.com

Weston A. Price Foundation
Offers numerous essays about the health, nutrition, and the nutritional philosophy of Dr. Weston A. Price. The best information you'll find on human nutrition.
Internet: www.westonaprice.org

Enzyme University
Everything you ever wanted to know about enzymes and digestion.
Internet: www.enzymeuniversity.com

Power Health
Web site of Dr. Stephen Byrnes. Teaches you "how to make naturopathy, natural nutrition, and alternative medicine a vital force in your life."
Internet: www.powerhealth.net

Doctors' Prescription for Healthy Living
Website of a magazine that covers Garden of Life and other excellent formulas extensively with timely newsworthy reports.
Internet: www.freedompressonline.com

Designs for Health Institute
Essays and information about health.
Internet: www.dfhi.com

ORGANIZATIONS

Weston A. Price Foundation
The Weston A. Price Foundation is one of the finest health and wellness organizations in the World. The teachings of this organization are based on the principals of one of my nutritional heroes Dr. Weston Price.
I would encourage anyone interested in health and human nutrition to become a member of this great organization.
PMB 106-380, 4200 Wisconsin Ave., NW, Washington, DC 20016
Tel: 202/333-4325
Internet: www.westonaprice.org

Price-Pottenger Nutrition Foundation	A great organization with a storied history. Based on the teachings of the great pioneers Drs. Price and Pottenger, PPNF is an exceptional resource for health and wellness. P.O. Box 2614, La Mesa, CA 91943-2614 Tel: 619/462-7600 Fax: 619/433-3136
Designs for Health Institute	Designs for Health Institute provides advanced training in clinical nutrition for health practitioners or those interested in becoming a nutritionist. Designs for Health conducts seminars around the country. I have personally been trained through this organization. 5345 Arapahoe Ave., Boulder, CO 80303 Tel: 303/415-0229 Fax: 303/415-9154 Internet: www.dfhi.com

BOOKS

Nourishing Traditions	Sally Fallon and Mary Enig, PhD. New Trends Publishing. Washington, DC. 1999
Stephen Byrnes' Online Whole Food Cookbook	Stephen Byrnes www.powerhealth.net
Reaching for Optimal Wellness	Dr. Joseph Mercola www.mercola.com
The Milk Book	William Campbell Douglass Second Opinion Publishing. Atlanta, GA. 1994
Your Body's Many Cries for Water	Dr. F. Batmanghelidj Global Health Solutions. Vienna, VA. 1995
Breaking the Vicious Cycle	Elaine Gottschall The Kirkton Press. Baltimore, Ontario, Canada. 2000
Enzyme Nutrition	Edward Howell Avery Publishing Group. Wayne, NJ. 1985
Native Nutrition	Ronald Schmid Healing Arts Press. Rochester, VT. 1995
Nutrition and Physical Degeneration	Weston A. Price Price-Pottenger Foundation. Los Angeles, CA. (1997) [1939]
Know Your Fats	Mary Enig Bethesda Press. Bethesda, MD. 2000

References

1 Van Winkle. E. "The toxic mind: the biology of mental illness and violence." *Medical Hypotheses*, 2000; 55(4): 356-368
2 Sydenham T. Edition of the Sydenham Society 1848; 1: 29.
3 Walker, M. "Medical journalist report of innovative biologics: Homeostatic Soil Organisms support immune system functions from the ground up." *The Townsend Letter for Doctors & Patients*, August/September 1997.
4 Ibid.
5 Downey, M. "Let them eat dirt." *Toronto Star*, January 10, 1999, F1.
6 Anonymous. "Down in the dirt, wonders beckon." *BusinessWeekonline*, December 3, 2001.
7 Downey, M., op cit.
8 Pignataa C, Budillon G, Monaco G, Nani E, Cuomo R, Parrilli G, and Ciccimarra F. "Jejunal bacterial overgrowth and intestinal permeability in children with immunodeficiency syndromes." *Gut* 1990; 31: 879-882.
9 Csordas A. Toxicology of butyrate and short-chain fatty acids. In: *Role of gut bacteria in human toxicology and pharmacology*, M. Hill, ed. (Bristol: Taylor & Francis Inc.) (p 286 (1995)
10 Hunnisett, A., et al. "Gut fermentation (or the 'autobrewery') syndrome: a new clinical test with initial observations and discussion of clinical and biochemical implications." *J Nut Med*, 1990;1:33-38.
11 Melñikova V.M., et al. "Problems in drug prevention and treatment of endogenous infection and dysbacteriosis." *Vestn Ross Akad Med Nauk*, 1997; (3):26-9.
12 Eaton, K.K., et al. "Abnormal gut fermentation: Laboratory studies reveal deficiency of B vitamins, zinc, and magnesium." *J Nutr Biochem*, 1993:635-637.
13 The diseases and conditions discussed in this overview are covered in greater detail by fact sheets and information packets. The statistics reported in this fact sheet come from *Digestive Diseases in the United States: Epidemiology and Impact*, edited by James Everhart, M.D., MPH., NIH Publication No. 94-1447. For copies of fact sheets, information packets, or the Digestive Diseases in the U.S., you may contact the National Digestive Diseases Information Clearinghouse (NDDIC), 2 Information Way, Bethesda, MD 20892-3570.
14 Anderson, R. "Mucoid plaque." Internet source: www.cleanse.net, accessed October 15, 2002.
15 Halpern, G.M., et al. "Analysis of the effect of various commercial nutraceutical preparations on the immune system." *Progress in Nutrition*, 2002; 4(S1). In press.
16 Ibid.
17 Ibid.
18 Ibid.
19 Ibid.
20 Rothschild, P.R. "Ambulatory treatment of chronic digestive disorder with malabsorption syndrome with Primal Defense™." *Progress in Nutrition*, 2002; 4(S1). In press.
21 Epstein, S.S. "Losing the war against cancer: who's to blame and what to do about it." *International Journal of Health Services*, 1990; 20(1): 53-71.
22 Epstein, S.S. "Evaluation of the national cancer program and proposed reforms." *American Journal of Industrial Medicine*, 1993; 24: 109-133.
23 Epstein, op cit., 1990.
24 United Press International (UPI). "Cancer now the leading killer of middle-aged studies show." *Los Angeles Times*, December 26, 1990.
25 Davis, D., et al. "Decreasing cardiovascular disease and increasing cancer among whites in the U.S. from 1973 through 1987." *Journal of the National Cancer Institute*, February 1994; 271: 431-437.
26 Laino, C. "With cancer rates up, environment is blamed." *Medical Tribune*, April 29, 1993; 34(8).
27 Konno, S. "Maitake D-fraction: Apoptosis inducer and immune enhancer." *Alternative & Complementary Therapies*, April 2001:102-107.
28 Chang R. "Functional properties of edible mushrooms." *Nutr Rev*, 1996; 54(11 Pt 2):S91-93.
29 Kliewer, E.V. & Smith, K.R. "Breast cancer mortality among immigrants in Australia and Canada." *Journal of the National Cancer Institute*, 1995;87(15):1154-1161.
30 Angier, N. "Move abroad can change breast cancer risk." *The New York Times*, August 2, 1995: A8.
31 Frassetto, L., et al. "Diet, evolution and aging—the pathophysiologic effects of the post-agricultural inversion of the potassium-to-sodium and base-to-chloride ratios in the human diet." *Eur J Nutr* 2001;40(5):200-213.
32 Bobkov, V.A., et al. "[Changes in the acid-base status of the synovial fluid in rheumatoid arthritis patients]." *Ter Arkh*, 1999;71(5):20-22.

33 Halpern, G.M., et al., op cit.

34 Rothschild, P.R. & Garcia Huertas, J. "Ambulatory naturo-pathic treatment of rheumatoid arthritis with FYI™ caplets." *Progress in Nutrition*, 2002; 4(S1). In press.

35 Gurwitsch, A.G. "Über Ursachen der Zellteilung." *Arch Entw Mech Org*, 1922;51:383-415.

36 Popp, F.A., et al. "Evidence of non-classical (squeezed) light in biological systems" *Physics Letters A,* 2002;293 (1-2):98-102.

37 Meyerowitz, S. *Wheat Grass: Nature's Finest Medicine*. Barrington, MA: Sproutman Publications, 1999.

38 Kohler, G.O. "The relation of the grass factor to guinea pig nutrition." *Journal of Nutrition*, 1937;15(5):445.

39 Cannon, M. & Emerson, G. *Journal of Nutrition*, 1939;18:155.

40 Randall, S.B., et al. "Distribution of the grass juice factor in plant and animal materials." *Journal of Nutrition*, 1940;20:459.

41 Scott, M.L. *Proceedings Cornell Nutrition Conference*, 1951:73.

42 Lindeberg, S. & Lundh, B. "Apparent absence of stroke and ischaemic heart disease in a traditional Melanesian island: a clinical study in Kitava." *J Intern Med*, 1993;233:269-275.

43 Murray, M. & Pizzorno, J. *Encyclopedia of Natural Medicine*, Rocklin, CA: Prima Publishing, 1998.

44 Dewailly, É., et al. "High organochlorine body burden in women with estrogen receptor-positive breast cancer." *Journal of the National Cancer Institute*, February 2, 1994; 86(3): 232-234.

45 Buikstra, J.E. The Lower Illinois River Region: A Prehistoric Context For the Study of Ancient Diet and Health. In: Cohen MN and GJ Armelagos (eds): *Paleopathology at the Origins of Agriculture*. Orlando, Academic Press, 1984, pp. 217-230.

46 Goodman A.H., et al. "Health changes at Dickson Mounds, Illinois." In: Cohen M.N. & G.J., Armelagos (eds): *Paleopathology at the Origins of Agriculture*. Orlando, Academic Press, pp. 271-305.

47 Ramisz, A., et al. "Epidemiological studies on Trichinellosis among swine, wild boars and humans in Poland. " *Parasite* 2001;8(2 Suppl):S90-1.

48 Bjorland, J., et al. "Trichinella spiralis infection in pigs in the Bolivian Altiplano." *Vet Parasitol*, 1993;47(3-4):349-54.

49 Jensen, B. *Nature Has a Remedy*. (Escondido, California: Bernard Jensen,1978), p.140.

50 Jensen, B. *Goat Milk Magic: One of Life's Greatest Healing Foods* (Escondido, California: Bernard Jensen, 24360 Old Wagon Road, Escondido, CA 92027, 1994), p. 96.

51 Gilbere, G. "The road to reversing MCS/EI is paved with good intestines." *Townsend Letter for Doctors & Patients* 210: 104.105, January 2001.

52 Douglass, W. C. *The Milk of Human Kindness Is not Pasteurized* (Lakemont,Georgia: Copple House Books, Inc., 1985).

53 Enig, M.G. "Health and nutritional benefits from coconut oil: an important functional food for the 21st century." Presented at the AVOC Lauric Oils Symposium, Ho Chi Min City, Vietnam, 25 April 1996.

54 Murray, M. "Encyclopedia of Nutritional Supplements." Rocklin, CA: Prima Publishing, 1996, pp. 235-278.

55 Tham, D.M., et al. "Clinical review 97: Potential health benefits of dietary phytoestrogens: a review of the clinical, epidemiological, and mechanistic evidence." *J Clin Endocrinol Metab*, 1998; 83(7): 2223-35.

56 Murray, M., op cit., p. 258.

57 Wagman, A.S. & Nuss, J.M. "Current therapies and emerging targets for the treatment of diabetes." *Curr Pharm Des*, 2001;7:417-450.

58 Healy, M. "Enormous rise predicted in diabetes case." *USA Today*, October 25, 2001:9D.

59 Groop, L.C. "Insulin resistance: The fundamental trigger of type 2 diabetes." *Diabetes Obes Metab*, 1999; 19(suppl.): S1-S7.

60 Le Poncin, M. Presentation at *2nd International Conference on New Directions in Affective Disorders*, Jerusalem, September 3-8, 1995.

61 Barefoot, J.C. & Schroll, M. "Symptoms of depression, acute myocardial infarction, and total mortality in a com-munity sample." *Circulation*, 1996; 93: 1976-1980.

62 McCully, K. "Atherosclerosis, serum cholesterol and the homocysteine theory: a study of 194 consecutive autopsies." *American Journal of Medical Science*, 1990);299:217-221.

63 Davis, D.L. & Bradlow, H.L. "Can environmental estrogens cause breast cancer?" *Scientific American*, October 1, 1995.

64 Bradlow, H.L., et al. "16a-hydroxylation of estradiol: a possible risk marker for breast cancer," p. 138, vol. 464 in *Endocrinology of the Breast: Basic and Clinical Aspects*. (Angeli, A., et al, eds.) Annals of the New York Academy of Sciences, New York, 1986.

65 Bradlow, H.L., et al. "Re: estrogen metabolism and excre-tion in oriental and caucasian women." *Journal of the National Cancer Institute*, 86(21): 1643-1644

66 Taioli, E., et al. "Ethnic differences in estrogen metabo-lism in healthy women." *Journal of the National Cancer Institute*, 1996; 86: 617.

67 Tarpila, S., et al. "The effect of flaxseed supplementation in processed foods on serum fatty acids and enterolac-tone." *Eur J Clin Nutr* 2002;56(2):157-165.

68 Maillard V., et al. "N-3 and N-6 fatty acids in breast adi-pose tissue and relative risk of breast cancer in a case-control study in Tours, France." *Int J Cancer*, 2002;98(1):78-83.

69 Joint Research Unit for Neurogastroenterology and Nutrition INRA-Université Toulouse III, Nutrition, Food and Food Safety Department, Toulouse Research Centre.

70 Murray, M.T. & Pizzorno, J.E. op cit.

71 Clayman, C. [medical editor]. *The American Medical Association Family Medical Guide*. New York, NY: Random House: 1994, p. 588.

72 Ibid.

73 Ibid.

74 Shapiro, J.A., et al. "Diet and rheumatoid arthritis in women: a possible protective effect of fish consumption." *Epidemiology*, 1996 May, 7(3):256-63.

75 Whitaker, J. *The Prostate Report: Prevention and Healing*. Potomac, MD: Phillips Publishing, Inc., 1994.

76 Lange, P.H. "Is the prostate pill finally here?" *The New England Journal of Medicine*; October 22, 1992; 327(17): 1234-1236.

77 United States Department of Health and Human Services. *Treating Your Enlarged Prostate*. Rockville, MD: United States Department of Health and Human Services, February 1994. AHCPR Publication 94-0584.

78 Lange, P.H. "Is the prostate pill finally here?" *The New England Journal of Medicine*; October 22, 1992; 327(17): 1234-1236.

79 Morley, J.E. "Management of impotence." *Postgraduate Medicine*, 1993; 93: 65-72.

80 Feldman, A., et al. "Impotence and its medical and psychological correlate: results of the Massachusetts Male Aging Study." *The Journal of Urology*, 1994; 151: 54-61.

81 Kruzel, T. "Treating impotence naturally." *Nutrition Science News*, 1997; 2(7): 354-356.

82 Buck, A.C., et al. "Treatment of chronic prostatitis and prostatodynia with pollen extract." *Brit J Urol*, 1989;64:496-499.

83 Kamijo, T., et al. "Effect of Cernitin pollen extract on experimental nonbacterial prostatitis in rats." *Prostate*, 2001;49:122-131.

84 Rudin, D.O. & Felix, C. *Omega-3 Oils*. Honesdale, PA: Paragon Press, 1996, p. 216.

85 Stoll, A.L. "Omega 3 fatty acids in bipolar disorder: a preliminary double-blind, placebo-controlled trial." *Arch Gen Psychiatry*, 1999; 56: 407-412.

86 Razin, S. "The minimal cellular genome of mycoplasma." *Indian J Biochem Biophys*, 1997;34(1-2):124-130.

87 CFS National Radio Program, Nov. 21st, 1999.

88 Pelletier, K. *Mind as Healer, Mind as Slayer*. New York, NY: Dell Publishing Co., Inc., 1977, p. 6.

89 Peteet, J.R. "Psychological factors in the causation and course of cancer." *Cancer, Stress, and Death*, [ed. Day, S.B.] New York and London: Plenum Medical Book Company, 1989: 63-77.

90 Riley, V. "Psychoneuroendocrine influences on immunocompetence and neoplasia." *Science*, 1981; 212: 1100-1108.

91 Leedham, B. & Meyerowitz, B.E. "The mind and breast cancer risk." In: *Reducing Breast Cancer Risk in Women*, [ed., Stoll, B.A.]. Netherlands: Kluwer Academic Publishers, 1995: 223-229.

92 Greer, S., et al. "Psychological response to breast cancer; effect on outcome." *Lancet*, 1979; ii: 785-787.

93 Levy, S.M., et al. "Immunological and psychosocial pre3dictors of disease recurrence in patients with early-stage breast cancer." *Behav. Med.* 1991; 17: 67-75.

94 *British Medical Journal*, 1995; 311: 1527-1530.

95 Leedham, B. & Meyerowitz, B.E. "The mind and breast cancer risk." In: *Reducing Breast Cancer Risk in Women*, [ed., Stoll, B.A.]. Netherlands: Kluwer Academic Publishers, 1995: 223-229.

96 Leedham, B. & Meyerowitz, B.E. "The mind and breast cancer risk." In: *Reducing Breast Cancer Risk in Women*, [ed., Stoll, B.A.]. Netherlands: Kluwer Academic Publishers, 1995: 223-229.

97 Lozano, P., et al. "The economic burden of asthma in US children: estimates from the National Medical Expenditure Survey." *J Allergy Clin Immunol*, 1999;104(5):957-963.

98 Clark, N.M., et al. "Childhood asthma." *Environ Health Perspect*, 1999; 107 Suppl 3(-HD-):421-429.

99 Broughton, K.S., et al. "Reduced asthma symptoms with n-3 fatty acid ingestion are related to 5-series leukotriene production." *Am J Clin Nutr*,1997;65:1011-1017.

100 Hodge, L., et al. "Consumption of oily fish and childhood asthma risk." *MJA*, 1996;164:137-140.

101 Cignarella, A., et al. "Novel lipid-lowering properties of *Vaccinium myrtillus L.* leaves, a traditional antidiabetic treatment, in several models of rat dyslipidaemia: a comparison with ciprofibrate." *Thromb Res*, 1996;84(5):311-322.

102 Morita, K. & Nakano, T. "Seaweed accelerates the excretion of dioxin stored in rats." *J Agric Food Chem*, 2002;50(4):910-917.

103 Kelly, G.S. "*Rhodiola rosea*: a possible plant adaptogen." *Altern Med Rev*, 2001;6(3):293-302.

Index

Acid Defense™, 223
Acne, 108, 245-246
ADD, *see* Attention Deficit Disorder/ Attention
    Deficit/Hyperactivity Disorder
Addiction, 35, 237, 253
ADHD, *see* Attention Deficit Disorder/ Attention
    Deficit/Hyperactivity Disorder
AIDS, 42, 44, 68, 69, 74, 201, 237
Allergies, 41, 44, 48, 49, 54, 75, 77, 79, 80, 93, 108, 132,
    159, 246
    food, 50, 51, 65, 80, 121, 127, 128, 131, 133, 148, 201,
        214ff.
    seasonal, 258ff.
        See also Hay fever
Alzheimer's disease, 35, 179-180
Angina pectoris, 80, 190-191
Ankylosing spondylitis, 229
Anxiety, 34, 35, 48, 199, 237-238, 250, 271
Arthritis, 21, 54, 55, 60, 84, 85, 86, 88, 94, 99, 113, 114, 121,
    163, 212, 229, 230, 232, 247
    osteoarthritis, 229, 269
    rheumatoid, 10, 21, 41, 50, 51, 61, 75, 77, 79, 80, 81, 85,
        87, 115, 119, 159, 173, 226, 229-230, 232, 243, 250,
        253, 255
Asthma, 41, 42, 51, 54, 60, 61, 226, 243, 246, 253, 258-259
Arteriosclerosis, 137, 191
Atherosclerosis, 136, 191, 192, 233
Atopic dermatitis (dermatitis, eczema), 42, 108, 170, 245, 246
    See also Skin health
Attention Deficit Disorder (ADD)/Attention
    Deficit/Hyperactivity Disorder (ADHD), 195-196
Autism, 196
Autoimmune disease, 44, 49, 50, 51, 52, 53, 54, 55, 60, 74,
    75, 77, 78, 80, 81, 83, 84, 86, 129, 131, 138, 139, 159,
    173ff., 204, 226

Back pain, 65
    See also Inflammatory conditions
Behavioral disorders, 49
Benign prostatic hypertrophy (BPH), 57, 232-233, 234
Biblical diet, *see* Maker's Diet
Bladder cancer, *see* Cancer, bladder

Blood pressure, elevated (hypertension), 78, 113, 114, 115,
    121, 122, 136, 143, 147, 159, 176, 191, 247, 250, 253,
    254, 255, 268, 271
Blood sugar imbalances, 59, 78, 116, 122, 133, 147, 160, 167,
    174, 176ff., 271
Bowel disorders, *see* Functional bowel disorders
Brain health, 49, 105, 117, 125, 131, 133, 161, 179ff.
Brain, cancer, *see* Cancer, brain
Breast cancer, *see* Cancer, breast
Bursitis, *see* Inflammatory conditions

Cancer, 18, 42, 44, 53, 59, 69ff., 84, 85, 96, 99, 113, 114,
    115-116, 120, 121, 134, 135, 136, 137, 138, 140, 142,
    160, 170, 176, 182ff., 192, 204, 208, 226, 253-254, 268
    bladder, 182
    brain, 75, 182
    breast, 49, 59, 69, 87, 116, 134,
        171, 182, 211-212, 253, 268
    cervical, 268
    colon/colorectal, 49, 50, 69, 90, 125, 141, 142, 182, 268
    endometrial, 49, 182
    esophageal, 222
    gallbladder, 268
    kidney, 69
    leukemia, 58, 77, 81, 182, 183, 265
    liver, 59, 87, 171
    lung, 59, 69, 87, 182, 201
    lymphoma, 69, 182, 183, 265
    melanoma, 69, 182, 183
    ovarian, 70-71, 182, 268
    prostate, 140, 182, 236, 268
Candida, 17, 21, 22, 48, 49, 53, 60, 61, 67,
    68, 127, 162, 185ff.
Candidiasis, 21, 44, 48, 68, 80, 171, 185ff.
Cardiac arrhythmias, 54, 80
Cardiovascular disease (CVD), 59, 115, 190ff.
Celiac disease, 17, 94, 199
CFIDS, *see* Chronic fatigue syndrome
CFS, *see* Chronic fatigue syndrome
CHD, *see* Coronary heart disease
Chemical sensitivities, see Multiple chemical sensitivities
Chemotherapy, 71, 74, 75, 76, 77, 133, 234

Children's health, 41-42, 44ff., 54, 106, 127, 134, 146, 195ff., 246, 258-259
Cholesterol, elevated, 52, 58, 59-60, 78, 80, 121, 132, 136, 191-192, 271
Chronic fatigue immune deficiency syndrome (CFIDS), *see* Chronic Fatigue Syndrome
Chronic fatigue syndrome (CFS), 10, 21, 41, 44, 49, 54, 60, 62, 79, 80, 82, 107, 189, 201ff., 243
Clear Energy™, 214, 235, 257, 279
Cold and Flu Defense™, 205
Colds, 40, 65, 85, 108, 145, 175, 204ff., 264ff.
Colitis, 17, 19, 22, 55, 60, 61, 64, 80, 106, 159, 160, 162, 171, 199
Colon/colorectal cancer, *see* Cancer, colon/colorectal
Colostrum, 82, 132-133, 278-279
Congestive heart failure, 190, 191
Constipation, 34, 35, 39, 46, 48, 49, 50, 55, 56, 60, 61, 62, 80, 88, 141, 142, 160, 163, 171, 175, 186, 198, 217
Coronary heart disease (CHD), 59-60, 190-191, 192
Crohn's disease, 9, 17ff., 41, 43, 49, 51, 55, 56, 80, 106, 129, 159, 160, 162, 163, 199, 277
Cystic fibrosis, 17, 196
Cystitis, see Urinary tract infection

Dementia, 179-180
Depression, 34, 48, 62, 121, 133, 147, 186, 199, 237, 238, 241, 247, 250, 253, 254
    postpartum, 238, 241
Dermatitis, *see* Atopic dermatitis
Detoxification, 22-23, 29, 40, 53, 56, 65, 79, 107, 130, 171, 172, 175, 189, 196, 204, 208ff., 271
Diabetes, 73, 80, 113, 114, 115, 116, 121, 122, 135, 137, 142, 147, 159, 160, 170, 233, 268, 271
    Type I, 173
    Type II, 59, 176-177
Diarrhea, chronic, 17, 61, 65, 94, 186, 198, 199, 200, 217
Digestive disease, 49-50, 198ff.
Diverticulitis , 49, 61, 108, 199
Dyspepsia, 34, 163, 198, 217

Ear, nose and throat problems, 54
Eclampsia, 54
Eczema, see Atopic dermatitis
Endometrial cancer, *see* Cancer, endometrial
Endometriosis, 186, 211
Epstein Barr virus, 265
Erectile dysfunction (impotence), 233, 253
Estrogen, 49, 114, 211-212
Eye problems, 21, 54, 186

Female health, 211ff.
Fibrocystic breast disease, 211
Fibromyalgia, 49, 54, 201ff., 243
Flu (influenza), 40, 53, 65, 73, 85, 146, 175, 204ff., 242, 264, 265, 266
For Your Inflammation™, see FYI™
Fruits of Life™, 161-162, 279
Functional bowel disorders, 19, 29, 55, 56, 64, 77, 93, 106, 162, 217ff.

Fungal Defense™, 189, 190, 278
FYI™ (For Your Inflammation™), 41, 84ff., 155ff., 183, 204, 278

Gallbladder disease, 21, 49, 268
Gallstones, 268
Garden of Life, 29, 38ff., 95, 97, 100, 146, 277
Gastritis, 80
Gastrointestinal esophageal reflux disease (GERD), 50, 222ff.
    See also Heartburn
Gastrointestinal health, 20, 32, 36, 38, 39, 48, 89, 170, 224, 251, 281
Goat's milk protein powder, 127ff., 149, 152, 165, 278
Goatein™, 107, 128ff., 149, 278
Gout, 85, 229, 269
Grave's disease, 173
Gulf War syndrome, 44, 243

Hay fever, 42, 246, 253
    See also Allergies, seasonal
Headache, 21, 49, 64, 65, 83, 88, 121, 126, 201
Health maintenance, general, 69, 108, 128, 220ff.
Heart disease, 59-60, 69, 70, 76, 86, 98, 99, 115, 116, 120, 121, 122, 125, 134, 135, 136, 137, 138, 159, 160, 163, 226, 233, 243, 254, 268, 271
Heartburn, 19, 48, 147, 158, 190, 222-223
    See also Gastrointestinal esophageal reflux disease
Heavy metal poisoning, 24, 73, 172, 196, 208, 239
Hemorrhoids, 49, 90, 142, 163
Hepatitis
    B, 53, 265, 266
    C, 53, 265, 266
    viral, 44
Herpes simplex (HSV-1 and HSV-2), 52, 53, 204, 264, 266
Homeostatic soil organisms™ (HSOs™), 9, 10, 28, 29, 39ff., 73, 83, 88, 94, 204, 245, 266, 277, 259
Homocysteine, elevated, 192-193
HSOs, see Homeostatic soil organisms
Human herpesvirus-6 (HHV-6), 204, 265, 266
Hypertension, see Blood pressure, elevated
Hypoglycemia, 49, 50, 177, 271

Immune disorders, see Autoimmune disease
Immune health, 70, 91, 133, 224ff.
Impotence, see Erectile dysfunction
Inflammation, 18, 21, 43, 48, 60, 64, 70, 78, 84ff., 93, 94, 121, 136, 145, 163, 165, 173, 175, 199, 204, 217, 226, 229, 232, 234, 246, 247, 258, 259
Inflammatory bowel disease (IBD), 20, 55, 56, 64, 77, 162, 243
Inflammatory conditions, 21, 77, 81, 85, 86, 87, 88, 159, 163, 199, 226ff.
Influenza, see Flu
Insomnia, 21, 34, 49, 75, 81, 88, 105, 133, 249ff., 253, 271
    See also Sleep disorders
Irritable bowel syndrome (IBS), 17, 19, 34, 39, 41, 49, 50, 51, 56, 60, 61, 62, 79, 93, 106, 129, 142, 160, 162, 163, 170, 171, 199, 217

Joint
    disorders, 16, 21, 60, 79, 85, 87, 173, 229ff., 247, 269
    pain, 21, 49, 60, 79, 83, 186, 201

Leaky gut syndrome, 49, 50, 129, 186, 217, 246
Learning disorders, 49, 195
Leukemia, *see* Cancer, leukemia
Liver disease, 49, 269
Lung cancer, *see* Cancer, lung
Lupus, *see* Systemic lupus erythematosus
Lymphoma, *see* Cancer, lymphoma

Maker's Diet/Biblical diet, 10, 20, 29, 65, 112ff., 124,
    177, 193, 196
Male health, 232ff.
Melanoma, see Cancer, melanoma
Memory loss, 56, 58, 161, 171, 179, 181, 186, 201, 272
Menopause, 211, 268
Mental disorders, 48, 237ff.
Multiple chemical sensitivities (MCS), 44, 128-129,
    186, 189, 214-215
Multiple sclerosis, 99, 173, 196, 201
Myalgic encephalomyelitis (ME), 201
Myasthenia Gravis, 173
Mycoplasma infections, 242ff.

Nausea and vomiting, 15, 16, 32, 34, 35, 49,
    61, 75, 81, 94, 199

Obesity, 115, 120, 136, 137, 138, 146, 176, 268-269, 271-272
    See also Weight management
Omega-Zyme™, 92ff., 152, 155, 156, 157, 189, 278
Osteoarthritis, *see* Arthritis, osteoarthritis
Osteoporosis, 115, 132, 136, 137, 142, 146, 155, 156, 157,
    162, 167, 211
Ovarian cancer, *see* Cancer, ovarian
Ovarian cysts, 211

Parkinson's disease, 35, 179-180, 243
Perfect Food™, 65, 99, 100, 104ff., 171, 172, 189, 272, 278
Pervasive Developmental Disorders (PDD), 20, 196
Phobias, 237-238
PMS, *see* Premenstrual syndrome
Postpartum depression, see Depression, postpartum
Poten-Zyme™ fermentation process, 41, 52, 73-74, 77, 78, 86,
    94, 99, 104, 277, 278, 279
Premenstrual syndrome (PMS), 186, 211, 212
Primal Defense™, 39ff., 51-52, 55ff., 80, 155, 156, 157, 183,
    189, 204, 277
Prostate cancer, see Cancer, prostate
Prostatitis, 48, 233, 234, 236
Psoriasis, 61, 62, 81, 108, 245, 246-247
    See also Skin health

Respiratory health, upper, 258ff.
RevivAll™ Classic, 277
RevivAll™ Female Vitality Formula, 211, 279
RevivAll™ Male Vitality Formula, 233, 234, 279
Rheumatoid arthritis, see Arthritis, rheumatoid
RM-10™, 41, 75ff., 155, 156, 157, 183, 204, 277

Schizophrenia, 237, 238-239
Scleroderma, 80, 81, 173
Shingles, 264
Sinus infection, 60, 83
Sinusitis, 61, 105, 259
Skin health, 57, 60, 64, 80, 86, 88, 104, 108, 129, 132, 133,
    139, 171, 172, 186, 245ff.
    See also Acne; Atopic dermatitis; Psoriasis
Sleep disorders, 34, 40, 65, 78, 79, 172, 201, 249ff., 269
    See also, Insomnia
Soil organisms, *see* Homeostatic soil organisms
Springs of Life™, 146, 149, 155, 156, 157, 171, 278
Stress, 22, 24, 46, 50, 56, 105, 120, 147, 186, 222, 237, 238,
    247, 250, 253ff., 272
Stroke, 21, 70, 113, 114, 115, 122, 125, 190, 191, 193, 194,
    226, 232, 268
Super Seed™, 142, 155, 156, 157, 163, 190, 211, 278
Syndrome X, 122, 176
Systemic lupus erythematosus, 41, 44, 51, 77, 80, 81, 86, 173

Thyroid gland disease, 54, 105, 138, 270, 271
Triglycerides, elevated, 57, 59-60, 80, 121, 136, 176, 193, 271

Ulcers, 19, 49, 73, 162, 163, 199, 253, 255
Ulcerative colitis, see Colitis
Upper respiratory health, see Respiratory health, upper
Uterine fibroids, 211
Urinary Tract Infection (UTI), 25, 48, 67, 94, 262ff.

Vaginitis, 48, 49
    See also Female health
Violent, impulsive behavior, 239, 241
Viral diseases, 264ff.
Viral Hepatitis, *see* Hepatitis, viral
Vomiting, *see* Nausea and vomiting

Weight management, 50, 93, 105, 107, 138, 141, 171, 186,
    255, 268ff.

Zero Gravity™, 270, 271-272, 279